Applying Linguistics in Health Research, Education, and Policy

Trends in Applied Linguistics

Edited by
Ulrike Jessner

Volume 34

Applying Linguistics in Health Research, Education, and Policy

---

Bench to Bedside and Back Again

Edited by
Brett A. Diaz and Robert W. Schrauf

DE GRUYTER
MOUTON

ISBN 978-3-11-152435-1
e-ISBN (PDF) 978-3-11-074480-4
e-ISBN (EPUB) 978-3-11-074486-6
ISSN 1868-6362

Library of Congress Control Number: 2022942124

Bibliographic information published by the Deutsche Nationalbibliothek
The Deutsche Nationalbibliothek lists this publication in the Deutsche Nationalbibliografie; detailed bibliographic data are available on the internet at http://dnb.dnb.de.

© 2024 Walter de Gruyter GmbH, Berlin/Boston
This volume is text- and page-identical with the hardback published in 2023.
Cover image: Cover design: Martin Zech, Bremen, using a photo
by Roswitha Schacht/morguefile.com
Typesetting: Integra Software Services Pvt.

www.degruyter.com

Preface

In the first season of Netflix's comedy *The Chair*, embattled English professor Bill Dobson is asked to work with the campus communications office in order to craft a letter of apology to his students for an offensive joke he used during a lecture. He refuses, stating, "I don't co-write." I imagine I was not the only applied linguist who heard this line, laughed a bit at the seemingly out-of-touch academic, and then said to myself, "That just wouldn't work in applied linguistics!" For many of us in the field, researching with colleagues, and, yes, in many cases, co-writing with them is central to our work and an aspect of our field that we both value and enjoy. Further, and as illustrated in the following chapters, we also know that working on teams is crucial in health research, education, and policy. In fact, moving from "bench to bedside and back again" with a team of health professionals and language experts is, in almost all respects, an *essential* aspect of applied linguistics work on health and healthcare-related issues.

In many ways, the book you are holding right now or reading on your computer screen is a product of these types of collaborations. In this case, the group formed in the summer of 2019 when Brett Diaz connected a group of researchers interested in presenting at an American Association for Applied Linguistics (AAAL) symposium with the same title as this book. Brett asked me to be the discussant on that panel along with the presenters: Emily Feuerherm, Peter Torres, and Abdesalam Soudi. I know we all were particularly excited by the specific focus of the symposium on the applied part of our work. As Brett wrote at the time, he wanted the symposium and discussion to be "as much about who as what." In other words, as we prepared our presentations and discussion points, he wanted us to emphasize not just the results of our work but, as Brett later wrote in the proposal for this volume, "the paths scholars take in applying their linguistic specializations." With this focus, we were all happy and excited to receive acceptance for AAAL 2020. Then, as is now a common story, COVID-19 delayed not just our conference symposium but also the work on this edited book that Brett was planning to use the symposium to jumpstart. Our initial conference plans were on hold, and like everyone else in the field, we had to recalibrate how we do conferences as well as how we perform all aspects of our professional lives, from teaching to research collaborations. With luck and hard work, AAAL was able to organize an online conference in March of 2021, and the symposium was accepted again for inclusion. The online, recorded presentations and discussion may have limited how we collaborated on the symposium, but the conversations and knowledge building about applied linguistics and health research presented during the symposium were as engaging for both presenters and audience members as they would have been in person. In the meantime, in the intervening year, Brett recruited additional chapter contributors for this book. I mention this brief timeline of the collaboration on the symposium and edited book in order to emphasize the fits and starts that occur in most research and writing collaborations. In addition, the extended timeline needed for this book project also illustrates the perseverance and dedication needed to make research collaborations work under any conditions, and the excellent and varied chapters in the book, including the single-authored chapters, reveal the contributions that result from such extended and deeply engaged research collaborations.

This is not to say that the personal, reflexive, and collaborative aspects of applied linguistics research is simple or easy. The final chapter of this volume is a dialogue among chapter authors and lays out many of the frustrations and benefits of doing this work in collaboration with health professionals and community organizations. In particular, one of the fundamental tensions in applied linguistics – the desire to help solve "real-world problems" while also contributing to theoretical understandings of language, communication, and identity – appears in many of the chapters and the final chapter discussion. This balance is tricky and, perhaps, inevitable. Doctors and nurses want to know the best way to ask patients about their symptoms, health policy writers want to know the correct verbs to use when writing instructions for drug prescriptions, and medical translators want to know exact, one-to-one translations of key medical terminology. Health professionals often do not feel they have the time in their workdays to struggle with the complexities of language and want straightforward answers that we, as applied linguists, feel might leave out or ignore too much about how and what languages do. In addition, applied linguists working in health contexts often feel helpless in relation to bigger structural issues such as rising healthcare costs, hospital closures, and deteriorating public health infrastructure, all of which were exacerbated by COVID-19.

Despite the complexities and difficulties working on health research in applied linguistics, this book is an argument for why this research is so important and why these inter-disciplinary collaborations are so essential. In her opening keynote address at the International Association of Applied Linguistics (AILA) triennial world congress in 2021, Professor Diane Larsen-Freeman noted this about interdisciplinary research collaborations in applied linguistics: "To deal with a truly complex world we need transdisciplinary, maybe post disciplinary thinking . . . where the overarching definitions of knowledge are being broken down." She cited as an example, a recent job posting at Northeastern University in the United States for an Assistant/Associate Professor in Environmental Cognition where the Psychology Department, Department of Marine and Environmental Science, and the School of Public Policy would share the position. Larsen-Freeman argued that these types of collaborations across academic fields and disciplines represent "the sort of thinking, I believe, [that] may save us."

In the same way, the focus in the following chapters on the interdisciplinary paths different researchers took in addressing their particular issues should continue to be at the core of future applied linguistics work. COVID-19 and the faltering responses of governments and communities throughout the world has made it clear that it is impossible to approach our work as applied linguists in health research alone as the isolated academic, thinking alone in our metaphorical tower. Researching in teams and, in many cases, co-writing as part of that team are simply required aspects of work in the field. Luckily, we have books like the current volume to continue pointing the way forward to this inter and post-disciplinary future.

Paul McPherron
Hunter College, City University of New York
September 8th, 2021

Contents

Preface —— V

Robert W. Schrauf
Introduction —— 1

Section 1: Applied linguistics and health/medical education

Abigail Konopasky, Anthony R. Artino, Jr., Clara Hua, Alexis Battista
Chapter 1
Functional linguistics and health professions education: An exploration of individual and group reflection processes —— 21

Caroline H. Vickers, Ryan A. Goble
Chapter 2
From cultural competence to discourse competence: Discourse analysis and the education of bi/multilingual health care professionals —— 57

Section 2: Applied linguistics, translation, and health

Boyd H. Davis, Ching-Yi Kuo, Margaret Maclagan
Chapter 3
Children learning about dementia in Taiwan: Using gist translations to clarify adult opinions —— 87

Robert W. Schrauf
Chapter 4
Research translation as situated practice —— 117

Section 3: Applied linguistics and public health

Peter Joseph Torres
Chapter 5
Modality and interpretative spaces in policies —— 143

Brett A. Diaz
Chapter 6
Discourses at work in elderly, health policy communication: Uncovering aspects of semantic preference and prosody in the rural opioid epidemic —— 169

Patria C. López de Victoria Rodríguez, Elba L. González Márquez, Krystal Colón Rivera
Chapter 7
Responding to crisis, responding to needs: Older adults seeking medical care in the aftermath of storms —— 193

Section 4: **Applied linguistics and health interventions**

Emily M. Feuerherm, Bonnie McIntosh
Chapter 8
Beyond "Limited English Proficient" in health care policy, practice, and programs —— 225

Lisa Mikesell
Chapter 9
Designing health interventions on transdisciplinary research teams: Contributions of LSI scholarship —— 247

Brett A. Diaz
Conclusion —— 275

Contributor information —— 291

Index —— 295

Robert W. Schrauf
Introduction

Health applied linguistics – the what and the who

Applied linguistics is a discipline grounded in the conviction that language is both a medium of social life and itself a social action. To the social and institutional world of health and illness, health applied linguists bring a unique form of scholarly attention and analysis: a close look at *how people* – providers, patients, caregivers, family members, administrators, public health personnel – *do health and illness* – diagnosis, treatment, caregiving, prevention, and public health – *in talk and text*. This volume presents a wide-ranging sample of current research in health applied linguistics across four contexts: medical education, public health, health interventions, and cross-cultural projects.

Pursuing this kind of research, however, requires a deep appreciation of the everyday experience of professionals and patients, and the endeavor becomes an inherently collaborative one. Hence, health applied linguists usually become networked into the very cultures they investigate, and these commitments shape who they become as researchers and scholars. Thus, beyond presenting new and interesting research, this volume also seeks to make salient the settings and collaborations of the contributors, to create a sense of *who* health applied linguists are and how they got there. To that end, each contributor has included more extensive descriptions of her or his collaborations in their chapters, and all contributors participated in a group discussion of their experiences as health applied linguists – captured and edited in the last chapter of the volume.

As a result, the volume is written for a varied readership. Obviously, other health applied linguists will find familiar themes and new applications of current methodologies. Scholars and social scientists in cognate fields of health communication and the social sciences of medicine (e.g., medical sociology, medical anthropology, health psychology) will see their work cited and recognize new findings in their research topics. Graduate students interested in health and illness may find especially interesting the lived realities of applied research in health settings. We also hope the volume finds its way into the hands of one or the other busy health professionals who work in the areas covered by the chapters – but certainly into the hands of researchers in academic medicine.

Robert W. Schrauf, The Pennsylvania State University

https://doi.org/10.1515/9783110744804-001

The remaining paragraphs of this introduction include a brief account of applied linguistics as a discipline, followed by a section which describes health applied linguistics itself and contextualizes the volume alongside other current publications. The third section articulates more explicitly the purposes and organization of the volume, and the final section summarizes the chapters, drawing attention to the theories and methods of each, as well the specific settings and collaborations of each set of authors.

1 What is applied linguistics?

Mapping academic fields can be challenging because they often seem to expand beyond their borders – more so in the cases of inherently interdisciplinary fields like applied linguistics. However, despite the overlap around the edges, each discipline retains a core emphasis, concern, or method. One of the more widely cited definitions of the applied linguistics is found on the homepage of the Association Internationale de Linguistique Appliquée/International Association of Applied Linguistics (AILA, 2022), and I take the liberty of bullet pointing its components.

"Applied Linguistics is
- an interdisciplinary and transdisciplinary field of research and practice dealing with practical problems of language and communication
- that can be identified, analysed, or solved by applying available theories, methods, and results of Linguistics or
- by developing new theoretical and methodological frameworks in Linguistics to work on these problems."

Point for point, this definition captures the core features of applied linguistics.

"*. . . .an interdisciplinary field.*" Obviously, linguistics provides the principal frame of reference, or in the phrasing of Candlin and Sarangi (2004: 2), linguistics is the "superordinate partner." Nevertheless, as we shall see, applied linguists draw on theories and research literatures from numerous other areas. For example, the discipline has deep and long-standing investments in research on second language acquisition, language pedagogy, and language teacher training, and applied linguists in these areas regularly cite and contribute to theory and research from cognitive and educational psychology, psycholinguistics, and education itself. Closer to home, *health* applied linguists work with clinicians, patients, caregivers, and scientists in a variety of institutional contexts associated with community, clinical, and public health. Notably, such interdisciplinarity goes well beyond theory and literature and involves extensive and sometimes long-lasting collaborations with professionals and experts to address multidimensional social issues.

"... *dealing with practical problems of language and communication."* General characterizations of applied linguistics often emphasize its orientation to solving "real-world problems" (Brumfit 1995: 27), linking language to "decision-making in the real world" (Simpson 2011: 1), and a "specific, problem-oriented way of 'doing linguistics' related to the real-life world" (Knapp and Antos 2014: xi). What kinds of 'real-world problems' are these? One way to sample the interests of applied linguists is to review the lists of special interest groups in regional or national conferences, and I reproduce below the relevant list of research 'strands' from the American Association for Applied Linguistics (AAAL, 2022). (Note that the category descriptors are my own, and that the special interest group designations follow the categories).

Language (aspects): language cognition and brain research; phonology/phonetics and oral communication; pragmatics; reading, writing and literacy; second language acquisition and attrition; vocabulary and lexical studies

Language pedagogy: assessment and evaluation; bilingual, immersion, and minority education; educational linguistics; second and foreign language pedagogy; teacher education and beliefs

Analytic methods: Analysis of discourse and interaction; corpus linguistics; text analysis (written discourse); sociolinguistics; research methodology

Language and Social issues: anti-racism, decolonization, and intersectionality; language and ideology; language and the law; language and technology; language, culture, and socialization; language, gender, and sexuality

Languages and Language Varieties: language planning and policy; language maintenance and revitalization; translation and interpretation.

A glance at these category labels and the associated special interest groups reflects (in my ordering) a scalar continuum of *language*. At the top of the list, there is an emphasis on individual aspects *within* language – the componential and relatively scaled phenomena of phonology/prosody, morphology, syntax, lexis, pragmatics, and discourse – brought into focus via representations in the brain *or* contextualized in highly-localized oral and written productions *or* pedagogically chunked in language teaching. At the bottom of the list, there are larger wholes –languages (plural) and discourses as the media of interactional life, social issues, ideology, and political interests.

"... *that can be identified, analyzed, or solved by applying available theories, methods, and results of Linguistics."* Clearly, although the topics listed above concern language and communication, there is a subtle and persistent focus on language itself as the medium – albeit at various levels. Again, linguistics is the 'superordinate partner.' Linguistics, however, is an expanding discipline with porous borders, and applied linguists make common cause in that expansion. Hence, new theories and methods are ever evolving.

". . . or by developing new theoretical and methodological frameworks in Linguistics to work on these problems." Across the many subfields of applied linguistics, there is a constant flow of new theory, but of particular concern for this volume are theories and methods associated with Language and Social Issues (the fourth category listed among the AAAL strands). The investigation of social practices and institutional orders (including health and illness) is largely dependent on theory and methods that fall under the broad umbrella of "discourse." These would include at least the following: discourse analysis proper, critical discourse analysis, conversation analysis, interactional sociolinguistics, the ethnography of communication, narrative analysis, and interactional linguistics.

Some common themes in these discourse traditions are these. First, broadly speaking, researchers in these areas treat language as an *analyzable, largely verbal, but inherently multimodal, semiotic system for human interaction*. Second, researchers who focus on social issues and institutions generally make at least three assumptions about language and language analysis.

1. *Talk and text are forms of social action*. This is an alternate formulation of the well-known position taken by the philosopher Austin in his *How to Do Things with Words* (Austin 1962). Austin argued that in speaking, people were not simply making reports about or commenting on the world but actively seeking to influence ongoing, shared social life. Applied linguists attend to *how* people design their talk and their texts to get things done in everyday contexts (Enfield & Sidnell 2017).
2. *Features of language and discourse at the micro-level of talk and text are crucially linked to meso- and macro-level institutional contexts and societal discourses*. That is, local text and talk reflect, realize, modify, constrain, and challenge larger regimes of discourse. In *Health and Risk Communication: An Applied Linguistics Perspective*, Jones (2013) notes that applied linguistics provides "a set of tools that allows the analyst to understand how broader voices and discourses in texts and talk are constructed at the level of discourse linguistic features and the micro-mechanics of social interaction."
3. *Institutional discourse involves specific vocabularies, genres, bodies of knowledge, rituals, ratified speakers, and defined 'others'* – as for example: clients, customers, patients, partners, associates, participants, students (for a brief summary, see Sarangi and Candlin 2011: 5–17). Applied linguistics and the

associated, discourse-centred methodologies have a robust tradition of empirical enquiry concerning institutional discourse.

The above characterization of language and these three fundamental tenets uniquely situate applied linguistics as an effective partner in the analysis of social life in collaboration with the social sciences concerned with human communication (e.g., communication, rhetoric, social psychology).

In sum, the description by the International Association of Applied Linguistics (AILA) reflects the key features of the discipline: *interdisciplinarity*, addressing *practical problems* in communication, that are identified, analyzed, or solved through *linguistic* (and discursive) theory and method. As we discuss the subfield of health applied linguistics in the paragraphs below, we will see these various themes worked out in current research.

2 Health applied linguistics

As the name implies, health applied linguistics focuses on language and communication in a vast array of institutional contexts through which illness is researched, diagnosed, and treated (e.g., labs, clinics, urgent care centers, hospitals, dispensaries); schools and centers in which practitioners are trained, certified, and organized (e.g., allied health professions training, graduate schools, colleges of nursing, medical schools, professional associations, licensure and certifying organizations, unions); across multiple professions (e.g., paramedics, technicians, social workers, psychologists, dentists, pharmacists, nurses, physicians, researchers); places where research is conducted and medical equipment designed and produced (e.g., laboratories, research and development firms, federal and private funding agencies, pharmaceutical companies, bioengineering firms, medical equipment manufacturers); government sectors responsible for public health and health product regulation (e.g., Departments of Health, Offices of Health and Safety; World Health Organization); private foundations and non-profits (e.g., Alzheimer's Association, American Heart Association, Diabetes Foundation; Doctors Without Borders, Red Cross, Red Crescent); and corporations through which healthcare is coordinated and financed (e.g., managed care corporations, insurance companies).

From the perspective of applied linguistics, the aforementioned contexts and collaborations are *brought into being via talk and text*, and we might ask how much of this terrain has been mapped by health applied linguistics. This latter question invites a literature review of the whole field, but such a task exceeds the space and goal of this introduction. Thus, to help situate this present volume, we offer the following sketch.

A brief review of the periodical databases such as *Linguistics and Language Behavior Abstracts* (LLBA) and the United States' *National Library of Medicine's PubMed* reveals a large and growing number of language- and discourse-oriented studies by applied linguists, communication scholars, social psychologists, and clinical linguists. There are now also numerous edited volumes on applied linguistics and specific health conditions (as for example, research on dementia: Davis 2005; Davis and Guendouzi 2013; Mates, Mikesell, and Smith 2013; Schrauf and Müller 2014; Plejert, Lindholm, and Schrauf 2017) or on communication contexts (as for example, doctor-patient communication: e.g., Heritage & Maynard 2005; Greenhalgh & Hurwitz 2004); monographs on specific topics (e.g., on risk and public health: e.g., Jones 2013); adolescent health communication (Harvey, 2013); discourse and mental health (Hunt and Brookes 2020); fatherhood and mental illness (Galasiński 2013); cancer (Semino, Demjén, Hardie, Payne, and Rayson 2017), and textbooks on applied linguistics and health (Harvey and Koteyko 2013).

Another class of literature is the disciplinary handbook, and these too have become more common in applied linguistics. A few of these include review chapters of health applied linguistics (e.g., Collins, Peters, and Watt 2011; Martin and Crichton 2020) which when read chronologically give a sense of the development of the field. Disciplinary handbooks devoted uniquely to health applied linguistics are still somewhat rare, and at the time of this writing, the seminal handbook was *The Routledge Handbook of Language and Health Communication*, edited by Hamilton and Chou (2014). This handbook is one of several volumes in a series entitled *Routledge Handbooks in Applied Linguistics*. It is designed as a "reference work covering key topics at the intersection of health communication and applied linguistics" (p. 1).

Indeed, the volume includes contributions by linguists, communication scholars, medical anthropologists, psychologists, sociologists, nurses, and physicians, and in the introduction Hamilton and Chou (both linguists) call attention to the benefits of this deep and extensive interdisciplinarity. In this regard, the editors highlight the "interdisciplinary fluency" necessary for collaboration across disciplinary and professional boundaries. Drawing on Wasson (2004: 45) from another context, they cite: "Researchers who inhabit both academic and applied worlds not only need to become fluent in the codes of each context, but they also need to develop the ability to translate each world's logic to the other" (quoted in Hamilton and Chou 2014: 5).

Nevertheless, the editors also explicitly emphasize a sustained focus on language itself as the unique contributions of applied linguistics (again, linguistics proves the "superordinate partner"). Commenting on contributions from cognate communication disciplines, the editors note: "While language plays a central role in these investigations, it is commonly viewed as facilitating exchange of information or enabling researchers' content analysis, rather than being an object of study in its own right" (p. 2). In fact, over two-thirds of the contributions demonstrate the utility of fine-grained linguistic and discursive analyses of text and talk.

A final genre of research literature is the edited volume. As noted above, there are a number of these dedicated to specific health conditions (e.g., dementia) or communicative practices (e.g., doctor patient communication), but there still seem few that offer a panoramic view of health applied linguistics as a field. However, Demjén's 2020a edited volume, *Applying Linguistics in Illness and Healthcare Contexts*, does precisely that. In this collection, thirteen empirical studies by applied linguists showcase the analytic diversity of the discipline. Methods include discourse analysis, conversation analysis, interactional sociolinguistics, narrative analysis, metaphor analysis, and corpus analysis. In the introduction, Demjén gathers these under the broad umbrella of "the discourse analytic tradition of applied linguistic analysis" (p. 5), and goes right to the heart of such analysis as follows:

> Linguistic analysis relies on systematic, replicable, and theoretically based methods of looking at what choices (e.g., in pronouns, metaphors, grammatical form, etc.) are made (consciously or not) in contrast with other choices that could have been made, how such choices patterns systematically, and what the implications might be. (2020b: 4)

This description succinctly captures the interpretive program of the *Language and Social Issues* research strand as listed by the American Association for Applied Linguistics (above). Again, at the very core of this program is the notion that "talk and text are forms of social action," which works in part by linking "features of language at micro-levels of talk and text to macro-levels of societal and institutional discourses" (see above, section 1).

Further, a unique emphasis in the Demjén volume is the explicit connection between research and practice. In every chapter, the authors explore the practical implications of their studies for actual healthcare, and again, it is impossible to miss the important links between applied linguists and their medical colleagues in institutional contexts.

The present volume follows in the tradition of these two endeavors (Hamilton and Chou 2014 and Demjén 2020a) by a wide sampling of health applied linguistics, by highlighting specifically linguistic and discursive methods in the analysis of data on health and illness, and by calling attention to the interdisciplinary and collaborative nature of the research process itself.

3 The dual purposes of this volume

As noted in Paul McPherron's preface, the guiding inspiration of this collection was to ask a range of scholars/scientists to contribute something of their best, recent work *and* to communicate something of who they are as health applied linguists and how that research emerged out of collaborations with others in the field. This twofold purpose is worked out in the volume as follows.

Like its predecessors reviewed briefly above, this volume presents new research ventures and deepening developments of established research programs; new methods and variations of existing methods; new applications of linguistic research to address clinical, public health, and research issues. On this account, the volume is divided into four sections along thematic lines: *health and medical education* (Konopasky and colleagues; Vickers and Goble), *translation and multilingual health projects* (Davis, Kuo, and Maclagan; Schrauf), *public health* (Torres; Diaz; López de Victoria, González Márquez and Colón Rivera), and *larger health interventions* (Feuerherm and McIntosh; Mikesell).

By design, however, the second purpose of this collection is to represent the *situated view* of applied linguists themselves– "situated" in the sense that the authors possess the linguist's habits of mind but move in collegial networks of medical professionals. Thus, while all chapter authors are connected with colleges or universities, and in that sense conduct their investigations as part of the research mission of their respective institutions, each one also has involvements with and commitments to the world of medicine: multidisciplinary collaborations; community-university partnerships; expert exchanges at key stages of data collection or analysis; direct research with patients or community members; and archival research on health policies, hospital charts, and other documents. As noted above, these commitments are at the core of doing health applied linguistics, and they require the "interdisciplinary fluency" mentioned by Hamilton and Chou (2014: 5). Again, along with the detailed summaries of each chapter, we include a paragraph outlining the setting and collaborations of each author.

Finally, the volume concludes with an epilogue that presents excerpts from a discussion by all contributors about their questions, instincts, curiosities, networks, and vision as health applied linguists – their professional world as it overlaps with the professional world of clinical practice, public health, and community. Thus, taken together, this introduction, the authors' comments on their collaborations in each of their works, and the final plenary discussion fill out the picture of the activities and collaborations of health applied linguists in a variety of contexts.

4 The chapters

In the following chapter summaries, each entry includes a brief review of the empirical study itself, a paragraph on the specific language focus and methods adopted by the investigators, and a brief discussion of the authors' research site and collaborations.

4.1 Section one: Health and medical education

The first section includes two chapters on medical education, or more precisely the specialized education and training of clinical personnel who become medical educators (Chapter One) and the ongoing language training of multilingual clinicians who work in their second languages (Chapter Two).

Chapter One is by Abigail Konopasky, Anthony R. Artino, Clara Hua, and Alexis Battista who are faculty members in a Health Professions Education program. The chapter is entitled "Functional Linguistics and Health Professions Education: An Exploration of Individual and Group Reflection Processes," and it addresses pedagogical practices of instructor feedback and student response following clinical instruction. In the first study, Konopasky et al. suspected that negative corrective feedback affected students' representations of the specificity, negativity, and cognitive processing of their task. Quantitative findings using lexical analysis software confirmed their predictions. In the second study, the authors analyzed teacher-student interactions during debriefings after simulation trainings. The authors addressed, not *what* students learned during debriefing, but rather the *how* of the debriefing, with a sustained focus on the social interactions of the *jointly constructed* reflection itself. Again, the linguistic analysis showed *how* reflection works – in this case by identifying the interactional functions of specifically linguistic elements of the instructor-student exchange.

Language Focus and Method. As the linguist in the studies, Konopasky worked from theory and method in systemic functional linguistics to guide her articulation of research questions and predictions. Specifically, she adopted two theoretical meta-functions of language to look at how reflection works: the *representational* function (language is used to represent experience) and the *interpersonal* function (language is used in acts of social interaction).

Collaboration and Site. As the authors note in their chapter, Health Professions Education (HPE) aims to equip accomplished clinicians with the knowledge and skills necessary to function as teachers and mentors for others in the world of medicine. Thus, HPE is about "teaching teaching" and involves a range of pedagogical foci: as for example, classroom and group instruction, hands-on skills acquisition, assessment practices, curriculum development, and interprofessional dynamics in medical interdisciplinary teams. Two authors of the article are faculty members in the Center for HPE at the Uniformed Services University of the Health Sciences and one is Associate Dean for Evaluation and Educational Research at the George Washington University School of Medicine and Health Sciences. Konopasky is a linguist with training in educational psychology, and Artino is an educational psychologist whose research focuses on self-regulated learning. The chapter documents their respective roles in the unfolding research, noting how and at what points they brought their specific skills and content knowledge to bear on the preparation and analysis of the data.

Chapter Two, by Caroline Vickers and Ryan Goble, examines a unique site of primary care in the United States, one in which the providers are bi- or multilingual in Spanish while the patient population is largely monolingual in Spanish. In "From Cultural Competence to Discourse Competence: Discourse Analysis and the Education of Bi/Multilingual Health Care Professionals," the authors locate moments of codeswitching during these consultations: brief interchanges in which the providers switch from Spanish to English while interacting with laptops (i.e., screens representing medical records in English), disability paperwork (in English), and accompanying family members (who speak English). These moves have the subtle yet real effect of rendering patients as non-participants, distancing them from their own medical information and health outcomes. The authors select these excerpts as "useful targets" for further sensitizing bi- and multilingual clinicians to the social implications of codeswitching during consultations, and they frame these efforts in terms of *language learning advising*.

Language Focus and Method. Vickers and Goble situate their work in a *discourse-based framework* designed to foster discourse competence among bi- and multilingual health care providers. At the level of data analysis, they work with tools and concepts from conversation analysis, and at the level of pedagogy, they address issues of advanced proficiency and pragmatic performance in professional medical settings. As noted, this latter pedagogical focus contributes to the wider field of Language Learning Advising (see references in the chapter).

Collaboration and Site. Vickers is a university-based researcher at California State San Bernardino, and she has developed a ten-year collaboration with clinicians, nurses, and support personnel at the multilingual clinic described above. Goble's methodological focus is on narrative and discourse analysis, and he is a graduate of the doctoral program at The University of Wisconsin - Madison.

4.2 Section two: Applied linguistics, translation, and health

This second section includes two chapters, one exploring the application of machine translation to qualitative data in Chinese, the other theorizing processes of bilingual data analysis, translanguaging, and publication of excerpts in multilingual, health-focused projects.

Chapter Three by Boyd Davis, Ching-Yi Kuo, and Margaret Maclagan is entitled "Children Learning about Dementia in Taiwan: Using Gist Translations to Clarify Adult Opinions." The chapter reports the results of an educational intervention in which the second author (Kuo) presented a brief power point about dementia to children in eight elementary schools in Taiwan followed by interviews with school administrators, school nurses, teachers, and parent classroom-volunteers about their attitudes towards the presentation of the information to their children. The chapter focuses specifically on the interviews, and in that context the authors demonstrate the utility, benefits, and drawbacks of machine translation followed by gist editing of the interview transcripts. They note that gist translations allow them to identify the genre and field of the text, as well as some degree of social interaction. "However, we can only infer tenor, or participant relationship, author's provenance and stance, social role relationship, or social attitude" (p. 99, this volume). Nevertheless, the chapter offers a rich exploration on just how such inferences might be made, based on both the interviews themselves and on the literatures treating pragmatics in translation and interpersonal pragmatics.

Language Focus and Method. Although the content focus of this chapter concerns attitudes of Taiwanese school administrators, teachers, nurses, and parents toward a curricular intervention about dementia, the chapter works as a kind of test case for whether and how machine-gist translations can be analyzed pragmatically. Thus, as noted above the authors carefully situate their efforts in literatures on translation and intercultural/interpersonal pragmatics.

Collaboration and site. The co-authors of this chapter comprise a truly international research team. Davis, emerita from the University of North Carolina – Charlotte in the United States has a long-standing and productive research program devoted to language and dementia, with particular emphasis on pragmatics. Maclagan is a retired professor in speech pathology from the University of Canterbury in Christchurch, New Zealand, and Kuo is a licensed professional counselor from Taiwan.

Chapter Four by Robert Schrauf is entitled, "Research Translation as Situated Practice." The chapter is a methodological reflection on applied linguists working with multilingual data in health applied contexts. Drawing on multiple cross-cultural projects on language, aging, and Alzheimer's disease, Schrauf reflects on both the craft of translation itself as a key dimension of linguistic and cultural analysis and on the applied linguist who practices that craft through deep immersion in the source and target languages. He adopts Silverstein's (2003) model of translation as the accomplishment of *indexical equivalence* between source and target texts and traces how researchers develop and deepen such indexical knowledge through materially situated acts of transcription early in a project and re-transcription over the course of a project. Similarly, other linked, situated, research activities involve extensive translanguaging, as for instance multilingual coding and qualitative analysis. Final (and formal) translations of source language excerpts for publication in the target language are then re-situated in the quite different worlds of clinical medicine and public health.

Language Focus and Method. As noted, Schrauf frames translation in terms of metapragmatics and the inherently indexical character of language. This approach attends to how a speaker's (or writer's) phonological, prosodic, syntactic, lexical, and discursive selections invoke cultural meanings and social distinctions for the immediate purposes of talk (or text), thus 'indexing' often multiple contexts for strategic purpose(s).

Collaboration and site. For health applied linguists, this chapter is primarily inward-looking – at our own research practices – rather than outward-looking toward clinical and public health contexts. However, reflection on the behind-the-scenes translation of excerpts for publication opens a window onto the much larger issue of dissemination-of-research-results by health applied linguists and the multi-scalar engagements that dissemination entails: for example, with our medical collaborators, health funders, journal readerships, and the public.

4.3 Section three: Applied linguistics and public health

Section Three gathers three chapters. Two of these address public policy about the opioid crisis in the United States. Both combine corpus analysis and discourse analysis and are thus examples of mixed methods studies. The third is a qualitative study of medical help seeking among older adults in the wake of Hurricane María in Puerto Rico in 2017.

In Chapter Five, entitled "Modality and Interpretive Spaces in Policies," Peter Torres examines 233 policies promulgated in the state of California on opioids from the 1970's through 2020. Torres focuses on modals (can, could, might, must, should, will, would, shall) because, while they are standard features of policy language, modals can also be a source of confusion and ambiguity at the level of policy implementation. He tracked change over time quantitatively in the frequencies of restrictive vs. permissive modals. The qualitative, discourse analytic portion of the study involved coding for the "to whom" of the policies – the stakeholders addressed by the documents – and the actions they were to undertake. Torres found that, from the 1970's to the present, as fatality rates increased, there was an observable shift toward restrictive language in policy documents. In conclusion, he points out that the "mining of modals" from an appropriate corpus reveals for policymakers the general tone of policies (restrictive; permissive).

Language Focus and Method. A key contribution is the methodological demonstration of Torres' *corpus-based discourse analysis* (CBDA) for analyzing policies. He characterizes the two components of CBDA as follows. Corpus analysis "provides a quantitative textual analysis of specific grammatical features," and discourse analysis "allows researchers to interpret the set of possibilities that motivate and explain the patterns that emerged from the corpus analysis" (p. 146, this volume). In addition, he demonstrates the significance of a close grammatical analysis of policy documents, drawing on a long tradition of analysis of verbal modals (e.g., deontic, epistemic auxiliaries).

Collaboration and site. This chapter fits squarely in a university-based research enterprise and derives from indirect involvement with public health personnel. Dissemination of the policy-related results depends on publication venues with likely targets being the growing periodical literature in health policy and administration.

From another angle, Brett Diaz in Chapter Six, also addresses policy and the opioid crisis via a corpus-assisted discourse analysis. However, he shifts the focus to the language of agents-on-the-ground who are responsible for implementation. The chapter is entitled, "Discourse at Work in Elderly, Health Policy Communication: Uncovering Aspects of Semantic Preference and Prosody in the Rural Opioid Epidemic." His corpora include both text (policies) and talk (agency directors, protective services case managers). Critically, he compares the patterns of similarity and dissimilarity of three terms – *opioid, protective, older* – and finds that agency directors and case managers seem to have a more varied repertoire of ways to talk about the epidemic than policy authors. He traces these differences in agents' personal accounts of how they believe themselves to be perceived in their communities and in their nuanced characterizations of what people want and need. Interestingly, agents rarely refer to actual policies.

Language Focus and Method. In this chapter, Diaz develops the method of *corpus-assisted discourse analysis* in which he adapts and characterizes an assemblage of corpus tools *as* discourse analytic tools. Thus, he sees the steps of identifying key words and characterizing their collocational patterns both in terms of semantic preference and semantic prosody (both corpus tools) as dimensions of stance-taking (a powerful discourse analytic tool). He then engages close readings (i.e., traditional discourse analysis) of key words in their preferred collocational contexts to reveal subtle differences both within and across his subcorpora.

Collaboration and Site. Diaz's work may also be characterized as university-based research, albeit grounded in community-based networking and ethnographic interviews. Though not extensively explored in this chapter, his data extend to personal and professional histories of his participants, their self-identification as members of rural societies, and their dedication to serving older adults beyond the opioid crisis. In short, via an ethnographic approach, the interpersonal relationships that he developed with his participants ground his interpretation (sensemaking) of his data.

Chapter Seven is entitled, "Responding to Crisis, Responding to Needs: Older Adults Seeking Medical Care in the Aftermath of Storms" by Patria López de Victoria Rodríguez, Elba González Márquez, and Krystal Colón Rivera. The storm in question is Hurricane María in Puerto Rico in September 2017, and the authors examine three cases drawn from a larger dataset of interviews with older adults, caregivers, and medical personnel. First, the discourse-analytic approach is at once micro-analytic (focused on how participants enact and perform small-scale, everyday, help-seeking activities) and meso- and macro-analytic (focused on how participants situate these activities in larger institutional and sociopolitical contexts). Second, the authors conceptualize *agency*, not as a characteristic of individual persons, but rather as distributed and concatenated across networks of persons and organizations. Third, they treat *language* as a medium for social action: a participants' resource or tool for accomplishing help seeking goals in interactions with others. The cases are selected to show both failed and frustrated agency as well as successful and collaborative agency.

Language Focus and Method. The authors employ a *discourse analytic ethnographic lens* that treats the language of participants as inherently *performative* and *indexical* – reflecting the foundational tenet that "language is social action." Further, their analysis focuses on the "linguistic resources (prosodic, morphosyntactic, lexical, discursive, and pragmatic) that [participants] use to describe, characterize, and interactively manage the search for material resources, the coordination of familial, social, and professional social networks, and their interface with health personnel" (p. 195, this volume).

Collaboration and Site. This project is another example of university-based research. López de Victoria Rodríguez is a faculty member at a local campus of the University of Puerto Rico in the town in which the research took place. A unique feature of the project is the extensive involvement of undergraduate research assistants in data collection, data management, and analysis. These students are local residents, and hence they are conducting linguistic and social science research in/on their own community. Further, given the focus on response to, and recovery from Hurricane María, the principal investigator and her assistants are at once: linguist-ethnographers, community members, and *survivors* of the very events that form the substance of their study. This research then is a compelling example of engaged scholarship.

4.4 Section four: Applied linguistics and health interventions

Section four focused on two interventions. The first is an example of participant-based action research in response to the Flint, Michigan water crisis. The second describes the involvement of an applied linguist in transdisciplinary teams developing clinical interventions.

In Chapter Eight, entitled "Beyond 'Limited English Proficient' in Health Care Policy, Practice, and Programs," investigators Emily Feuerherm and Bonnie McIntosh describe the development and delivery of an ESL-based, health literacy intervention addressing the concatenated emergencies of the Flint Water Crisis and COVID-19. The Flint Water Crisis refers to the discovery in 2014 of elevated levels of lead in the drinking water of city residents, with cascading illness complications especially for children. The dangers were disproportionately visited on urban African American and immigrant populations, and the government response was slow, misguided, and counterproductive. The intervention was the product of a university-community partnership including community leaders, the applied linguist (Feuerherm) and a health care management scholar & community partner (McIntosh). The team collaboratively designed, advertised, and delivered the curriculum which combined ESL pedagogy with principles and practices related to health literacy. In circumstances of COVID-19 lockdown, the curriculum was piloted in both Spanish and English over the internet program Zoom.

Language Focus and Method. This project showcases the application of language pedagogy (a topic at the very heart of applied linguistics) to the amelioration of a community health issue. Feuerherm and McIntosh draw on three specific academic traditions: health policy (with an emphasis on health advocacy and policy implementation); theory, pedagogy, and delivery of ESL in community contexts; and multilingual adaptation of health literacy instruction and materials.

Collaboration and site. The authors of the chapter are two university-based scholars. Feuerherm is an applied linguist at the University of Michigan in Flint, and McIntosh is a community partner, and both scholars involved their research assistants in the project. Crucially, from the very beginning, community members in Flint were also recruited to the development and design of the intervention. These included San Juana Olivares, the director of the Genesee County Hispanic Latino Collaborative, and a project advisory board consisting of representatives of eleven local, community organizations (e.g., health, education, business). These latter provided information on local resources, advice and review of the research plans, and helped with recruitment of participants. Importantly, Feuerherm and McIntosh framed the conception and conduct of the entire project in terms of Community-Based Participatory Action Research, and in the chapter, they evaluate their efforts and offer suggestions for future research from within this framework.

Chapter Nine by Lisa Mikesell is entitled "Designing Health Interventions on Transdisciplinary Research Teams: Contributions of LSI Scholarship." Mikesell presents three examples from her own work that show how scholars in Language and Social Interaction have contributed to intervention development before, during, and after the design stage itself. The first two examples are drawn from a project to design a decision tool for patients considering bone marrow transplant versus chemotherapy for certain kinds of cancer. *Before* the design stage, LSI scholars examined patients' and clinicians' assumptions, meanings-in-context, and sense of the actual problem and found that, while clinicians perceived an information gap (i.e., patients needed to know more about the possible outcomes), the patients experienced an intersubjectivity gap (i.e., patients didn't hear doctors' explanations as applicable to the real-life outcomes that they experienced). *During* the design process, applied linguists analyzed discussion sessions of an advisory panel, and found that discursive devices that would trigger participant contributions would improve communication. Finally, as example of the contributions of LSI analysis *after* an intervention has been developed, Mikesell documents a project involving an online tracking tool through which parents with children taking ADHD medications could report daily reactions and interactions in real time. The linguists found that online tracking may have triggered a lack of trust and threatened the doctor-patient relationship. Linguists recommended that clinicians ask open-ended questions that would be more likely to invite parent narratives.

Language Focus and Method. Rooted in traditions of ethnography of communication, discourse analysis, and especially conversation analysis, Language and Social Interaction is the study of how humans use language in social contexts to accomplish actions and negotiate interpersonal relations. Linguistic and discursive analyses are based on a thorough understanding of institutional context, work-related practices, and the perspectives of actors in those settings.

Collaboration and Site. As a scholar in the Department of Communication, affiliated with the Institute for Health, Health Care Policy, and Aging Research and the Cancer Institute of New Jersey, Mikesell has developed long-standing collaborations with clinicians at the Robert Wood Johnson Medical School at Rutgers. Clearly, successful collaboration in such circumstances requires a thorough knowledge of, and respect for, others' expertise, a wholehearted commitment to both the practical and higher goals of the project, and a willingness to develop deep understandings across professional boundaries.

4.5 Conclusion

The last chapter of the volume is a series of reflections by the contributors to the volume. In a discussion moderated by the first editor (BD), contributors were asked to talk about their professional histories as health applied linguists and to share their perspectives on the trajectory of the field. The conversation was a deeply satisfying one for the participants, and we hope that readers of this volume will find themselves reflected here – or invited to join.

References

AILA, Association Internationale de Linguistique Appliquée/International Association of Applied Linguistics. (2022, May 4). What is AILA? https://aila.info/
AAAL, American Association for Applied Linguistics. (2022, May 4). AAAL Call for Proposals, Strands. https://www.aaal.org/2023-call-for-proposals##
Austin, John L. 1962. *How to do things with words*. Cambridge, MA: Harvard University Press.
Brumfit, Christopher J. 1995. Teacher professionalism and research. In Guy Cook & Barbara Seidlhofer (Eds.), *Principle and practice in appled linguistics*. Oxford, UK: Oxford University Press.
Candlin, Christopher N. & Srikant Sarangi. (eds.). 2011. *Handbook of communication in organisations and professions*. Berlin, Boston: De Gruyter Mouton.
Candlin, Christopher N. & Srikant Sarangi. 2004. Making applied linguistics matter. *Journal of Applied Linguistics*, (1) 1–8. https://doi.org/10.1558/japl.2004.1.1.1
Collins, Sarah, Sarah Peters & Ian Watt. 2011. Medical communication. In James Simpson (ed.), *The Routledge handbook of applied linguistics*, 96–110. New York: Routledge. https://doi.org/10.4324/9780203835654
Davis, Boyd H. & Jacqueline Guendouzi (eds.). 2013. *Pragmatics in dementia discourse*. Newcastle upon Tyne: Cambridge Scholars Publishing.
Davis, Boyd H. (ed.). 2005. *Alzheimer talk, text, and context: Enhancing communication*. New York: Palgrave MacMillan.
Demjén, Zsófia (ed.). 2020a. *Applying linguistics in illness and healthcare contexts*. New York: Bloomsbury Academic.
Demjén, Zsófia. 2020b. Introduction. In Zsófia Demjén (ed.), *Applying linguistics in illness and healthcare contexts*, 1–14. New York: Bloomsbury Academic.
Enfield, Nick J. & Jack Sidnell. 2017. *The concept of action*. New York: Cambrdge University Press.
Galasiński, Dariusz. 2013. *Fathers, fatherhood and mental illness: A discourse analysis of rejection*. Basingstoke: Palgrave.

Greenhalgh, Trisha & Brian Hurwitz (eds.). 2004. *Narrative research in health and illness.* London: BMJ Books.
Hamilton, Heidi & Wen-ying Sylvia Chou (eds.). 2014. *Routledge handbook of language and health communication.* Abingdon: Routledge.
Harvey, Kevin. 2013. *Investigating adolescent health communication: A corpus linguistics approach.* New York: Bloomsbury Academic.
Harvey, Kevin & Nelya Koteyko. 2013. *Exploring health communication: Language in action.* London, New York: Routedge Taylor & Francis.
Heritage, John & Douglas W. Maynard (eds.). 2005. *Communication in medical care: Interactions between primary care physicians and patients.* Cambridge, UK: Cambridge University Press.
Hunt, Daniel & Gavin Brookes. 2020. *Corpus, discourse, and mental health.* New York: Bloomsbury Academic.
Jones, Rodney H. 2013. *Health and health risk communication: An applied linguistics perspective.* Abingdon, Oxon: Routledge.
Knapp, Karlfried & Gerd Antos. 2011. Introduction to the handbook series: Linguistics for problem solving. In Christopher N. Candlin & Srikant Sarangi (eds.), *Handbook of communication in organisations and professions*, v–xv. Berlin, Boston: De Gruyter Mouton. https://doi.org/10.1515/9783110214222.3.
Martin, Gillian & Jonathon Crichton. 2020. Intercultural communication in health care settings. In Jane Jackson (ed.). *The Routledge Handbook of Language and Intercultural Communication 2E*, 503–520. London, New York: Routledge.
Mates, Andrea W., Lisa Mikesell & Michael Sean Smith (eds.). 2013. *Language, interaction and frontotemporal dementia.* Sheffield, UK: Equinox Publishing.
Plejert, Charlotta, Camilla Lindholm & Robert W. Schrauf (eds.). 2017. *Multilingual interaction and dementia.* Multilingual Matters.
Sarangi, Srikant & Christopher N. Candlin. 2011. Professional and organisational practice: A discourse/communication perspective. In Christopher N. Candlin & Srikant Sarangi (eds.), *Handbook of communication in organisations and professions*, 3–58. Berlin, Boston: De Gruyter Mouton. https://doi.org/10.1515/9783110214222.3
Schrauf, Robert W. & Nicole Müller. (eds.). 2014. Dialogue and dementia: Cognitive and communicative resources for engagement. New York: Taylor and Francis.
Semino, Elena, Zósfia Demjén, Andrew Hardie, Sheila Payne & Paul Rayson. 2017. *Metaphor, cancer and the end of life: A corpus-based study.* New York: Routledge.
Silverstein, Michael. 2003. Translation, transduction, transformation: Skating "glossando" on thin semiotic ice. In Paula G. Rubel & Abraham Rosman (eds.). *Translating cultures: Perspectives on translation and anthropology*, 75–105. New York: Berg.
Simpson, James (ed.). 2011. *The Routledge handbook of applied linguistics.* Abingdon: Routledge.
Wasson, Christina. 2004. Review of 'Linguistics, language and the professions: education, journalism, law, medicine, and technology. *Language in Society*, *33*, 121–124.

Section 1: **Applied linguistics and health/medical education**

Abigail Konopasky, Anthony R. Artino, Jr., Clara Hua,
Alexis Battista

Chapter 1
Functional linguistics and health professions education: An exploration of individual and group reflection processes

1 Introduction

A rapidly growing area in health research is *health professions education* (HPE), a field concerned with better understanding and supporting teaching and learning across the health professions (e.g., nursing, medical, and pharmacy education). Put more succinctly, the broad object of HPE research is "the problem of guiding a layperson to become a professional" (van Enk and Regehr 2018, p. 342). There has been a veritable explosion of HPE Master's degree programs in the past 20 years, with only seven globally in 1996 increasing to 121 in 2014 (Tekian and Harris 2012; Tekian et al. 2014). These programs prepare health professionals (often already clinical faculty themselves, differentiating these programs from other masters programs often pursued directly after an undergraduate degree) as teachers, curriculum developers, assessors, and, critically for applied linguistics scholars, researchers (Tekian & Artino Jr 2013). Accompanying this surge in HPE Master's programs has been an increase in the amount of HPE research published annually: pharmacy education publications grew from 104 in 2000 to 598 in 2018 (Sweileh et al. 2018) and medical education publications grew from 279 in 1960 to

---

Acknowledgments: We would like to thank Ryan Boyd for his help exploring the literature around LIWC measures.

Disclaimer: The views expressed herein are those of the authors and do not necessarily reflect the official policy or position of the Uniformed Services University of the Health Sciences, the United States Department of Defense, the National Naval Medical Center, or the Henry M. Jackson Foundation for the Advancement of Military Medicine, Inc.

Abigail Konopasky, Alexis Battista, Uniformed Services University of the Health Sciences and Henry M. Jackson Foundation for the Advancement of Military Medicine, Inc.
Anthony R. Artino, George Washington University School of Medicine and Health Sciences
Jr., Clara Hua, National Naval Medical Center

https://doi.org/10.1515/9783110744804-002

3,760 in 2010 (Lee et al. 2013). There is also growth recently in the number of "Altmetrics events" for HPE articles, like Mendeley saves, tweets on Twitter, and posts on Facebook, suggesting an increasing interest across a variety of audiences in this research (Maggio et al. 2017).

This growing body of HPE research seeks to better support teaching, learning, and assessment across the many, varied, and complex contexts in which health professionals learn – from more traditional classrooms to hospital wards or clinics to simulated learning environments. This research spans developmental stages – from basic science in high school and college to training in medical, nursing, pharmacy, or other allied health professional schools to ongoing professional development for licensed clinicians. HPE scholars take a variety of research design approaches, from more in-depth qualitative analyses to broader quantitative analyses to mixed methods approaches bringing in a variety of data sources (Yonge et al. 2005; Lee et al. 2013; Sweileh et al. 2018). HPE scholars tackle a wide variety of topics and problems, including clinical teaching, assessment methods, feedback to learners, curriculum design and evaluation, and interprofessional team education (Tekian and Artino Jr 2013; Varpio et al. 2017). HPE, then, is a growing and vibrant research field addressing important problems in healthcare.

Moreover, in HPE, more than in many other academic fields, practitioners and "discipline-trained researchers" actively work together, practicing what van Enk and Regehr (2018) call "use-inspired basic research" (p. 341). At HPE conferences, teachers and researchers (and teacher-researchers) collaborate to develop tools to better understand and support teaching and learning in the health professions (van Enk & Regehr). This collaborative and productive atmosphere can be an engaging and inspiring space for linguists, who bring with them a plethora of methods, theories, and perspectives that could advance the field of HPE. As one of few trained linguists in HPE, the first author, Abigail Konopasky, has not only felt welcomed, but has at times felt inundated with invitations to collaborate with researchers and practitioners.

Yet, few scholars or practitioners in HPE make use of linguistic tools (see Konopasky et al. 2019 for an informal review of some of this research). Those who do, however, are offering considerable value to the field. Jeff Bezemer and his team's use of conversation analysis and sociolinguistics to understand operating room discourse, for instance, has provided important insights into patient safety (Bezemer et al. 2016; Bezemer et al. 2017). The automated linguistic analysis research (using Linguistic Inquiry and Word Count, LIWC) of Molly Carnes and her group on how gender affects medical school admissions and National Institutes of Health grant allocation has strengthened the literature on gender inequity in the health professions in the United States (Isaac et al. 2011; Kaatz et al. 2015). These programs of research are built on linguistic methods, exploring the insights we can gain from the language health professionals use. In addition to these research programs driven primarily by linguistic research methods, other research has used linguistic methods alongside more traditional HPE methods like surveys and thematic analysis of interviews (Ginsburg et al. 2016; Cleary et al. 2020; Rachul and Varpio 2020; Ramani et al. 2020). In these approaches to HPE research, linguistic methods often act to fill in the gaps left by traditional methods.

One particular family of linguistic approaches that we have found useful in HPE is (systemic) functional linguistics, a theory approaching discourse through three distinct *metafunctions* of language: interpersonal (enacting relationships), representational (representing experience), and textual (organizing discourse; Martin and Rose 2003, pp. 3–4). Functional linguistics is a useful framework for better understanding the various contexts, developmental stages, and teaching and learning problems in HPE research. For instance, Woodward-Kron and colleagues (2011) focus on the interpersonal function, exploring how non-native speaking medical trainees' use of questions as they interacted with patients shifted over the course of their training. This allowed them to trace their improvement in patient history taking. In another example, Konopasky and colleagues (2020), working with the representational function, examine the ways physicians evaluate their emotions and certainty about a clinical situation during a clinical reasoning exercise. These functional linguistic tools revealed some of the effects of more challenging clinical reasoning cases that other analyses and instruments had not. Functional linguistics, then, while not yet widely used, offers promise for HPE research.

One area of HPE research where we think functional linguistic tools can be particularly helpful is learner written or oral *reflection* (see Locher 2017, for an application of functional linguistics to reflection in medicine), an approach many health professions instructors use to support learning. In this chapter, we explore how functional linguistic tools might help us to better understand the processes of reflection in HPE. We begin with a brief discussion of reflection and reflective practice, explaining in more detail what it is and how it is used in health professions environments. We then present two secondary analyses of previously published data (Cleary et al. 2015; Battista 2017) using functional linguistic tools. The first is a quantitative analysis of the individual oral reflections of 69 students in their first and second years of medical school. The second is a detailed qualitative analysis of a single group oral reflection (often called a "debrief") after two emergency medical technicians and their instructor participate in a simulated learning experience. In both cases, we demonstrate how linguistic analysis reveals important aspects of the learning environment not accessible by traditional HPE methods alone. We conclude by discussing the implications of this research and some suggestions for future directions for linguistics research in HPE.

1.1 Reflection in health professions education

Over the past decade, healthcare educators have started to incorporate reflection into healthcare education. While there are multiple models of reflection and many concepts of how to perform reflective practice, an accepted definition is the following:

> Reflection is the process of engaging the self in attentive, critical, exploratory, and iterative interactions with one's thoughts and actions, and their underlying conceptual frame, with a view to changing them and with a view on the change itself. (Nguyen et al. 2014)

In other words, reflection is an active exercise where health professionals critically think through their values and actions to improve their practice. Even though reflection seems to be a "thinking" exercise, reflective practice is almost always done through language. These exercises occur in group settings where the group talks through their thoughts or through an individual writing prompt (Smith 2011; Chaffey et al. 2012). Either way, these reflection practice options reinforce the idea that reflection is rooted in language and linguistics.

Reflection in healthcare education spans multiple levels of education from undergraduate (a category that includes medical school, despite the fact that it follows a four-year university degree) to postgraduate and multiple professions including medicine, nursing, and allied health professions which include physiotherapists, occupational therapists, pharmacists, therapists, social workers, and psychologists (Fragkos 2016). Reflection across these various contexts, while divergent depending upon the profession's goals and responsibilities, is similar in that the overarching goal of reflective practice is to implement positive changes in clinical practice through improved self-awareness. Reflection has been widely studied and is shown not only to be linked with higher grades (Stephens et al. 2012), but to aid in developing clinical knowledge and skills, particularly with more complex learning problems (Paget 2001; Jayatilleke and Mackie 2013; Schei et al. 2019). Reflective practice can also improve self-directed learning and motivation (Koshy et al. 2017), improve attitudes when studying complex material (Winkel et al. 2017), and contribute to professional identity formation and values development (Wald 2015; Schei et al. 2019). Based on these findings, it is no surprise that reflective practice has earned a permanent place in multiple healthcare curricula.

While sometimes practiced in a less structured way, one common approach is in a group setting where students are guided by a facilitator through a process of deconstructing their feelings and knowledge about a critical situation that occurred. Delaney and colleagues describe a five-stage curriculum, each with its own set of questions: narrative, deconstruction, identification of underlying values, relevance of assumptions, and new theories into practice and ongoing evaluation (Delany and Watkin 2009). Other ways of organizing reflective activities include utilizing a guided prompt to write and process a certain feeling or event, watching a video podcast and then writing a reflective statement, and other reflective tools such as journals, diaries, and videos (Tsingos-Lucas et al. 2016). Thus, reflective learning and practice are heavily rooted in language, both oral and written, as healthcare learners explore knowledge, values, and feelings. We should note that reflective practice is not without its criticism, particularly regarding whether the *assessment* of it changes its fundamental nature, shifting from reflection to surveillance and regulation (Hodges 2015; Ng et al. 2015). Nonetheless, it remains widely used.

Below we explore two reflective learning and practice contexts: the first individual and the second in a group. Both are drawn from existing studies (Cleary et al. 2015; Battista 2017), and we demonstrate how using functional linguistic tools to *reanalyze* the data brings additional insights that cannot be obtained with traditional analytic tools in HPE like surveys or thematic coding. Each study also takes a distinct approach to reflection. In the first, a study of first- and second-year medical student learners, reflection is conceived of as part of a larger cycle of *self-regulated learning* that can help students to improve their practice. In the second, a study of emergency medical technicians learning an ultrasound procedure, reflection occurs as part of *simulation-based learning*, where instructors and learners traditionally "debrief" after participating in a hands-on simulation of clinical practice. We examine the self-regulated learning process through the representational metafunction and the simulation-based learning process through the interpersonal metafunction. These functional linguistic tools deepen our understanding of both self-regulated and simulation-based learning processes.

2 Study 1: Self-regulated learning and reflection: The effects of simple corrective feedback

Self-regulated learning (SRL) is a process by which individuals monitor and regulate their thoughts, feelings, actions, and the environment as they engage in goal-directed activities (Boekaerts et al. 2000). In HPE, educators and researchers have long acknowledged that successful students tend to be those who effectively self-regulate. That is, across multiple contexts, high-performing students strategically engage in learning and clinical activities; adapt and flex when faced with learning challenges; and critically reflect on their own performance and areas for improvement. Effectively self-regulated learners are also especially adept at proactively setting goals, planning their activities, and monitoring their successes and failures through metacognition, which is the degree to which individuals monitor, control, and regulate their own thinking (Pintrich et al. 2000). What is more, proactive, self-regulated learners often seek external feedback from more experienced individuals, such as teachers or other learners. From a regulatory perspective, externally provided feedback is important because it helps learners determine whether and how they will *reflect* on and improve their current and future approaches to learning or clinical performance (Sargeant et al. 2009).

Although external feedback is considered a key component of SRL, when feedback is limited to corrective or task feedback (e.g., simply telling students that their answer is correct or incorrect), learners are less likely to engage in *adaptive* reflection, such as analyzing their errors or rethinking how they might approach the task differently. In fact, for some students, such assessment-based feedback may even cause them to disengage or withdraw from the activity (Zimmerman 2000; Hattie and Timperley 2007). However, in HPE contexts, little is known about how the regulatory and reflective responses of medical trainees might shift during specific clinical tasks following corrective feedback.

Cleary et al. (2015) set out to address this literature gap by examining shifts in medical students' SRL processes during two iterations of a case-based diagnostic reasoning activity. The original study asked two primary research questions. First, do novice medical trainees show significant declines in their self-efficacy and strategic thinking as they engage in multiple iterations of a challenging clinical reasoning task? And second, if changes in students' strategic thinking are observed, what are the primary types of responses that students exhibit following the corrective task feedback?

Findings from this study revealed statistically significant declines in students' self-efficacy beliefs (i.e., their confidence to perform specific behaviors) and in the quality of their strategic thinking, as measured by strategic planning and metacognitive monitoring questions, over the multiple iterations. In particular, when students could not arrive at the correct diagnoses and received corrective feedback that their answer was wrong, they started focusing on irrelevant aspects of the case and ineffective diagnostic reasoning processes. They also exhibited large drops in their task-specific confidence. These results highlight the notion that when medical learners do not experience success – and when they receive simple corrective feedback during that practice – they may experience maladaptive shifts in both their motivation and their strategic focus during reflection.

We chose to do linguistic reanalysis of these study data for two reasons: first, to support the original study's results through *triangulation*, bringing in another analytic approach to the same data to see if it yields the same results; and second, to further explore the *quality* of learners' reflections as measured by whether or not they are reflecting on cognitive processes, which may reflect stronger diagnostic reasoning (Cleary et al. 2020). We chose to use the automated linguistic analysis tool, LIWC (mentioned above in the context of Carnes' and colleagues' work). This allowed us to further explore two concepts that emerged in the original study—specificity and negativity of reflections—and one that prior study measures were *not* able to explore–the types of cognitive processes on which participants reflected. While not exclusively composed of functional tools, the linguistic dimensions LIWC encompasses are robust (Tausczik and Pennebaker 2010). We were interested primarily in the representational metafunction of these medical learners' reflections: did their representations of their experience change after simple corrective, assessment-directed feedback? Specifically, based on the prior study, we asked the following three research questions:

1. Do participants' representations of the specificity of their task change after simple corrective feedback?
2. Do participants' representations of the negativity of their task change after simple corrective feedback?
3. Do participants' representations of cognitive processing in their task change after simple corrective feedback?

3 Study 1 methods

We begin by reviewing the methods of the original study and then discuss our reanalysis with LIWC.

3.1 Participants and study context

In 2011 and 2012, 342 second-year medical students were invited to complete the study: 71 students (21%) volunteered to participate, and data were analyzed on 69 (20%) complete records. The study was conducted in the context of an Introduction to Clinical Reasoning course offered at the F. Edward Hébert School of Medicine, Uniformed Services University of the Health Sciences. At the time of the study, the university offered a traditional four-year curriculum: two years of basic science courses followed by two years of clinical rotations (clerkships). This study was part of a larger project conducted and was approved by Uniformed Services University's Institutional Review Board. Prior to participation in the study, all student volunteers provided written informed consent.

3.2 Procedures

During the final month of the course, the second author individually administered a diagnostic reasoning task to participants during a 25–30 minute session outside of normal class time. The participants were instructed to read a one-page description of a case depicting diabetes mellitus. The scenario was identified as a difficult case based on consensus among a group of medical educators at Uniformed Services University who had previously developed and pilot tested the case.

All participants were given the opportunity to use a post-encounter form as a guide to developing an accurate diagnosis. The participants were familiar with the components of the post-encounter form (e.g., summary statement, problem list, differential diagnosis) because they had received training on how to use this form as part of the 10-month Introduction to Clinical Reasoning course. Following their initial attempt to provide the correct diagnosis, the examiner provided simple corrective feedback: "Sorry, your most likely diagnosis is incorrect." The participants were then given the opportunity to complete another post-encounter form as they engaged in a second iteration of the same clinical reasoning activity. Following their second attempt at generating a most likely diagnosis, the students were given a similar corrective feedback statement.

To evaluate shifts in students' reflections, as measured by SRL processes during the multiple iterations, an SRL microanalytic interview was administered to the participants at different points during the task. The reflective microanalytic questions paralleled the temporal dimensions of the task. For example, given that goal setting and strategic planning are forethought phase processes (i.e., they happen *before* the activity), questions targeting these processes were administered *prior* to each iteration of the task. Moreover, given that metacognitive monitoring is a performance phase process (i.e., it happens *during* the activity), this measure was administered *during* both the first and second iterations of the task. All sessions were audio recorded and transcribed. See Cleary et al. 2015 for a detailed description of study procedures.

3.3 Original study measures

Goal setting. We administered a single-item, microanalytic measure to assess participant goals for the diagnostic reasoning task (Cleary et al. 2015). Participants were asked, "Do you have a goal (or goals) in mind as you prepare to do this activity? If yes, please explain."

Strategic planning. We administered a single-item, microanalytic measure to assess participant plans for approaching the diagnostic reasoning task (Cleary et al. 2015). Participants were asked, "What do you think you need to do to perform well on this activity?"

Metacognitive monitoring. We administered a single-item microanalytic question to examine the extent to which the participants focused on strategic processes during each of the two iterations of the clinical reasoning task. Across both iterations, the participants were stopped after they wrote down their first differential diagnosis and asked, "As you have been going through this process, what has been the primary thing you have been thinking about or focusing on?" If the participants provided a response, they were asked, "Is there anything else you have been focusing on?"

3.3.1 LIWC measures

In order to further explore the effect of simple corrective feedback on learners' reflection, we used three sets of LIWC measures in this current study to compare goal setting, planning, and metacognition *before* simple corrective feedback with goal setting, planning, and metacognition *after* simple corrective feedback. The three sets of LIWC measures were specificity, negativity, and cognitive processing (Pennebaker et al. 2001).

First, we used LIWC to measure the differences in specificity that Cleary et al. (2015) found through hand coding. Drawing from linguistic work, our *specificity* measure was made up of the following LIWC markers: (a) words six letters or more long (more of these are hypothesized to be more specific; Piantadosi et al. 2012), (b) analytic thinking words (the LIWC user manual says a higher number of these words "reflects formal, logical and hierarchical thinking" [Pennebaker et al. 2001, p. 21]; also see Boyd Blackburn & Pennebaker 2020), (c) words from the LIWC dictionary (using *fewer* words from the dictionary reflects *more* specificity as they will be less common words; Malvern et al. 2004; Markowitz and Hancock 2016), and (d) words representing biological processes (we hypothesized that more of these would be more specific since the task was to reflect on *medical* diagnosis).

Second, we used LIWC to measure the increase in negativity and decrease in self-efficacy that Cleary and colleagues found in hand coding. We constructed this *negativity* measure by combining the automated LIWC negation (the negation markers *not* and *n't*) and negative emotion (words associated with negative emotions like *wrong, problem,* and *bad*) markers.

Third, moving beyond the prior study, we wanted to explore whether participants' reflections on their thinking changed after simple corrective feedback. We hypothesized that LIWC's cognitive processing markers – insight, causation, discrepancy, tentativeness, certainty, and difference – would be used *less* after simple corrective feedback as participants' motivation to work through the diagnostic problem decreased (see Table 1 for examples of cognitive processing markers from our data).

Table 1: Examples of LIWC Cognitive Processing Words from the Study One Data.

Cognitive Processing Category	Explanation	Examples from the Data
Insight	Words related to learning or understanding (Pennebaker et al., 2001)	identify, find, know, think
Causation	Words indicating a causal relationship	cause, make, how, effect
Discrepancy	Words indicating a difference, often between some real and ideal state	could, would, lack, problem
Tentativeness	Words suggesting hesitation or lack of certainty	try, might, seem, probably
Certainty	Words suggesting being sure or definite	sure, all, clear, obvious
Difference	Words indicating lack of similarity, often using negation	but, without, other, different

3.3.2 Data analysis

To determine if simple corrective feedback affected the quality of participants' reflection, we performed three multivariate analyses of variance (MANOVAs). A MANOVA is a test that allows us to compare a number of variables at a time without the loss of statistical power that would come by running each comparison separately (Warner 2012). The first MANOVA compared the four specificity variables before and after simple corrective feedback, the second the two negativity variables, and the third the seven cognitive processing variables.

3.4 Approach to linguistic collaboration

To develop and carry out this linguistic reanalysis, Konopasky – a linguist who has done work in generative grammar, critical discourse analysis, and functional linguistics and who also has training in educational psychology – worked together with Artino – a medical education scholar who does work on SRL and learning theories and is trained in educational psychology. First, we both reread the original study (Cleary et al. 2015), noting limitations, gaps, and opportunities for further research that could potentially be addressed through linguistic methods.

Second, we came together to discuss our thoughts, focusing in on two key goals: (1) *automating* some of the hand coding that had been done to understand participants' strategic planning and metacognitive monitoring, and (2) expanding the analysis of participants' reflection beyond task specificity and difficulty to the *quality of reflection*, asking what kinds of cognitive processes they were engaging in. We determined that LIWC would allow us to explore automation and, given its robust cognitive processing measures, quality of reflection.

Third, we worked together to develop research questions to address our goals and Konopasky drew from the literature to develop three measures made up of LIWC variables to answer these questions.

Fourth, Konopasky cleaned the participant transcripts from the original study for use with LIWC so that they did not contain any interviewer language and so that reflections from each of the two time points were in a separate file.

Finally, after running the data through LIWC and importing it into SPSS, Konopasky and Artino worked together to determine which inferential statistical tests to run, deciding on the MANOVA.

We approached the writing process in a similar fashion, with each of us bringing in constructs, observations, and literature from our own disciplines (educational psychology, medical education, linguistics). Our discussions focused on how the linguistic concepts we had chosen to work with (specificity, negation, and cognitive processing words) informed the field of undergraduate medical education where our research was located. Given the context of this volume, we also discussed how to best describe the educational concepts we were working with (self-efficacy, goal setting, strategic planning, metacognitive monitoring) for an applied linguistic audience.

3.5 Study 1 findings

The MANOVA results comparing multiple variables revealed statistically significant differences in reflection before and after simple corrective feedback in specificity (we provide these figures for those who want to track the statistics, but it is not needed to understand our findings: Pillai's trace = .17, F = 3.27, df = [4, 65], p <.05) and cognitive processing (Pillai's trace = .19, F = 2.53, df = [6, 63], p <.05). There was no significant difference in negativity (Pillai's trace = .07, F = 2.48, df = [2, 67],

$p = .09$). Follow-up univariate analyses (i.e., looking at each variable one by one) for specificity indicated that, while differences were in the direction expected (fewer six-letter, analytic, and biological words and more dictionary words after simple corrective feedback), the only significant difference was in six-letter words, with a small effect size (see Table 2). Follow-up univariate analyses for cognitive processing indicated that the only significant differences were in insight and discrepancy words, both of which went down after simple corrective feedback, as predicted, and both with medium effect sizes. While not statistically significant, potentially due to inadequate power, certainty words also appeared to go down, while causation, tentativeness, and difference words went up (see Table 3). Although there were no significant differences in negativity after simple corrective feedback, Table 4 offers descriptive statistics showing that, while negation words went up, negative emotion words went down.

Table 2: Univariate Effects for Specificity.

	Before Corrective Feedback		After Corrective Feedback		$F(4, 65)$	p-value	η^2_p
	Mean (%)	SD	Mean (%)	SD			
Six-Letter	25.3	8.7	21	8.1	11.7	.001	.15
Analytic	58	29	53	29	1.1	.297	.02
Dictionary	90.7	5.4	91.2	6.3	.2	.629	0
Biological	7.4	5.8	6.9	4.2	.6	.43	0

Table 3: Univariate Effects for Cognitive Processing.

	Before Corrective Feedback		After Corrective Feedback		$F(6, 63)$	p-value	η^2_p
	Mean (%)	SD	Mean (%)	SD			
Insight	7.9	5.1	6.1	4.1	5.7	.02	.08
Causation	1.9	2	2.2	2.1	.7	.407	.01
Discrepancy	3.4	3	2.3	2.6	5.6	.021	.08
Tentativeness	5.4	3.8	6.4	3.8	2.9	.093	.04
Certainty	2.1	2.4	1.6	2.5	2.4	.244	.02
Difference	4.2	3.6	4.7	4.1	.7	.406	.01

Table 4: Descriptive Statistics for Negativity.

	Before Corrective Feedback		After Corrective Feedback	
	Mean (%)	SD	Mean (%)	SD
Negation	3.1	4.5	4.2	3.4
Negative Emotion	2.6	3.1	2.2	2.5

3.6 Study 1 limitations

There were several limitations to this study. First, as a reanalysis of existing data, the study was not designed to elicit rich linguistic reflections. Some participant reflections were quite short (e.g., "I don't know") and they were not prompted to expand on their contributions. In other collaborative work, Konopasky, Artino, and Battista have designed the research to better support linguistic analysis, leading to richer data (Cleary et al. 2020; Konopasky et al. 2020a; Konopasky et al. 2020b). Second, in limiting the analyses to only those tools provided by LIWC, we were not able to use a full range of functional linguistic tools. For instance, while LIWC captured many aspects of negative affect through words like *trouble* or *bad*, self-appraisals like, "I still don't know the answer," were not captured. In context, and with the use of the amplifier *still*, it is clear that this learner is frustrated. This is something we could have examined had we hand coded. Study 2, below, draws on a fuller range of linguistic tools, examining a group debriefing after a simulation to explore how reflecting *in a group* affects the reflective process and the potential learning from it.

3.7 Study 1 discussion

Our examination of undergraduate medical learners' reflections on their goals, planning, and metacognitive monitoring supported the original study's (Cleary et al., 2015) findings that simple corrective feedback resulted in student reflections being less specific. Our examination also expanded on this study, finding that student reflections contained fewer cognitive processing words after simple corrective feedback. Our findings for negativity were inconclusive. The seemingly simple feedback that a learner's diagnosis was incorrect led to declines in how specific their reflections were and how much talking about thinking (i.e., cognitive processing words) they did. This further adds to the reflection literature, indicating that feedback focused purely on poor performance rather than specific areas of improvement can negatively affect the quality of student reflection and thinking (Hattie and Timperley 2007; Shute 2008; Archer 2010).

This study also broadens the ways HPE scholars may *conceive* of reflection, expanding our toolkit for studying this vital area. As a functional linguist who has done work with verbal process types and agency (e.g., considering how the quality of being an agent is different for, say, a verbal verb like *say* versus a material verb like *do*; Konopasky & Sheridan 2016), Konopasky approached the study with questions about the types of thinking (e.g., expressing certainty, noting difference, asserting causation) participants were reflecting on and whether they were reflecting on thinking at all, or instead on other aspects of experience (like feeling frustrated). In this way, trained linguists can bring further richness and depth to existing educational and psychological constructs, making them more useful and powerful.

Our research also adds to the field of HPE by developing an automated analytic approach to learner reflection through LIWC. Reflection is a widely used practice in undergraduate medical education, both to support student learning and to offer instructors insight in student thinking (Smith 2011). Yet, to our knowledge, these uses of reflection all involve instructors individually analyzing what students write or say. While this individual attention to reflection is a critical part of the instructor-student relationship, LIWC could allow medical education programs to review large numbers of learner written or transcribed reflections to determine if learners are struggling – becoming less specific, using fewer cognitive processing words, or (if borne out in further studies) becoming more negative. This could signal the need for support *before* learners' motivation or self-efficacy decreases, perhaps affecting their performance, emotional state, or professional identity formation. Yet, as with all assessment of reflection, this approach could lead to less learner trust in the process, engendering an atmosphere of surveillance (Hodges 2015; Ng et al. 2015). These are critical considerations for the field.

The inclusion of linguistic analytic methods like LIWC also fulfills the function of analytic triangulation. While the original study by Cleary and colleagues offered strong evidence for shifts in learners' self-regulatory processes, the addition of the linguistic measure strengthens the study by addressing the same problem with different methods (Patton 2014, p. 316). Comparing the results of two distinct analytic approaches to the same data can both strengthen conclusions and offer future directions for study where these approaches do not align. For instance, while our negation measure may not have shown significance because of a lack of statistical power, the descriptive analysis indicating that learners' negative *emotion* words did not decrease suggests future research directions. Perhaps simple corrective feedback does not increase the expression of negative emotions, for instance, but leads to learners simply sharing fewer emotions. Investigation of the source of this lack of significance could lead to a better understanding of reflection and negative emotion. What is more, the use of linguistic methods allows researchers to examine so-called nonanalytic approaches to clinical diagnosis. In other words, physicians-in-training are not consciously aware of many of their own cognitive and behavioral activities during diagnostic reasoning (Mamede et al. 2007), and so non-intrusive tools like LIWC are quite valuable, giving researchers some access to these nonanalytic processes.

4 Study 2: Simulation-based learning and reflection: What the interpersonal metafunction reveals about a group debriefing session

Simulation is defined as, "A technique that creates a situation or environment to allow persons to experience a representation of an event for the purpose of practice, learning, evaluation, testing, or to gain understanding of systems or human actions" (Lopreiato 2016). It involves a wide range of activities, including learning a specific technique or procedure, such as how to give medications or perform a medical procedure. Other simulations are more complex and present participants with a medical problem to identify and then solve, while interacting with actors or patient simulators designed to respond in the ways actual patients or healthcare providers would. These scenario-based simulations are grounded in narratives which help set boundaries for, and guide participants' activities (Battista 2017).

Simulations are regularly used across HPE contexts, including in the undergraduate and postgraduate curricula for physicians, dentists, nurses, pharmacists and other allied health specialists (e.g., paramedics, respiratory therapists; Cook et al. 2011). Some of the most common reasons simulations are employed, include, a) improving healthcare provider performance in crisis events (Gaba et al. 2001); b) its use in lieu of practicing on actual patients to support patient safety (Ziv et al. 2003; Bradley 2006; Ziv et al. 2009); and c) as a solution to challenges associated with contemporary medical education (Issenberg et al. 2009).

Simulations are viewed as learner centered, whereby learners interact with the simulation and other simulation activities to transform and discuss their experiences, internalize what they have learned and make connections with their prior knowledge (Dieckmann et al. 2007; Battista 2015; Dieckmann et al. 2016; Battista 2017). They foster learner centered actions in large part because they enable social interactions among students, instructors, simulated participants (e.g., simulated patient, simulated clinician), and facilitators (individuals who lead or help ensure the simulation is implemented according to plan; Lopreiato 2016) as they work collectively towards a shared goal (e.g., participation in a simulated medical emergency; Dieckmann et al. 2007).

Implementation of simulations involves at least three stages: a preparatory phase called a pre-simulation briefing, a simulation phase, and a post-simulation reflection, often called a debrief (Tyerman et al. 2019). Pre-simulation briefings immediately precede the simulation and are intended to orient participants to the simulation environment; the objectives and logistics are clarified, roles are assigned, expectations established and boundaries surrounding confidentiality and privacy for creating a safe learning environment are discussed (Rudolph et al. 2006).

During the simulation stage, individuals or groups are asked to suspend their disbelief, as if they were in the clinical setting, and manage clinical situations or procedures while simultaneously engaging with a simulated patient or clinicians. Learning is supported through direct practice as well as through socially mediated learning activities such as instructor-led modeling, peer interactions (Tolsgaard et al. 2009) or direct or telephone support from instructional faculty (Parker and Myrick 2012; Piquette et al. 2014), much of which is achieved via language. Additionally, attention is given to simulating the physical, social, and cultural practices of healthcare, enabling participants to learn the language, practices, and cultural norms of healthcare (Dieckmann et al. 2007; McNiesh 2015; Battista 2017).

In the following post-simulation debriefing stage participants, instructors, a facilitator, and others who partook in or observed the simulation, review and reflect on the actions taken during the simulation (Fanning and Gaba 2007). Debriefing is a structured process involving reaction, analysis and summary phases (Rudolph et al. 2006). The reaction phase allows participants to express their initial emotional reactions to the simulation, and helps them make the transition from the simulation to the debriefing. The analysis phase focuses on specific gaps in participants' performance; facilitators or instructors provide feedback and discuss how participants can close that gap. Lastly, participants summarize what they learned and how they envision acting on that learning in the future.

While simulation-based research continues to examine each of these stages, most studies examining debriefing have focused primarily on whether or not reflection improves learning outcomes such as knowledge retention or improved performance (Raemer et al. 2011). For example, several studies suggest that debriefing can lead to improvements in rescuer performance in life-threatening situations, and improvements in performance metrics, including knowledge and specific procedural skills (Dine et al. 2008; Edelson et al. 2008; Tannenbaum and Cerasoli

2012; Cook et al. 2013). However, Raemer and colleagues (2011) noted that there was limited research into the actual practice of debriefing and how it supports learning. They suggested examining when and where debriefings are conducted, what training facilitators and instructors might need, and which structured approaches are best for different types of simulations and the varying skill levels of learners. Furthermore, Edelson and Lafond (2013) suggest that there is much diversity in how debriefing sessions are conducted. Factors that influence debriefing quality include, who conducts them (e.g., skilled debrief facilitator) and whether or not participants perceive that it is "safe" to contribute.

Another challenge includes examining how the different stages–pre-simulation briefing, simulation participation, and debriefing–influence and intersect with each other. We chose to look at the debriefing data from this prior study (Battista 2017) through a *linguistic* lens because in the original study from which these data were drawn, we explored how participants achieved their goals during practice and what influenced their participation. Here, we also wanted to explore participants' debriefing reflections to better understand how the combined activities (i.e., simulation participation, debriefing) supported learning. When we began our analysis of the transcribed debrief sessions, we realized that simply accounting for how or what participants indicated they learned was overly reductive and that the social interactions between the study participants, debrief facilitator, and the clinical instructor were more than a simple back and forth exchange where knowledge was *imparted* to learners. Rather, we noted that the reflection was jointly *constructed* by all of the parties (i.e., learners, facilitator, instructor). Having prior experience partnering with a linguist to examine how different simulation contexts might influence reflection (see, for example, Cleary et al. 2020), we wondered if linguistic tools could help us examine how participants jointly constructed the debriefing session when the Debriefing with Good Judgment approach is used.

Debriefing with Good Judgment, one of the most commonly employed debriefing approaches, helps participants scrutinize the actions they took during the simulation while also examining what prior frames, beliefs and knowledge informed their choices (Rudolph et al. 2007). It posits that all choices are informed even if the participant isn't immediately aware of what informs them. Its theoretical underpinnings include cognitive psychology, social psychology and anthropology, and it argues that true growth and change cannot occur without examining what underlies action. In practice the approach follows the familiar sequence of reaction, analysis and summarizing. Yet, during the analysis phase, Debriefing with Good Judgment uses language emphasizing participants' actions and assumptions and instructors' explicit descriptions of what they believed happened and how. For example, rather than stating that a participant did something incorrectly, facilitators using this model may instead state, "I noticed X. I was concerned about that because Y. I wonder how you saw it?"

We draw on the *interpersonal metafunction* of language to better understand this, using the Debriefing with Good Judgement approach and asking the following questions:
1. How do the learners, instructor, and facilitator use Mood markers (words and clauses signaling the interpersonal metafunction, e.g., *should*, to indicate obligation) in a debriefing session?
2. What do these patterns suggest about how participants, instructors and facilitators jointly construct the debriefing process?

4.1 Study 2 methods

We begin by reviewing the methods of the original study and then discuss our reanalysis using the concept of the interpersonal metafunction from SFL (i.e., clause as exchange; Halliday and Matthiessen 2014) to explore the interactions among participants, facilitator, and instructor.

4.1.1 Participants and study context

The purpose of the larger study from which these data were drawn was to better understand how learning was supported in skills-based simulations (i.e., those teaching one specific procedure or skill) and scenario-based simulations (i.e., those encouraging problem solving and bound by a narrative). To do so, we analyzed various data sources – including participant reflections in the post-simulation debriefing session – to map the activity in each type of simulation. The guiding research questions were: a) How do student healthcare professionals engage in skills- and scenario-based simulations? and b) what kinds of connections do participants in skills- and scenario-based simulations make to their simulation practice when engaging in a post-simulation debrief? The study employed a prospective case study design to allow for input from multiple data sources (e.g., video recorded participation, audio recorded debriefing sessions, written journals). We chose the Extended Focused Assessment for Sonography in Trauma (EFAST) as the exemplar skill, a common ultrasound exam, and we designed skills- and scenario-based simulations with similar features to teach the skill. In terms of participants, we identified 10 student healthcare professionals who were naive to EFAST and who were unlikely to have access to additional ultrasound practice through the duration of the study. We also recruited physician instructors who specialized in conducting the EFAST in clinical practice and who regularly taught the exam to novices and also had expertise and training in debriefing.

4.1.2 Data analysis

The initial analysis focused on mapping the activity of the two simulation contexts (i.e., skills and scenarios) through video analysis, followed by post-simulation debriefing sessions. For this reanalysis, we purposely selected a high-quality debriefing session that included two learners, one debrief facilitator, and one clinical instructor. The debriefing length was 25 minutes 31 seconds, and the audio recording was transcribed verbatim. To determine debrief quality a trained rater reviewed and rated the debriefing sessions using the Debriefing Assessment for Simulation in Healthcare rater short form tool. The tool assesses six elements: (1) establishing and (2) maintaining a safe and engaging learning environment, (3) structuring the debriefing in an organized way (e.g., reactions, analysis, summary), (4) promoting engaging discussions, (5) identifying and addressing performance gaps, and (6) helping participants establish plans for future performance (Brett-Fleegler et al. 2012). The Debriefing Assessment for Simulation in Healthcare evaluates the strategies and techniques used to conduct debriefings and is based on evidence and theory about how people learn and change in experiential contexts (Brett-Fleegler et al. 2012).

We coded elements of Halliday and Matthiessen's (2014) system of *Mood* – "the primary interpersonal system of the clause" (p. 113) – that we thought might offer insight into how the interpersonal aspect of the debrief was affecting participants. Table 5 lists the codable elements that comprise Mood and gives a phrasal summary of each element with examples from the data. The relevant Mood Elements are the following: interrogative clauses; positive and negative polarity items; modal markers of probability, usuality, obligation, or inclination; modal commitment; and modal responsibility (Halliday & Matthiessen; Thompson 2013). Martin and Rose (2003) frame these Mood elements as *negotiation* of the exchange between speakers and as *appraisal* – a claim about attitudes – of aspects of the exchange. We were interested in how the facilitator, instructor, and learners negotiated the debriefing process and their appraisals of their own and others' roles in the simulation and the debriefing.

Table 5: Coded Mood Elements.

Mood Element	Explanation	Examples from the Data
Subject/ Modal Responsibility	The element responsible for the clause's function	**I** [self] thought towards the end **we** [learners] could get the hang of it at the end of each session. And then **you** [generic] would go away for a week and forget. (participant 6)
Interrogative	Any type of question (yes/no or WH-)	*Yes/no*: **Did** you feel like you had forgotten some things from last week? (facilitator) *WH-*: I'm curious, while you are working together, **what** are you thinking about? (facilitator)
Polarity	Quality of all finite clauses – either positive or negative	*Negative*: I did**n't** really do that [twist the probe] today. (participant 6) *Positive*: (after reconsideration) I think I **did** it [twist the probe] briefly today. (participant 6)
Modal Markers	Markers of degree between positive and negative poles	*Probability*: So **maybe** speed would be what I say that I got better at. (participant 6) *Usuality*: **Sometimes** I would think back on it and do a quick mental review of the quadrants. (participant 7) *Obligation*: [Paying attention to depth to realize] Oh, you **need** to go more shallow. (participant 7) *Inclination*: Reach out and I **will** schedule a time (debriefer)
Modal Commitment	Degree to which the speaker stands behind the utterance	*High commitment*: I think you [learners] **definitely** are much more comfortable with it [ultrasound]. (instructor) *Low commitment*: [in response to facilitator statement] I can **kind of** see that. (participant 7)
Modal Responsibility	Degree of subjectivity of utterance – often lowered via generic	*High responsibility*: I thought it was easier **for me** this week. (participant 7) *Low responsibility*: Once **you** know the general area, **it**'s pretty easy to figure it all out. (participant 6)

This table is drawn from Halliday and Matthiessen (2014) and Thompson (2013).

After coding all participants' utterances for these Mood markers, we examined sequences of exchanges initiated by a facilitator question, seeking *patterns* in Mood elements. We memoed on and discussed these patterns to better understand them (Saldaña 2015). Given our focus on the interpersonal metafunction and the *joint* construction of the debrief, we focused on how the four participants used Mood to negotiate the debriefing process, appraising the situation and eliciting reactions or contributions from others.

4.1.3 Approach to linguistic collaboration

While the functional linguistic tools used in this study (Mood markers) and analytic approach (qualitative) were quite different from Study 1, the approach to collaboration was similar. For this analysis, Konopasky worked with Battista, a health professions educator and simulation researcher who does work on social learning theories and is also trained in educational psychology. Both reread the original study (which has been submitted for publication) and decided to work on a debriefing transcript because it gave us an opportunity to look at a different kind of reflection than study 1 and because there has been little work in the simulation literature on debriefing language. We felt this could offer insight into the debriefing *process* (versus the product – i.e., surveys or assessments after the debrief) that could help support instructors.

After choosing our transcript (based on the assessment tool – see above), Battista briefed Konopasky on some of the unanswered questions about debriefing in the simulation literature. We determined that, although many scholars agree that the social interaction that occurs in a debriefing reflection is valuable, there is little research on precisely *how* that social interaction might support high quality reflection and learning. Thus, we decided to focus our linguistic investigation on the *interpersonal* aspect of the debrief, exploring how the participants jointly construct the reflection.

Next, Konopasky went back to the functional linguistics literature, with a focus on the interpersonal metafunction. There, the Mood element is described as the grammatical system facilitating interpersonal exchange (Halliday & Matthiessen 2014), so that became our focus. Konopasky then went through the transcript, noting every instance of the Mood elements in Table 5 and coding them for which type of element they were. She then went back through the transcript to look for *patterns*: places where certain types of Mood markers tended to be followed by other types. In so doing, she discerned six patterns, which she shared with Battista. Working together and using Battista's knowledge of both simulation generally and this particular debriefing reflection, we narrowed it down to four patterns that are meaningful to learning in the simulation context, reported below.

4.2 Study 2 findings

We identified four patterns in Mood elements that might explain how participants jointly constructed debriefing. Three of these patterns show how participants jointly constructed a safe environment for sharing and increased the focus or specificity of the reflection and the last suggests ways joint construction can result perhaps in discomfort and less focused reflection.

4.2.1 Finding 1: "Yeah, Yeah": How participants used positive polarity to improve reflection

All four participants – facilitator, instructor, and learners – made more statements with positive polarity than negative and frequently emphasized their agreement with others' positive statements with "yeah" or "yes." What seems like a simple part of joint reflection – agreement – actually had a powerful effect on learners' reflections. One pattern we noted was that when participants affirmed another's contribution with "yeah," this was followed by either (a) a more focused appraisal of the situation by that same contributor or (b) another participant adding *their* appraisal of the situation, whether similar or different. In the example below, for instance, participant 7 uses positive polarity to agree with participant 6:

(1) PARTICIPANT 6: *I mean it's kind of a – like a comfort thing on our perspective initially is that doing it together, chances are if one of us forgets something, the other will remember it.*

PARTICIPANT 7: *Yeah.*

PARTICIPANT 6: *And then once we sort of did you know, went through one FAST exam, between the two of us like alternating, each view is kind of like, "Yeah, they could probably do it. So, like just go off and practice on your own." That was kind of my thought.*

Here, participant 7's positive appraisal of participant 6's reasoning for working together supports a more focused and detailed assessment by participant 6 of how they decided to work initially as a pair and then split up. While most of these supportive "yeah" assessments were used by the two learners, the instructor occasionally used this as well. In one exchange, for instance, she uses it to support the learners' tentative implication that they could ask patients to disrobe to do an ultrasound: **"Yeah**, don't be afraid."

Participants also use these positive polarity markers to support their own reflection, using them as a way to make space for their appraisal:

(2) PARTICIPANT 6: *I was playing around with the gain a little bit, but that was mostly just making sure you had the correct orientation with the dot and then that you were far enough or not too far to see the size of the screen that you wanted.*

PARTICIPANT 7: **Yeah, yeah**, *I felt today that probably the area I most improved is with the breadth of it, like the weight, the scale*

In this example, participant 7 uses positive polarity not only to note a shared appraisal of the situation, but to give further detail on it, in fact even *disagreeing* with participant 6 about the primary area of improvement. In this way, positive polarity was used to signal surface shared appraisal while making space for a different appraisal.

4.2.2 Finding 2: "I noticed . . .": How the facilitator used high modal responsibility and interrogative mood to support quality of reflection

Following the Debriefing with Good Judgment model (Rudolph et al. 2007), the facilitator explicitly noted what *she* observed before directing questions towards the learners. In other words, she took high modal responsibility, as in this exchange:

(3) FACILITATOR: ***I heard** several conversations between the three of you about the dot indicator and making sure that it was pointed in the right direction. And also you talked a lot about depth. In thinking about it, like **what** were things you feel like you worked the hardest on and really had focused on today? **What** might that would you say were some of the big things you were focusing on?*

PARTICIPANT 6: ***For me [responsibility]**, it was **just, like [low commitment]** getting the picture to look better. So, like if I was able to for the most part find the organs, right, and then just as far as making – I was trying to make the picture look more easily decipherable so that you know right away that it's – that's where that is based on like the depth. I was playing around with the gain **a little bit [usuality]**, but that was **mostly [usuality]** just making sure you had the correct orientation with the dot and then that you were far enough or not too far to see the size of the screen that you wanted.*

The modal responsibility the facilitator takes in noting what she *heard* the learners focusing on was followed by a *wh*-question about the learners' observation of their own focus. This led the learner to explicitly take modal responsibility and frame it around his own experience ("for me"). Participant 6 actually disagreed with the facilitator's claim about a focus on depth, stating instead that it was about "getting the picture to look better," whether that was through depth or through "the correct orientation." Yet the participant disagrees only to a certain degree, framing his claim with low commitment ("just, like") and marking it as not accounting for all cases ("a little bit," "mostly").

Another function of learners' use of low commitment (via modal markers like *kind of, sort of,* and *might*) and high responsibility (via phrases like *I think* and *to me*) appears to be to support the other learner in sharing their voice and making their own commitment about the situation. At one point, for instance, the facilitator notes that the learners chose to work together for a while before separating to their own stations and asks them both to reflect on it. Participant 6 is the first to respond, followed by 7 and both make space for the other's opinion via modality:

(4)　PARTICIPANT 6: *Participant 7 and I worked together for a while on a lot of things. So, I think we're **just kind of** –*

　　　PARTICIPANT 7: *We're used to working as a team. So it's **probably** more natural **I guess** that way, or at least to start off that way and **like** reorganize our bearings, or such **at least for me**, that's what it was.*

There are a series of exchanges on this topic and, throughout, both learners carefully mark their contributions modally to allow each other to contribute uniquely.

4.2.3 Finding 3: "It was really difficult": How the facilitator and instructor used low modal responsibility to support learners' confidence

In contrast to the high modal responsibility that the facilitator took when noting what she had observed, there were several instances where either the facilitator or instructor used a subject other than "I" to take *low* modal responsibility. In these cases, they were trying to reassure the learners that an unexpected detail about or difficulty with the simulation was quite common. For instance, when participant 7 is sharing the strategies she used when she could not get a good view of the heart, the facilitator and instructor respond simultaneously, talking over each other to say, "**It** was pretty hard" and "**It** was really difficult" respectively. While there is no verbal response from participant 7, these sorts of claims about how things generally "are" from these two experienced practitioners were intended to reassure them.

4.2.4 Finding 4: "I don't know how else you can improve": How learners used low modal responsibility and negative polarity to create distance

While the facilitator and instructor used low modal responsibility to support learners' confidence, the learners themselves used it to create some distance between themselves and the task. Thompson (2013) refers to this as "objectivizing" a point of view to make it appear to be a general state of affairs or a property of the situation itself rather than the speaker's point of view. In talking about what "you" do or simply what "happens" in these types of situations, learners shift the agency from themselves to any reasonable person in a similar situation. For instance, in the example below, the debriefer cues an "I" answer by asking a second-person "you" question about how they might improve next time, but participant 6 responds with negative polarity and low responsibility:

(5) PARTICIPANT 6: *Well, I **don't** really know what else, how else **you** can improve as far as like doing the EFAST better other than just getting the definitive results in a faster time period that is still comfortable for the patient and **you** still are able to explain what you're doing and everything like that. Just because at least in my mind, me, if it's a real trauma scenario, **you** want to be able to find what's ailing the patient as fast as possible.*

In this response, participant 6 does not take responsibility for what he might improve upon. Instead, he notes that the only reasonable expectation for *anyone* in such a situation would be an increase in speed as opposed to any improvement in technique.

4.3 Study 2 limitations

There are several limitations in this study. First, we only selected one debriefing session associated with skills-based simulations. Thus, we cannot determine whether the features we are finding are part of all debriefings or only those associated with skills-based practice sessions. Additionally, our choice of debriefing sessions rated as high quality may reveal certain behaviors that may not be present in lower quality debriefings. Further analysis of other debriefing sessions may yield different patterns. Additionally, there is no comparison among debriefing models because this study employed only the debriefing with good judgement approach. Future efforts could include examining other models.

4.4 Study 2 discussion

Our examination of how learners, instructors, and facilitators co-construct this post-simulation debriefing session reveals a complex picture of *how* facilitated debriefing contributed to learners' reflection on their actions and provides support for the Debriefing with Good Judgement model (Rudolph et al. 2007).

It expands our understanding of the system of debriefing which goes beyond a simple description of learning through dialogue framed by participation in a simulation experience. Rather, this analysis points to higher order functions as underpinning the learning behavior of reflection, such as the use of positive polarity which led to increased focus. The use of high modal responsibility and *wh*-interrogatives helped facilitators and learners gain a shared understanding of students' motivations while in the simulation, an explicit goal of Debriefing with Good Judgement. The analysis also extends our understanding of *how* all participants can play a role in jointly maintaining a psychologically safe environment – historical views and practices have primarily emphasized that the responsibility of maintaining psychological safety is the role of the facilitator and/or instructor.

These findings also generated some conflict regarding the goals of debriefing: when the instructor and facilitator said, "it's really difficult," they are helping support learners' confidence rather than passing judgement. This support and lack of judgment is an important expectation of debriefing or feedback. The finding of use of high modal responsibility ("I saw," "I heard") by the facilitator is likely a direct result of the structure of the Debriefing with Good Judgment model, wherein "I" is intended to minimize judgement and maintain safety for participants. Thus, linguistic analysis may offer a way to evaluate and test not only this model, but potentially others, such as Debriefing for Meaningful Learning (Dreifuerst 2012).

The language data generated from simulation-based learning activities – the pre-simulation briefing, utterances during simulation, and post-simulation debriefings, to name a few – provide numerous opportunities for examining how learning is constructed, measuring learner outcomes, and evaluating simulation debrief models. For example, in this study, the linguistic analysis not only sheds light on how co-construction occurred, but also provided evidence that the Debriefing with Good Judgment Model was working as intended (Rudolph et al. 2007). With so many debriefing and feedback models in use, and linguistic analysis could help address calls to understand which models work best (Raemer et al. 2011). Given that simulations can support novice to expert learners' education and training, the development of assessment approaches to reliably distinguish between participants of various levels is critical. Here, conjunctions like *and, but,* and *because* indicate that a speaker is connecting multiple statements together, which is typically seen in more advanced practitioners and can be indicators of cognitive complexity (Konopasky et al. 2019). Functional linguistic tools also offer an opportunity to examine how teams of healthcare professionals work together to make diagnoses and treat patients, something that is studied in both simulated and actual clinical environments (Konopasky et al. 2020a; Ramani et al. 2020). Ultimately, functional linguistics offers a novel methodological approach to studies employing simulation and those directly examining simulation as a learning strategy.

5 Discussion

Below we discuss the implications these studies have for reflective practice in medicine, HPE research design, and collaboration between linguists and those in health professions fields.

5.1 Implications for reflective practice

These studies have important insights for reflective practice in HPE. Study 1 shows that simple corrective feedback affects the quality of reflections, leading to less specificity and less use of cognitive processing words. While LIWC was unable to code phrases such as "I *still* don't know" as potentially "negative," participants did seem to be frustrated and discouraged after being told only that they had the wrong diagnosis. Simply labeling a response as incorrect appears to make it difficult for learners to fully engage with feedback. This supports work on reflection showing the importance of the *kind* of feedback and guidance instructors or mentors offer students (Delany and Watkin 2009; Tsingos-Lucas et al. 2016). To support deeper reflection, HPE instructors should carefully consider the kind of feedback they provide.

Study 2, meanwhile, demonstrates how a group-led reflective debriefing can support student reflection Students in the debrief were supported in exploring their thought processes, which allowed for better processing of information. This aligns with Winkel's (2017) finding that reflection allows for improved attitudes when studying complex material. Further linguistic analysis could help us to better understand the ways group reflection participants support each other interpersonally in approaching this complexity.

5.2 Implications for HPE linguistic research design

In addition to offering insight into reflection in HPE, this chapter has implications for design of research across different HPE contexts. In the first study, participants were undergraduate medical learners who had just completed a clinical reasoning course. They were offering short, performance-based reflections to a study researcher in a structured context while receiving minimal feedback.

In this learning context, we were interested in the ways learners represent their experiences (what Halliday and Matthiessen [2014] call the *experiential* component of the representational metafunction) and what those representations might indicate about their approach to and feelings about this task. Contexts like this – structured reflection on a specific task – are common across the health professions as academic programs prepare learners with the strategies and knowledge needed to approach real-world clinical problems and assess them on their progress. In these contexts, functional linguistic tools like the transitivity system (the grammatical system allowing us to divide experiences into nominals, predicates, and other circumstantial elements) and conjunction (cohesive devices linking elements like *and* or *but*) offer further opportunities for better understanding learners' approaches to tasks and how best to support them.

In the second study, in contrast, the participants are emergency medical technicians learning how to do an ultrasound assessment. They were reflecting as a group, led by a trained debriefing facilitator, where the goal was not to provide corrective feedback, but to reflect on what they learned, how they best learned, and how they might approach similar learning tasks in the future (in fact, they were preparing to come *back* in a week and further improve their EFAST skills). While there were guiding prompts, they were open-ended and encouraged discussion among the participants (students, instructor, and facilitator) while everyone (not just the learners) reflected on and compared their experiences in the simulation. These responses were much longer, and the reflection was far more conversational than in study 1. In this learning context, we were interested in the ways learners used language to enact interpersonal relationships through their reflection (i.e., the interpersonal metafunction; Halliday & Matthiessen). More open-ended debriefing reflections like this one are also common across the health professions, particularly in simulation. They also play a major role in the growing field of interprofessional education, where clinicians from a variety of fields – medicine, nursing, pharmacy, social work, etc. – are learning to operate together as a team (Pomare et al. 2020). In these types of learning contexts, linguists should consider drawing on frameworks exploring the interpersonal dimensions further, including pragmatics, or even discourse and conversation analysis. In designing linguistic studies of HPE, the learning context should be carefully considered so that the team can choose the appropriate analytic tools.

5.3 Implications for collaboration

The secondary analyses reported on in this chapter argue strongly for *collaboration* among linguists and HPE researchers. In both studies, Konopasky was able, as a linguist, to see opportunities for understanding and assessment in these learning contexts that the researchers trained in educational psychology were not. This resulted in a potentially automated type of reflection analysis from study 1 and an articulated description of the process of reflection from study 2. Yet, this collaboration did not follow the model that is perhaps typical in HPE, where, for instance, a research team presents a methodologist with research questions and then the methodologist offers the appropriate analytic choices (note that while this model *is* common, it does not make the most of the potential partnership with a methodologist). Instead, the linguist and HPE researchers worked together to better understand each other's domains (functional linguistic tools and reflection) so that they could *jointly* construct a set of questions. This type of collaboration is more time consuming, but ultimately more productive. It was also helpful that the linguist in this case did have overlapping training with the HPE researchers (in educational psychology) and was beginning her own research career in HPE. These sorts of interdisciplinary collaborations can bear the fruit not only of useful studies, but also of interdisciplinary *scholars* who can think in more diverse ways about the field of HPE.

6 Conclusion

While different sets of linguistic tools and different analytic techniques were used in each secondary analysis, both significantly added to our understanding of reflection processes in the context of HPE. In study 1, a *quantitative* linguistic analysis using LIWC allowed us to strengthen the original study's finding that specificity decreases after simple corrective feedback while enriching the original study by adding the dimension of cognitive processes and examining how representation of them changes after that feedback. In study 2, a *qualitative* linguistic analysis with a focus on the Mood system offered insight into how the facilitator, instructor, and learners jointly create a psychologically safe learning environment to explore the learning experience for each of the participants. Study 1's quantitative approach allowed us to begin to generalize about the effect of simple corrective feedback on reflection experiences, but it did not provide a deeper understanding of the process of feedback and reflection. Meanwhile, study 2's qualitative approach enabled us to more deeply explore the process of debriefing reflection, but the small sample size did not allow us to generalize beyond these learners. While it can be a challenging undertaking for a team of researchers due to its complexity, a mixed methods approach – designing a study incorporating qualitative *and* quantitative measures – may be useful for further studies of reflection. Moreover, other domains of linguistics, including discourse and conversation analysis, should be explored as lenses for the diverse array of HPE research contexts and questions.

References

Archer, Julian C. 2010. State of the science in health professional education: effective feedback. *Medical education* 44. Wiley Online Library: 101–108.
Bandura, Albert. 2006. Guide for constructing self-efficacy scales. *Self-efficacy beliefs of adolescents* 5: 307–337.
Battista, Alexis. 2015. Activity theory and analyzing learning in simulations. *Simulation & Gaming* 46. SAGE Publications Sage CA: Los Angeles, CA: 187–196.
Battista, Alexis. 2017. An activity theory perspective of how scenario-based simulations support learning: a descriptive analysis. *Advances in Simulation* 2. BioMed Central: 23.
Bezemer, Jeff, Alexandra Cope, Terhi Korkiakangas, Gunther Kress, Ged Murtagh, Sharon-Marie Weldon & Roger Kneebone. 2017. Microanalysis of video from the operating room: an underused approach to patient safety research. *BMJ Qual Saf* 26. BMJ Publishing Group Ltd: 583–587.
Bezemer, Jeff, Ged Murtagh, Alexandra Cope & Roger Kneebone. 2016. Surgical decision making in a teaching hospital: a linguistic analysis. *ANZ journal of surgery* 86. Wiley Online Library: 751–755.
Boekaerts, Monique, Paul R. Pintrich & Moshe Zeidner. 2000. *Handbook of self-regulation*. San Diego, CA: Academic Press.
Boyd, Ryan L, Kate G. Blackburn & James W. Pennebaker. 2020. The narrative arc: Revealing core narrative structures through text analysis. *Science advances* 6. American Association for the Advancement of Science: eaba2196.
Bradley, Paul. 2006. The history of simulation in medical education and possible future directions. *Medical Education* 40. John Wiley & Sons, Ltd: 254–262. https://doi.org/10.1111/J.1365-2929.2006.02394.X.
Brett-Fleegler, Marisa, Jenny Rudolph, Walter Eppich, Michael Monuteaux, Eric Fleegler, Adam Cheng & Robert Simon. 2012. Debriefing assessment for simulation in healthcare: Development and psychometric properties. *Simulation in Healthcare* 7: 288–294. https://doi.org/10.1097/SIH.0B013E3182620228.
Chaffey, Lisa J., Evelyne Johanna Janet de Leeuw & Gerard A. Finnigan. 2012. Facilitating students' reflective practice in a medical course: literature review. *Education for Health* 25. Medknow Publications: 198.
Cleary, Timothy J., Alexis Battista, Abigail Konopasky, Divya Ramani, Steven J. Durning & Anthony R. Artino. 2020. Effects of live and video simulation on clinical reasoning performance and reflection. *Advances in Simulation* 5. Springer Science and Business Media LLC. https://doi.org/10.1186/s41077-020-00133-1.
Cleary, Timothy J., Ting Dong & Anthony R. Artino. 2015. Examining shifts in medical students' microanalytic motivation beliefs and regulatory processes during a diagnostic reasoning task. *Advances in Health Sciences Education* 20. Springer: 611–626.

Cook, David A, Ryan Brydges, Benjamin Zendejas, Stanley J. Hamstra and Rose Hatala. 2013. Technology-enhanced simulation to assess health professionals: a systematic review of validity evidence, research methods, and reporting quality. *Academic Medicine* 88. LWW: 872–883.
Cook, David A., Rose Hatala, Ryan Brydges, Benjamin Zendejas, Jason H. Szostek, Amy T. Wang, Patricia J. Erwin & Stanley J. Hamstra. 2011. Technology-Enhanced Simulation for Health Professions Education: A Systematic Review and Meta-analysis. *JAMA* 306. American Medical Association: 978–988. https://doi.org/10.1001/JAMA.2011.1234.
Delany, Clare & Deborah Watkin. 2009. A study of critical reflection in health professional education:'learning where others are coming from.' *Advances in health sciences education* 14. Springer: 411–429.
Dieckmann, Peter, David Gaba & Marcus Rall. 2007. Deepening the Theoretical Foundations of Patient Simulation as Social Practice. *Simulation In Healthcare: The Journal of the Society for Simulation in Healthcare* 2: 183–193. https://doi.org/10.1097/SIH.0b013e3180f637f5.
Dieckmann, Peter, Tanja Manser, Theo Wehner & Marcus Rall. 2016. Reality and Fiction Cues in Medical Patient Simulation: An Interview Study with Anesthesiologists: *http://dx.doi.org/10.1518/155534307X232820* 1. SAGE Publications CA: Los Angeles, CA: 148–168. https://doi.org/10.1518/155534307X232820.
Dine, C. Jessica, Ronna E. Gersh, Marion Leary, Barbara J. Riegel, Lisa M. Bellini & Benjamin S. Abella. 2008. Improving cardiopulmonary resuscitation quality and resuscitation training by combining audiovisual feedback and debriefing. *Critical Care Medicine* 36. Lippincott Williams and Wilkins: 2817–2822. https://doi.org/10.1097/CCM.0B013E318186FE37.
Dreifuerst, Kristina T. 2012. Using debriefing for meaningful learning to foster development of clinical reasoning in simulation. *Journal of Nursing Education* 51. Slack Incorporated: 326–333.
Edelson, Dana P., Barbara Litzinger, Vineet Arora, Deborah Walsh, Salem Kim, Diane S. Lauderdale, Terry L. Vanden Hoek, Lance B. Becker & Benjamin S. Abella. 2008. Improving In-Hospital Cardiac Arrest Process and Outcomes With Performance Debriefing. *Archives of Internal Medicine* 168. American Medical Association: 1063–1069. https://doi.org/10.1001/ARCHINTE.168.10.1063.
Edelson, Dana P. & Cynthia M. LaFond. 2013. Deconstructing Debriefing for Simulation-Based Education. *JAMA Pediatrics* 167(6). 586–587. https://doi.org/10.1001/jamapediatrics.2013.325.
van Enk, Anneke & Glenn Regehr. 2018. HPE as a field: implications for the production of compelling knowledge. *Teaching and learning in medicine* 30. Taylor & Francis: 337–344.
Fanning, Ruth M. & David M. Gaba. 2007. The role of debriefing in simulation-based learning. *Simulation in healthcare* 2. LWW: 115–125.
Fragkos, Konstantinos. 2016. Reflective practice in healthcare education: an umbrella review. *Education Sciences* 6. Multidisciplinary Digital Publishing Institute: 27.
Gaba, David M., Steven K. Howard, Kevin J. Fish, Brian E. Smith & Yasser A. Sowb. 2001. Simulation-based training in anesthesia crisis resource management (ACRM): a decade of experience. *Simulation & Gaming* 32. Sage Publications Sage CA: Thousand Oaks, CA: 175–193.
Ginsburg, Shiphra, Cees van der Vleuten, Kevin W. Eva & Lorelei Lingard. 2016. Hedging to save face: a linguistic analysis of written comments on in-training evaluation reports. *Advances in Health Sciences Education* 21. Springer: 175–188.

Halliday, Michael A.K. & Christian Matthiessen. 2014. *An introduction to functional grammar.* Routledge.

Hattie, John & Helen Timperley. 2007. The power of feedback. *Review of educational research* 77. Sage Publications Sage CA: Thousand Oaks, CA: 81–112.

Hodges, Brian David. 2015. Sea monsters & whirlpools: Navigating between examination and reflection in medical education. *Medical teacher* 37. Taylor & Francis: 261–266.

Isaac, Carol, Jocelyn Chertoff, Barbara Lee & Molly Carnes. 2011. Do students' and authors' genders affect evaluations? A linguistic analysis of medical student performance evaluations. *Academic Medicine* 86. NIH Public Access: 59.

Issenberg, S. Barry, William C. Mcgaghie, Emil R. Petrusa, David L. Gordon & Ross J. Scalese. 2009. Features and uses of high-fidelity medical simulations that lead to effective learning: a BEME systematic review. *https://doi.org/10.1080/01421590500046924* 27. Taylor & Francis: 10–28. https://doi.org/10.1080/01421590500046924.

Jayatilleke, Nishamali & Anne Mackie. 2013. Reflection as part of continuous professional development for public health professionals: a literature review. *Journal of Public Health* 35. Oxford University Press: 308–312.

Kaatz, Anna, Wairimu Magua, David R. Zimmerman & Molly Carnes. 2015. A quantitative linguistic analysis of National Institutes of Health R01 application critiques from investigators at one institution. *Academic medicine: journal of the Association of American Medical Colleges* 90. NIH Public Access: 69.

Konopasky, Abigail, Divya Ramani, Megan Ohmer, Steven J. Durning, Anthony R. Artino & Alexis Battista. 2019. Why health professions education needs functional linguistics: the power of 'stealth words.' *Medical Education* 53. https://doi.org/10.1111/medu.13944.

Konopasky, Abigail & K.M. Sheridan. 2016. Towards a Diagnostic Toolkit for the Language of Agency. *Mind, Culture, and Activity* 23. https://doi.org/10.1080/10749039.2015.1128952.

Konopasky, Abigail, Steven J. Durning, Anthony R. Artino, Divya Ramani & Alexis Battista. 2020a. The Linguistic Effects of Context Specificity: Exploring Affect, Cognitive Processing, and Agency in Physicians' Think-Aloud Reflections. *Diagnosis*.

Konopasky, Abigail W., Divya Ramani, Megan Ohmer, Alexis Battista, Anthony R. Artino, Elexis McBee, Temple A. Ratcliffe & Steven J. Durning. 2020b. It totally possibly could be: how a group of military physicians reflect on their clinical reasoning in the presence of contextual factors. *Military medicine* 185. Bethesda, MD: 575–582.

Koshy, Kiron, Christopher Limb, Buket Gundogan, Katharine Whitehurst & Daniyal J. Jafree. 2017. Reflective practice in health care and how to reflect effectively. *International journal of surgery. Oncology* 2. Wolters Kluwer Health: e20.

Lee, Kyungjoon, Julia S. Whelan, Nancy H. Tannery, Steven L. Kanter & Antoinette S. Peters. 2013. 50 years of publication in the field of medical education. *Medical teacher* 35. Taylor & Francis: 591–598.

Locher, Miriam A. 2017. *Reflective writing in medical practice: a linguistic perspective.* Blue Ridge Summit, PA: Multilingual Matters.

Lopreiato, Joseph O. 2016. *Healthcare simulation dictionary.* Agency for Healthcare Research and Quality.

Maggio, Lauren A., Holly S. Meyer & Anthony R. Artino. 2017. Beyond citation rates: a real-time impact analysis of health professions education research using altmetrics. *Academic Medicine* 92. Wolters Kluwer: 1449–1455.

Malvern, David, Brian Richards, Ngoni Chipere & Pilar Durán. 2004. Comparing the Diversity of Lexical Categories: the Type-Type Ratio and Related Measures. In *Lexical Diversity and Language Development*, 121–151. Springer.

Mamede, Silvia, Henk G. Schmidt, Remy M.J.P. Rikers, Julio C. Penaforte & João M. Coelho-Filho. 2007. Breaking down automaticity: case ambiguity and the shift to reflective approaches in clinical reasoning. *Medical education* 41. Wiley Online Library: 1185–1192.

Markowitz, David M. & Jeffrey T. Hancock. 2016. Linguistic obfuscation in fraudulent science. *Journal of Language and Social Psychology* 35. SAGE Publications Sage CA: Los Angeles, CA: 435–445.

Martin, James R. & David Rose. 2003. *Working with discourse: Meaning beyond the clause*. Bloomsbury Publishing.

McNiesh, Susan G. 2015. Cultural Norms of Clinical Simulation in Undergraduate Nursing Education: *https://doi.org/10.1177/2333393615571361* 2015. SAGE PublicationsSage CA: Los Angeles, CA: 1–10. https://doi.org/10.1177/2333393615571361.

Ng, Stella L., Elizabeth A. Kinsella, Farah Friesen & Brian Hodges. 2015. Reclaiming a theoretical orientation to reflection in medical education research: a critical narrative review. *Medical education* 49. Wiley Online Library: 461–475.

Nguyen, Quoc Dinh, Nicolas Fernandez, Thierry Karsenti & Bernard Charlin. 2014. What is reflection? A conceptual analysis of major definitions and a proposal of a five-component model. *Medical education* 48. Wiley Online Library: 1176–1189.

Paget, Tony. 2001. Reflective practice and clinical outcomes: practitioners' views on how reflective practice has influenced their clinical practice. *Journal of clinical nursing* 10. Wiley Online Library: 204–214.

Parker, Brian C. & Florence Myrick. 2012. The pedagogical ebb and flow of human patient simulation: Empowering through a process of fading support. *Journal of Nursing Education* 51: 365–372. https://doi.org/10.3928/01484834-20120509-01.

Patton, Michael Q. 2014. *Qualitative research & evaluation methods: Integrating theory and practice*. Sage publications.

Pennebaker, James W., Martha E. Francis & Roger J. Booth. 2001. Linguistic inquiry and word count: LIWC 2001. *Mahway: Lawrence Erlbaum Associates* 71: 2001.

Piantadosi, Steven T., Harry Tily & Edward Gibson. 2012. The communicative function of ambiguity in language. *Cognition* 122. Elsevier: 280–291.

Pintrich, Paul R., Christopher A. Wolters & Gail P. Baxter. 2000. 2. assessing metacognition and self-regulated learning.

Piquette, Dominique, Maria Mylopoulos & Vicki R. LeBlanc. 2014. Clinical supervision and learning opportunities during simulated acute care scenarios. *Medical Education* 48. John Wiley & Sons, Ltd: 820–830. https://doi.org/10.1111/MEDU.12492.

Pomare, Chiara, Janet C. Long, Kate Churruca, Louise A. Ellis & Jeffrey Braithwaite. 2020. Interprofessional collaboration in hospitals: a critical, broad-based review of the literature. *Journal of interprofessional care* 34. Taylor & Francis: 509–519.

Rachul, Christen & Lara Varpio. 2020. More than words: how multimodal analysis can inform health professions education. *Advances in Health Sciences Education* 25. Springer: 1087–1097.

Raemer, Daniel, Mindi Anderson, Adam Cheng, Ruth Fanning, Vinay Nadkarni & Georges Savoldelli. 2011. Research regarding debriefing as part of the learning process. *Simulation in Healthcare* 6. https://doi.org/10.1097/SIH.0B013E31822724D0.

Ramani, Divya, Michael Soh, Jerusalem Merkebu, Steven J. Durning, Alexis Battista, Elexis McBee, Temple Ratcliffe & Abigail Konopasky. 2020. Examining the patterns of uncertainty across clinical reasoning tasks: effects of contextual factors on the clinical reasoning process. *Diagnosis* 7. De Gruyter: 299–305. https://doi.org/10.1515/DX-2020-0019.

Rudolph, Jenny W., Robert Simon, Ronald L. Dufresne & Daniel B. Raemer. 2006. There's no such thing as "nonjudgmental" debriefing: a theory and method for debriefing with good judgment. *Simulation in healthcare* 1. LWW: 49–55.

Rudolph, Jenny W., Robert Simon, Peter Rivard, Ronald L. Dufresne & Daniel B. Raemer. 2007. Debriefing with Good Judgment: Combining Rigorous Feedback with Genuine Inquiry. *Anesthesiology Clinics* 25. Elsevier: 361–376. https://doi.org/10.1016/J.ANCLIN.2007.03.007.

Saldaña, Johnny. 2015. *The coding manual for qualitative researchers*. Sage.

Sargeant, Joan M., Karen V. Mann, Cees P. Van der Vleuten & Job F. Metsemakers. 2009. Reflection: a link between receiving and using assessment feedback. *Advances in health sciences education* 14. Springer: 399–410.

Schei, Edvin, Abraham Fuks & J. Donald Boudreau. 2019. Reflection in medical education: intellectual humility, discovery, and know-how. *Medicine, Health Care and Philosophy* 22. Springer: 167–178.

Shute, Valerie J. 2008. Focus on formative feedback. *Review of educational research* 78. Sage Publications: 153–189.

Smith, Elizabeth. 2011. Teaching critical reflection. *Teaching in higher education* 16. Taylor & Francis: 211–223.

Stephens, Mark B., Brian V. Reamy, Denise Anderson, Cara Olsen, Paul A. Hemmer, Steven J. Durning & Simon Auster. 2012. Writing, self-reflection, and medical school performance: the human context of health care. *Military medicine* 177. Oxford University Press: 26–30.

Sweileh, Waleed M., Samah W. Al-Jabi, Sa'ed H. Zyoud & Ansam F. Sawalha. 2018. Bibliometric analysis of literature in pharmacy education: 2000–2016. *International Journal of Pharmacy Practice* 26. Oxford University Press: 541–549.

Tannenbaum, Scott I. & Christopher P. Cerasoli. 2012. Do Team and Individual Debriefs Enhance Performance? A Meta-Analysis: *http://dx.doi.org/10.1177/0018720812448394* 55. SAGE PublicationsSage CA: Los Angeles, CA: 231–245. https://doi.org/10.1177/0018720812448394.

Tausczik, Yla R. & James W. Pennebaker. 2010. The psychological meaning of words: LIWC and computerized text analysis methods. *Journal of language and social psychology* 29. Sage Publications Sage CA: Los Angeles, CA: 24–54.

Tekian, Ara & Anthony R. Artino Jr. 2013. AM last page: master's degree in health professions education programs. *Academic Medicine* 88. LWW: 1399.

Tekian, Ara & Ilene Harris. 2012. Preparing health professions education leaders worldwide: A description of masters-level programs. *Medical teacher* 34. Taylor & Francis: 52–58.

Tekian, Ara, Trudie Roberts, Helen P. Batty, David A. Cook & John Norcini. 2014. Preparing leaders in health professions education. *Medical teacher* 36. Taylor & Francis: 269–271.

Thompson, Geoff. 2013. *Introducing functional grammar*. Routledge.

Tolsgaard, Martin G., Amandus Gustafsson, Maria B. Rasmussen, Pernilla HØiby, Cathrine G. Müller & Charlotte Ringsted. 2009. Student teachers can be as good as associate professors in teaching clinical skills. *https://doi.org/10.1080/01421590701682550* 29. Taylor & Francis: 553–557. https://doi.org/10.1080/01421590701682550.

Tsingos-Lucas, Cherie, Sinthia Bosnic-Anticevich, Carl R. Schneider & Lorraine Smith. 2016. The effect of reflective activities on reflective thinking ability in an undergraduate pharmacy curriculum. *American journal of pharmaceutical education* 80. American Journal of Pharmaceutical Education.

Tyerman, Jane, Marian Luctkar-Flude, Leslie Graham, Sue Coffey & Ellen Olsen-Lynch. 2019. A Systematic Review of Health Care Presimulation Preparation and Briefing Effectiveness. *Clinical Simulation in Nursing* 27. Elsevier: 12–25. https://doi.org/10.1016/J.ECNS.2018.11.002.

Varpio, Lara, Carol Aschenbrener & Joanna Bates. 2017. Tackling wicked problems: how theories of agency can provide new insights. *Medical education* 51. Wiley Online Library: 353–365.

Wald, Hedy S. 2015. Professional identity (trans) formation in medical education: reflection, relationship, resilience. *Academic Medicine* 90. LWW: 701–706.

Warner, Rebecca M. 2012. *Applied statistics: From bivariate through multivariate techniques*. Sage Publications.

Winkel, Abigail Ford, Sandra Yingling, Aubrie-Ann Jones & Joey Nicholson. 2017. Reflection as a learning tool in graduate medical education: A systematic review. *Journal of Graduate Medical Education* 9. The Accreditation Council for Graduate Medical Education: 430–439.

Woodward-Kron, Robyn, Mary Stevens & Eleanor Flynn. 2011. The medical educator, the discourse analyst, and the phonetician: A collaborative feedback methodology for clinical communication. *Academic Medicine* 86. LWW: 565–570.

Yonge, Olive J., Marjorie Anderson, Joanne Profetto-McGrath, Joanne K. Olson, D. Lynn Skillen, Jeanette Boman, Ann Ranson Ratusz, Arnette Anderson, Linda Slater & Rene Day. 2005. An inventory of nursing education research. *International Journal of Nursing Education Scholarship* 2. De Gruyter.

Zimmerman, Barry J. 2000. Attaining self-regulation: A social cognitive perspective. In *Handbook of self-regulation*, 13–39. Elsevier.

Ziv, Amitai, Shaul Ben-David & Margalit Ziv. 2009. Simulation Based Medical Education: an opportunity to learn from errors. *https://doi.org/10.1080/0142159050012671827*. Taylor & Francis: 193–199. https://doi.org/10.1080/01421590500126718.

Ziv, Amitai, Paul Root Wolpe, Stephen D. Small & Shimon Glick. 2003. Simulation-based medical education: an ethical imperative. *Academic medicine* 78. LWW: 783–788.

Caroline H. Vickers, Ryan A. Goble
Chapter 2
From cultural competence to discourse competence: Discourse analysis and the education of bi/multilingual health care professionals

1 Introduction

A typical medical consultation involves an initial phase in which the health care provider interviews the patient to obtain the patient's health history, which constitutes the patient's narrative around a particular medical issue. This health narrative contributes 60–80% of the information that leads to a diagnosis (Peterson et al. 1992), and it is crucial to the development of a trusting relationship between the medical provider and the patient (Keifenheim et al. 2015). Therefore, health care providers must become skilled in the elicitation of patient narratives. All human interaction involves co-construction (Jacoby and Ochs 1995), but in a medical consultation in which the diagnosis is so heavily dependent on the patient's health history, health care providers need to be especially attentive to how they interpret patient contributions (Vickers et al. 2012).

Over the past ten years, we have worked with collaborators in Health Sciences and Nursing to examine the health history interview in bilingual medical consultations in a community clinic in Southern California in which the patients are monolingual Spanish users, and the providers use both Spanish and English. The medical consultations that we examine are language concordant in Spanish. We have found that the elicitation of health history narratives can become complicated when bi/multilingual health care providers conduct the medical consultation in a minoritized language but tend to code-switch to the majority language (Vickers and Goble 2011; Vickers et al. 2015; Vickers 2020). Our work has implications for training bi/multilingual health care providers to better serve patients who use a minoritized language.

This chapter will focus on the use of discourse analytic data for the purpose of training bi/multilingual health care providers involved in language concordant medical consultations. Our purpose is use data to point to crucial meaning

---

Caroline H. Vickers, California State University, San Bernardino
Ryan A. Goble, University of Wisconsin-Madison

https://doi.org/10.1515/9783110744804-003

making moments during the elicitation of the monolingual Spanish-speaking patient's health history narrative and to reflect on how these moments contribute to patient care outcomes. We will review findings from our own previous research and present data to demonstrate patterns of problematic interaction types that could be useful targets for training for bi/multilingual health care professionals.

1.1 Medical provider training

Health history narratives are successful when patients are able to convey to the health care provider their lifeworlds, and then health care providers are able to use that information to both build a relationship with the patient and to devise a diagnosis. As Mishler (1984: 14) asserted, during the health history narrative, the "voice of the lifeworld" is constantly reinterpreted by "the voice of medicine." This reinterpretation is essential to a diagnosis. However, as we have shown in our research, particularly Vickers et al. (2012), if the health care provider does not sufficiently listen to and understand the patient's lifeworld, the medical interpretation may be flawed, a deleterious patient care outcome. Therefore, it is critically important for health care providers to be aware of and attentive to patient contributions, to relinquish some interactional control and provide interactional space for patients to depict their lifeworlds.

Then the question becomes one of health care provider training. Discourse analytic work has shed light on many aspects of patient-provider interaction in the medical consultation (Barnes 2019, Robinson and Heritage 2014). Therefore, it becomes important to consider how best to make use of the insights gained from discourse analysis of patient-provider interaction to improve healthcare delivery.

Robinson and Heritage (2014: 202) recommend designing intervention studies based on conversation analytic findings, but as they state, "Medical sciences recognize that research involving this type of intervention involves a complex of activities, which fall into two broad parts," which include a preintervention and an intervention phase. They then recommend "Preintervention CA" as a step toward intervention studies. As they state, "Preintervention CA commonly involves noticings of discrete and contrastive practices that are deployed in some identifiable phase of (or medical activity within) the visit" (203).

Several researchers have used discourse analysis as a research method to study various issues related to health communication for training and assessing health care providers (Atkins 2019; Barnes 2019; Candlin and Roger 2013; Leahy and Walsh 2008; O'Grady 2016). Studies that focus on training have involved role-play scenarios. Atkins (2019) employed CA and corpus linguistics (CL) to study simulated consultation, or role-play, to educate and assess providers on patient-provider communication. Although Atkins acknowledged differences between role-play and real-time assessment, she asserted that "the study demonstrates how CL and CA methods can be usefully applied in analyzing simulated interactions, identifying key linguistic features and participation structures that may not easily be recognized in real-time assessment" (126). Alternatively, O'Grady (2016) promoted the use of "real-life clinical encounters" as the basis for discourse analytic approaches to training as role-play differs from real-life clinical interactions. From our vantage point, even given the limitations of role-play for training, either approach can be helpful for training bi/multilingual health care providers. Regardless, our purpose here is to ensure that such training includes some specific problematic interaction types that seem common in bilingual medical consultations. First, it is not uncommon for third-party family members to be present in such consultations, and so it is important to consider how a third-party participation framework impacts patient care outcomes, particularly when both the health care provider and the third-party are bi/multilingual and the patient is not. Second, given that two languages are involved in a bilingual medical consultation, it is essential to provide training on how notions of language normativity impact language choice and patient care outcomes.

1.2 Participation framework and narrative co-construction

As people interact, participants co-construct the participation framework (Goffman 1981) as well as whose contributions are more or less powerful. According to Goffman, the basic participation framework includes a speaker and a hearer as well as the potential for overhearers and eavesdroppers. Of course, interactions often have multiple speakers and multiple hearers. The combination of speakers and hearers and their identities in relation to the interaction become important in terms of whose contributions are ratified, or uptaken, as well as who has access to the speakers' contributions. Hutchby and O'Reilly (2010) showed how family therapy sessions that involved parents and children relegated children to "half-member" and non-participant status as parents and therapists failed to ratify them and instead authored their contributions during the therapy session. During health history narratives, such relegation to non-participant status happens when medical providers and third-party family members switch to a language the patient does not use (Vickers 2020; Vickers et al. 2015). In these cases, patients can completely lose control over their own health history narrative, which is clearly detrimental to patient care.

It is also vital to analyze how code-switching, or changing the language code in the course of an interaction, is related to the macro-level social structure within which the clinical consultations are embedded, especially because by using either Spanish or English, participants make their identities as members of particular macro-level groups within the macro-societal context relevant. Auer (2005) posed important questions concerning how studies of code-switching might consider the relationship between the micro and the macro. He asked, "first, what kind of identity predicates can the alternating use of two languages be an index of in conversation? And second, how, exactly, can such an index be shown to be interpretively relevant?" (p. 404). The micro-interaction and macro-societal aspects of the participation framework are important for bi/multilingual health care providers to consider as language choice is meaningful in terms of how patient identities are constructed and what becomes interpretively relevant in the medical consultation. Of particular concern is how health care providers' language choices affect patient care outcomes. For example, when a health care provider code-switches to a language the patient cannot understand, the patient becomes a non-participant.

1.3 Language normativity

The medical literature often calls for *cultural competence* in medical settings that serve minoritized patients. But like any ideology, cultural competence is not simply an abstract concept. Rather, it is based in practice. As Philips (2000) argued, language is a window into ideology. Stated policies, such as cultural competence, may not be practiced on the ground during the micro-interactional practice of patient care even when clinic policies are explicit about a mission of cultural competence (Vickers et al. 2015).

The value of English becomes clear in clinical consultation micro-interactions in which health care providers are bi/multilingual in the dominant language of the larger context and the minoritized language of the patient (Vickers 2020). Hill (1998) has argued that ideological notions about the relative value of language affect attitudes about the people who use those languages. For instance, Martinez (2008) demonstrated that language-concordant clinical spaces in the Texas borderlands privilege English over Spanish, which leads to worse health outcomes for Spanish-speaking patients. Notions of language hierarchy and language normativity are imperative to consider in language concordant medical consultations.

Furthermore, Vickers et al. (2013) looked at how the animation of powerful stances in English in Spanish-language clinical consultations illuminated ideological notions about the normativity of English. Indeed, Vickers and Goble (2011) and Vickers et al. (2012, 2015) have demonstrated that even in a clinical context that is quite consciously Spanish-speaking, the normativity of English is pervasive and factors into the co-construction of meaning in patient-provider interactions. Therefore, one important aspect of bi/multilingual health care provider training is understanding language normativity and hierarchy, and how ideological notions about language can affect clinical micro-interactions and patient care outcomes.

1.4 Non-English-speaking people and ideologies of incompetence

Language ideologies factor into notions of patient (in)competence. For example, health scholarship often refers to bi/multilingual patients whose second language is English and those who do not use English as *Limited English Proficient* (LEP) (Berkowitz and McCubbin 2005; Betancourt 2006; Carter-Pokras et al. 2004; Chapman and Berggren 2005; Egede 2006; Flores et al. 2005; Green et al. 2005; Holmes 2006; Leyva et al. 2005; Pamies and Nsiah-Kumi 2006; Pope 2005; Ramirez 2006; Wlison et al. 2005; Wynia 2006; Zsembik and Fennell 2005). This research contends that communication issues place so-called LEP patients at a high risk of poor quality of care and decreased health outcomes (Morales et al. 1999; Casey et al. 2004; Fiscella et al. 2002; Timmins et al. 2002; Jacobs et al. 2010; Schenker 2010). Health scholarship describes these communication issues as a health disparity resulting from a language *barrier*.

To work toward health equity, many studies have examined and assessed *culturally competent* healthcare delivery (Anderson et al. 2003; Brach and Fraser 2000; Edwards 2003; Hobgood et al. 2006; Rosa 2006; Rust et al. 2006; Taylor and Lurie 2004; Vega 2005). *Bridging the language barrier* is recognized as one component of such cultural competence. Several suggestions related to bridging the language barrier have been put forward in health scholarship, including cultural competence training (Anderson et al. 2007; Selig et. al. 2006), professional standardization of interpreter qualifications (Aranguri et al. 2006; Erdmann, J. 2008), and training on appropriate interpretive service utilization (Aranguri et al. 2006; Carter-Pokras et al. 2004; Ngo-Metzger et. al. 2007; Wilson-Stronks et al. 2008; Erdmann 2008; USDHHS, 2001).

It is important to note that this body of work generally assumes the normativity of English with the terminology *limited English proficient* and notions of *bridging the language barrier* and often points to ways to supplement the provider through interpretation services. In the United States, there is a pervasive ideology in which monolingual English is normative, and any notion that bi/multilingualism is many people's reality in the U.S. is invisible, making it acceptable for institutions to other the bi/multilingual experience. In the medical context, for example, the use of interpreters rather than access to language concordant health care providers to interact with language minoritized patients is common practice. Therefore, the idea of institutions actually structuring themselves as bi/multilingual seems quite radical in the U.S. context. The clinic that we studied here is quite progressive in the sense that all staff, documents, and many medical materials were bi/multilingual. The language concordance that we discuss here is good practice, but our purpose is to point out how an already good practice can be made more inclusive. Essentially, we will demonstrate that English is pervasive and intrusive at times in these Spanish concordant consultations, and how such English intrusions exclude the Spanish-speaking monolingual patient.

Some scholarship has called for increasing the representation of linguistic minorities in the health care professions (Brach and Fraser 2000; Flores 2005; USDHHS 2001; *CLAS* final report). Clarridge et al. (2008) asserted that *language concordance* is an essential physician intervention in moving toward minimizing health disparities of linguistically diverse patients. We agree that language concordance and increasing the representation of linguistic minorities are beneficial. However, as we will demonstrate in this paper, even in language concordant medical consultations, health care providers may code-switch in ways that affect patient care. Therefore, training for bi/multilingual health care providers serving patients who speak a minoritized language in the minoritized language is crucial.

1.5 A framework for bi/multilingual medical provider training

One area of research that is helpful in conceptualizing a framework for training for bi/multilingual health care providers is the professional practice of language learning advising (LLA), which is conceptualized as a meta-learning site where multicompetent individuals develop the capacity to autonomously attend to the cognitive, social, and affective dimensions of their bi/multilingual development (Carson and Mynard 2012; Ciekanski 2007; Morrison and Navarro 2012; Mozzon-McPherson 2007, 2012, 2015; Tassinari 2016). This professional practice, like medical consultations, involves eliciting narratives about language learners' current circumstances, needs, and goals to develop a plan for second language users to assume greater control over and responsibility for managing their interactions in which they use the target language. Therefore, methods for training advising practitioners are applicable to health care provider training.

Research on language learning advising is commonly undertaken by advisor practitioners or researchers in close partnership with advisors in multilingual settings to inform advisor training and professional development (Bisset and Gödeke 2015; Castro 2018, 2019; Ciekanski 2007, Crabbe et al. 2001; Morrison and Navarro 2012; Mozzon-McPherson 2012, 2013; Pemberton et al. 2001; Tassinari 2016; Watkins 2015). For example, Mozzon-McPherson (2013) deployed discourse analysis as a reflective tool for five language learner advisors to critically describe how language influenced the joint construction of meaning with advisees in their learning conversations. In effect, the advisors both created and contributed to the discourse analysis of data in this small-scale, localized study. They submitted written self-reflections and peer evaluations of how language was used in two audio-recorded advising appointments totaling two hours. In preparation for a debriefing discussion, Mozzon-McPherson then distributed the peer evaluations to advisors to analyze and observe similarities and differences in terms of communication. Finally, each advisor participated in an individual research interview.

Similarly, such research methods can facilitate a heightened awareness for bi/multilingual health care practitioners to understand the implications of using a non-English language in English-dominant settings and using English with those who primarily use a minoritized language. In particular, they can scrutinize moments of code-switching to a language that their patients do not understand when they engage in bureaucratic side talk (Vickers et al. 2013) or communicate with a bi/multilingual third-party family member (Vickers et al. 2015; Vickers 2020). They can observe how the formulation of questions afforded agency for patients to narrate their health circumstances, as well as health care providers' own contributions that subsequently shaped the narrative. Health care providers might reflect or give feedback on impressions of how language may position someone as more or less competent and autonomous in their ability to manage their own healthcare and follow-up.

Indeed, every professional practice has *stocks of professional knowledge*, which are established frameworks or conceptual models that serve as a knowledge base for conventional best practices and communicative norms, but they may not align with what unfolds interactionally *in situ* (Peräkylä and Vehviläinen 2003). Careful attention to discourse can elucidate mismatches between theory and practice and clarify assumptions about discourse thought to ideally characterize a given professional practice. Accordingly, we advocate for discourse-based health care provider training.

2 Data

The data for this chapter come from a corpus of transcribed audio-recorded Spanish language medical consultations between patients, three Spanish-English bi/multilingual nurse practitioners, and one Spanish-English bi/multilingual intake nurse. Study participants included one nurse (Laura[1]) and one intake nurse (Maria) who used Spanish as a first language and English as a second language, as well as one medical doctor and one nurse who used English as a first language. The data presented here include the medical provider who used English as a first language (Dr. Thomas) and the nurse who used English as a first language (Carrie). The code-switching patterns that we found held across three providers, except for the intake nurse, who rarely code-switched to English. However, the duties of the intake nurse were more routinized, which may explain why her interactions were different. Though she did collect health history information, the questions were the same each time and elicited discrete answers. The three health care providers who engaged in the more complex health history interactions related to the particular ailment concerning the patient that day were the purview of Carrie, Dr. Thomas, and Laura, who were all similar in their tendencies to code-switch during clinical micro-interactions that we examine in this paper.

The corpus was collected from October 2009 to July 2010 and includes approximately 150,000 words and 50 medical consultations. The medical consultations that we present in this paper were conducted in Spanish. After gaining informed consent from all participants, we set up portable digital audio recorders in the consultation rooms, and one of us was present in the consultation room during the consultation to take field notes.

There were a variety of participation frameworks in the consultations, including one-on-one interactions between bi/multilingual providers and monolingual Spanish-speaking patients, as well as one-on-one interactions between bi/multilingual health care providers and bi/multilingual patients. Furthermore, some consultations involved situations in which a third party was in the room, which included various combinations of monolingual Spanish-speaking and bi/multilingual third-parties interacting with bi/multilingual providers.

---

[1] All names are psuedonyms.

3 Methods

This analysis focuses on the history-taking phase of the consultation, which occurs at the beginning of the consultation after the provider enters the consultation room to greet the patient. The history-taking phase constitutes an interview in which the health care provider asks the patient questions related to their health. This provider-patient interview elicits a health narrative from the patient. In the analysis of the data, we employed conversation analysis (CA) to allow us to identify particular conversational sequences (Antaki 2011) during talk in interaction (Schegloff 2007) within the consultation. We were particularly attuned to how the patient and health care provider co-constructed (Jacoby and Ochs 1995) meaning within the medical consultation.

In addition, as CA framework allows for a turn-by-turn analysis of meaning making, it enabled us to examine the situated meanings created through code-switching (Auer 1998), which is of course common among bi/multilingual people. We further analyzed how code-switching related to the macro-level social structure within which the participants lived because the participants potentially made relevant their identities as members of particular macro-level groups by code-switching (Auer 2005; Cashman 2005; Gafaranga 2005; Zhang 2005). As Zhang argued,

> [. . .] through sequential analysis of naturally occurring data of talk-interaction, we are able to discover members' procedures for doing code-choice and codeswitching. We hope to have shown here that individual acts of speech and interaction at the microlevel allow participants to 'play out' the social structures relevant to the macrosociolinguistic setting in which particular speech events are situated'. (372)

Similar to Zhang, we attended to how language choice indexes macro-societal structures. Finally, we examined the shifting participation framework (Goffman 1981) that occurred during third-party interaction, identifying who was a ratified participant and authoring patient accounts. CA studies have utilized Goffman's participation framework to understand how institutional roles are interactionally achieved (Greatbatch 1988; Hutchby 1996). We, too, accounted for how the addition of a third party shifted the participation framework and the effect on patient care outcomes.

4 Using data for training

In what follows, we have selected particular excerpts from our data to illustrate a. targets for bi/multilingual health care provider training regarding language choice and b. targets for bi/multilingual health care provider training related to third-party interaction when a bi/multilingual family member is present.

We aim to demonstrate how health care provider interactional moves within the health history segment of the clinical consultation affect control over information and patient care outcomes, focusing on how English normativity contributes to control in the context of Spanish language concordant clinical consultations in English dominant Southern California. These consultations involve monolingual Spanish speaking patients, Spanish-English bi/multilingual health care providers, and Spanish-English bi/multilingual third-party family members. We are particularly interested in the impact of the health care provider code-switching from Spanish to English.

We will demonstrate that a pervasive language ideology with regard to the normativity of English and an ideology in which non-English speaking people are considered to be less capable are both at play in the co-construction of control. We argue that the implications of the data presented include the need to consider how language ideology and ideologies about the capabilities of non-English speaking people in English-dominant contexts affect health care experiences among language minoritized people Based on the data excerpts below, we will then suggest ways to implement training for health care providers serving people who use minoritized languages.

4.1 Excerpt 1: Language normativity and marginalization

The normativity of English was often indexed in the history-taking segment of the clinical consultation as the health care providers switched to English to interact with computerized health records (Goble and Vickers 2014; Vickers et al. 2013). In Excerpt 1, Carrie switches from Spanish to English as she reads information from the computer, which contains the patient, Rosana's, health records. The information on the computer is in English.

<T=0:18:29>
Excerpt 1: Rosana (R) and Carrie (C)

```
1. C; sacábamos sangre? (1.0,        1. C; did we draw blood? (1.0,
2.     MOUSE CLICK) hace              2.    MOUSE CLICK) has it been
3.     mucho?                         3.    awhile?
4. R; m:[::                           4. R; m:[::
5. C;    [oh looks like it (2 MOUSE   5. C;    [oh looks like it (2 MOUSE
6.       CLICKS) °let me see°         6.       CLICKS) °let me see°
7. R; no te[ngo memoria de esto       7. R; I don't [have memory of this
```

```
 8. C;          [y:es::              8. C;           [y:es::
 9.      hace: hac-yeah en febrero    9.      it ha:s ha-yeah in February
10.      (CLICK)[sacábamos sangre    10.      (CLICK)[we drew blood
11. R;           [mhm                11. R;           [mhm
12. C;   ((to computer)) °let's see  12. C;   ((to computer)) °let's see
13.      how that looked° (5.5, MOUSE 13.     how that looked° (5.5, MOUSE
14.      CLICKING) oh @that's okay@@@ 14.     CLICKING) oh @that's okay@@@
15.      °okay°:: mira bien..mire muy 15.     °okay°:: looks good..it all
16.      bien todo (1.0) (H)         16.      looks very good..(H) (1.0)
17.      okay Good(CLICK) °and what  17.      okay good (CLICK) °and what
18.      was that other test? (CLICK)18.      was that other test? (CLICK)
19.      we did? (TSK) two five°     19.      we did? (TSK) two five°
20.      CLICK) °two five (2 CLICKS) 20.      (CLICK) °two five (2 CLICKS)
21.      it's that one° (1.0) °same  21.      it's that one° (1.0) °same
22.      thing° (2.0, MOUSE CLICKING)22.      thing° (2.0, MOUSE CLICKING)
23.      ((to R)) no tiene           23.      ((to R)) you don't have
24.      colesterol ni nada          24.      cholesterol or anything
25. R;   no ((clears throat))        25. R;   no ((clears throat))
26. C;   nope..mira muy bien (TSK)   26. C;   nope..looks very good (TSK)
27.      okay..entonces..este comezón↑ 27.    okay..so then..this itch↑
28.      le duele el pecho?          28.      does your chest hurt?
```

In the case of Excerpt 1, the computer acts as a third interactant, as we discussed in Goble and Vickers (2014). As we argued in Vickers et al. (2013), Carrie makes the computerized health records, which are in English, relevant in line 5. Importantly, the entry of the health records into the conversation also seems to motivate Carrie's switch to English in line 5, making the fact that the health records are in English relevant to the interaction. The fact that the health records of this monolingual Spanish-speaking patient are stored in English on the computer, of course, indexes the normativity of English in the clinical context.

Throughout Except 1, the English interaction between Carrie and the computer renders Rosana as a non-participant (Hutchby and O'Reilly 2010). In line 7, Rosana answers Carrie's question in line 1, inquiring about whether they drew blood. Of course, Carrie had already referred to the computer in line 3 to answer her own question in English, which contradicted Rosana's memory. Clearly, Rosana is not in control over the narrative of her own health history here. The computer is clearly a third interactant here as we discuss in Goble and Vickers (2016).

In lines 9–10, Carrie acts as a translator between the information on the computer, which she had already relayed in English in line 5, and Rosana, which ratifies Rosana as a listener. In lines 12–14, Carrie switches to English, a move that seems to ratify the computer as a third interactant and positions Rosana as a non-participant in the English conversation between Carrie and the inanimate computer. Carrie then orients toward Rosana as a ratified participant in lines 15–16 as she relays Rosana's test results. In lines 17–22, the computer once again becomes ratified, and Rosana is rendered a non-participant, as Carrie switches to English to engage with the information on the computer screen. In lines 23–24, Carrie switches to Spanish, ratifying Rosana's role as a listener.

The code-switching in this excerpt makes Rosana's identity as a non-English speaking person relevant and constructs such an identity as a marginalized one as Rosana cannot access all the information conveyed during the consultation. Throughout Excerpt 1, Rosana becomes marginalized as Carrie switches to English to interact with the information, which is in English, on the computer screen. In the consultation, Carrie indexes Rosana's membership category as a marginalized non-English speaking person. Rosana's marginalization allows Carrie control over the information as accessed on the computer.

4.2 Excerpt 2: Language normativity and non-membership

Similarly, in Excerpt 2, Dr. Thomas indexes the normativity of English as she refers to disability paperwork in English to accurately fill in the health history of a monolingual Spanish-speaking patient, Dalia. As mentioned, such switches to English instigated by artifacts such as calendars, computerized records, and paperwork were not uncommon in the data. Indeed, these artifacts become third interactants.

In Excerpt 2, the patient, Dalia, had fallen while traveling and had surgery to repair the injury in a hospital in Mexico, which necessitated inserting plates and screws. The patient was reaching the point where she needed another surgery to remove the screws, which was necessary for her to resume the ability to bear weight on the limb, but she was uninsured. The purpose of her visit to the clinic was to gain the physician's determination that she was eligible for disability compensation because of her inability to work, which necessitated Dr. Thomas taking Dalia's health history and recording that history on the disability form.

<T=0:40:31>
Excerpt 2: Dr. Thomas (DT), Dalia (D), and husband (G)

```
1.   DT; vamos a ver..okay (4.5) (H)      1.   DT; let's see..okay (4.5) (H)
2.       esta es que: tengo que           2.       this is wha:t I have to
3.       estima:r↑..cuánto tiempo         3.       estima:te↑..how much time
4.       va a necesita:r                  4.       you're going to nee:d
```

```
5.  G;   una rec -                      5.  G;   a rec -
6.  DT;  más de recuperación            6.  DT;  more for recovery
7.  D;   m:: uh tengo mi ((xxx          7.  D;   m:: uh I have my ((xxx
8.       xxx)) este:..si:: ah: aquí     8.        xxx)) este:..i::f ah: here is
9.       está la copia de [ustedes      9.        the copy for [you all
10. DT;                  [okay:         10. DT;                 [okay:
11. D;   allí está=                     11. D;   there it is=
12. DT;  =yeah okay (3.0) hm: hm (3.0)  12. DT;  =yeah okay (3.0) hm: hm (3.0)
13.      this says tibial fracture      13.      this says tibial fracture
14.      (1.0) it's fibular @(Hx)=      14.      (1.0) it's fibular @(Hx)=
15. G;   =yeah                          15. G;   =yeah
16. DT;  (1.5) (Hx)                     16. DT;  (1.5) (Hx)
17. D;   ((xxx)) las placas..no?=       17. D;   ((xxx)) the plates..no?=
18. G;   =sí aquí está..es..fibular     18. G;   =yes here is..it's..fibular
19.      (Hx)@@ @@                      19.      (Hx)@@ @@
20. DT;  ((sounds frustrated; papers    20. DT;  ((sounds frustrated; papers
21.      shuffling)) course             21.      shuffling)) course
22.      unfortunately this. is         22.      unfortunately this. is
23.      a. different..piece. of.       23.      a. different..piece. of.
24.      paper.                         24.      paper.
25. D;   (paper audible)) oh::          25. D;   ((paper audible)) oh::
26. DT;  but it has the co:des:         26. DT;  but it has the co:des:
```

In lines 1–4, Dr. Thomas speaks to Dalia, informing her that the paperwork is instructing her to estimate the time for recuperation. Dalia then refers Dr. Thomas to the discharge paperwork she received from the hospital where she had surgery in Mexico in lines 6–9. Dr. Thomas then switches to English in lines 12–14 to indicate that the discharge paperwork indicates a tibia fracture rather than a fibular fracture, which she had assumed based on the health history she had taken earlier in the consultation. The inconsistency that Dr. Thomas discovered seems to motivate her to switch to English. Her sigh and laugh in line 14 indicate her possible confusion and frustration even though the paperwork from a Mexican medical facility was in Spanish.

In line 15, Dalia's husband, who speaks some English, begins to speak, saying "yeah" and sighing, and Dalia indicates in line 17 that the doctor can feel the plates, followed by the husband's pointing to the location of the plates in line 18, which is followed by laughter in line 19. Dr. Thomas switches to English again in line 21 and in a frustrated tone, indicates that she has a different piece of paper that has the codes. Dalia, who does not speak English, interjects "oh:" in line 25.

The fact that Dr. Thomas does not ratify Dalia and her husband's contributions in lines 17–18 tells us that they have lost control over the narrative. In this exchange, the bureaucracy animated in English trumps the physical evidence, rendering Dalia's physicality irrelevant to Dr. Thomas's determination of the injury. For Dr. Thomas, the definitive diagnosis of Dalia's injury rests in the codes on the bureaucratic paperwork, the professional terms that make Dalia's diagnosis real (Sarangi 2001).

In this rather tense exchange, we argue that Dalia is rendered a non-participant (Hutchby and O'Reilly 2010), indexing a membership category of non-membership in the professional bureaucracy, which strips Dalia over control over her own health narrative. The switch to English clearly cements Dalia's non-member status as it also renders her a non-participant. Dalia is further marginalized here because Dr. Thomas's decision-making processes, rooted in English-speaking bureaucratic rituals, are hidden from her. As Dr. Thomas animates her bureaucratic thought processes in English in this supposedly Spanish language concordant clinical consultation with Spanish-language medical records, Dalia is a non-participant. Bureaucratic rituals are often hidden from lay people anyway as they are non-experts, but when the bureaucratic is carried in a language the patient does not use, it adds another layer of opaqueness that is unnecessary.

4.3 Excerpt 3: Language normativity and lovable incompetence

In Excerpt 3, Carrie educates Luisa about diet in Spanish, and Luisa informs Carrie about her dietary habits. The conversation between Carrie and Luisa is rather egalitarian (Vickers and Goble, 2018) until Luisa's daughter intervenes. This excerpt involves a code-switch to English instigated by a bilingual third-party family member, which tends to occur in the data, as we have written about in previous work (Vickers et al. 2015; Vickers 2020).

<T=0:49:22>

Excerpt 3: Carrie (C), Luisa (L), and Daughter (D)

```
1. L;  yo no como..comidas grasosas    1. L;  I don't eat..fatty foods or
2.     ni nada [puro pesca:do↑         2.        [anything just fi:sh↑
3. C;         [goo:d goo:d             3. C;        [goo:d goo:d
4. L;  pescado es lo que como y        4. L;  fish is what I eat and
5.     los nopales y la lechuga=       5.     cactus and lettuce=
6. D;  =that's all she eats..a:ll      6. D;  =that's all she eats..a:ll
7.     day                             7.     day
8. C;  oh my go:sh..she must be        8. C;  oh my go:sh..she must be
9.     starving                        9.     starving
10.D;  y:es..and then she gets mad    10.D;  y:es..and then she gets mad
11.    and then she cries porque      11.    and then she cries porque
```

```
12.     dice..I'm still hungry [well      12.     dice..I'm so hungry [well
13.C;                          [yeah:     13.C;                       [yeah:
14.D;   'cause you don't eat -            14.D;   'cause you don't eat -
15.C;   ='cause you're eating nothing     15.C;   ='cause you're eating nothing
16.D;   yeah[::                           16.D;   yeah[::
17.C;        [porque porque no hay        17.C;        [because because there's
18.     mucha nutrición..en los           18.     not much nutrition..in cactus
19.     nopales no hay mucha:             19.     there's not mu:ch nutrition
20.     en la la lechuga=                 20.     in lettuce=
21.L;   =es por eso que me levanto        21.L;   =because of that I get up dos
22.     dos veces a orinar porque los     22.     times to urinate because the
23.     nopales se convierten en agua     23.     cactus convert to water
24.     en las noches                     24.     in the nights
25.C;   sí: sí porque tiene ha:mbre:      25.C;   ye:s yes because you're
26.     tiene que comer comida comida     26.     hu:ngry: you have to eat food
27.     ..[por ejemplo productos de       27.     food..[for example animal
28.D;      [@@                            28.D;          [@@
29.C;   animal como:..u:m..(TSK)..        29.C;   products li:ke..u:m..(TSK)..
30.     pollo..co:[mo:                    30.     chicken..i:[ke
31.L;              [pollo también..       31.L;              [chicken also..I
32.     como también=                     32.     eat too=
33.C;   =uhuh pero tiene que comer..      33.C;   =uhuh but you have to eat.. a
34.     poco de esto diario..okay?        34.     little of this daily..okay?
35.     (H) le gusta:: what else can      35.     (H) do you li::ke what else
36.     you eat? pescado es bueno..       36.     can you eat? fish is good..
37.     puede come::r↑..u::m              37.     you can eat ea::t↑..u::m
38.     (1.0)       re::s:↑ (.5) a        38.     (1.0)    bee:f↑ (.5) sometimes
39.     veces..okay? no no no::           39.     ..okay? not not no:t daily
40.     diario diario (H) pero dos        40.     daily (H) but two times a
41.     veces por semana puede            41.     week you can
42.     come:r:(.5) (H) u:m carne         42.     ea:t: (.5) (H)u:m bee:f
43.     de res::↑ (H) puede..comer        43.     (H) you can..eat
44.     cualquier cosa pero estas         44.     whatever thing but these
45.     cosas con mucha grasa↑ (H)        45.     things with a lot of fat↑ (H)
46.     entonces tiene que:: comer        46.     so you have to:: eat
47.     me::nos..pobrecita no está        47.     le::ss..poor thing you aren't
48.     comiendo nada por eso             48.     eating anything that's why
49.     perdiendo peso..porque            49.     you're losing weight..because
50.     está  tan confun[dida             50.     you're con[fused
51.L;                   [porque           51.L;              [because
52.     no n: n: porque                   52.     no n: n: because I don't
53.     no quiero:: (.5) (H)  que me      53.     wa::nt (.5) (H) my
54.     suba la azúcar porque             54.     sugar to rise because
55.     me di[cen..que si te sube la      55.     they [told me if my su
56.C;        [sí                          56.C;        [yeah
57.L;   azúcar↑ (.5) te puedes..te        57.L;   rises↑ (.5) you can.. you
```

```
58.      puede: k - puedes caer en       58.      ca:n k - you can fall into a
59.      coma si te sube mucho           59.      coma if it increases too much
60. C;   well es la verda::d pero        60. C;   well it's true:: but we're
61.      estamos dos cientos..no tiene   61.      two hundred..you don't have a
62.      coma hasta seis..cientos (H)    62.      coma until six..hundred (H)
63.      entonces [tenemos bastante      63.      so [we have really
64. L;            [hasta que::           64. L;        [until wha::t
65. C;   @@[@                            65. C;   @@[@
66. L;      [ah hasta que[::             66. L;      [ah until[::
67. C;                [lo:: siento       67. C;              [I'm sorry::
68.      que [esta persona que le        68.      that [this person scared you
69. L;       [no no                      69. L;       [no no
70. C;   asustó tanto                    70. C;   so much
```

In lines 1–2, Luisa indicates that she does not eat much fatty food and uses fish as an example in line 3. Carrie responds "good" in English to Luisa's Spanish contributions. It was not unusual for Carrie to respond in English to patients with words like "good" or "excellent," which indexes English normativity but aligns with Luisa's construction of reality. However, the daughter adds, "that's all she eats a::ll day" in lines 6–7. The lengthened vowel in "a::ll" emphasizes Luisa's unvaried diet of fish, lettuce, and cactus, which becomes evident as Carrie aligns with the daughter in lines 8–9, acknowledging that Luisa "must be starving" with prosodic emphasis. Here, Carrie and the daughter co-construct Luisa as incompetent in managing her dietary choices in a language Luisa does not use. Moreover, as we have discussed above, the language that Luisa does not use is the one that is normative in the procedures and bureaucratic rituals of the clinical context. Luisa's non-normativity as a non-English user, then, already marginalizes her in the same way Rosana and Dalia were marginalized in the previous excerpts.

As the daughter continues in line 10, she uses the habitual present tense in English to construct her mother as a consistently angry, hungry, sad person. The daughter and Carrie take control over the construction of the mother's narrative through line 16, constructing the mother as an incompetent person. It is notable here that Luisa does not have access to this emergent English narrative around her eating habits and temperament since Luisa does not use English, which renders her a non-participant in her own identity construction.

Carrie switches to Spanish in line 17 to educate Luisa about the lack of nutrition in cactus and lettuce. Luisa then provides explains her need to urinate in the night in 21–24, but Carrie alins with Luisa's diet in lines 25–27, asserting that she needs to eat "comida comida" (food food), again making Luisa's identity as incompetent in managing her diet relevant. The daughter's laughter in line 28 seems to align with Carrie. In lines 29–34, Carrie suggests that Luisa eat chicken and some meat and continues with dietary advice through line 50 without asking Luisa what she actually eats.

In lines 51–59, Luisa resists Carrie's dietary advice indicating that she is following the advice of the hospital providers who treated her previously. Luisa is trying to control the narrative surrounding her dietary choices and asserts that not managing her diet properly could result in a coma. As Bauman and Briggs (1990) state, "institutional structures and mechanisms confer legitimate authority to control texts" (77). However, Carrie reasserts Luisa's incompetence in lines 61–63, noting that Luisa is not familiar with the blood sugar level that would induce a coma and the illegitimacy of her claims regarding the hospital providers in lines 68 and 70. Carrie speaks over Luisa to say that she is sorry that the providers in the hospital scared her so much, indexing Luisa's incompetence even as Luisa resists with "no no" in line 69.

Vickers (2020) argued that the interactions presented in Excerpt 3 rendered Luisa as a lovable incompetent (Goffman 1981). Carrie and the daughter take control over Luisa's narrative and co-construct her choices as incompetent ones and her reasoning as flawed. Importantly, much of Luisa's membership categorization as a lovable incompetent occurs in a language that Luisa cannot understand. By the time Luisa becomes a participant in her own identity construction in Spanish in line 21, she has already lost control over her narrative and has been constructed as a lovable incompetent who is starving herself.

5 Implications for training

The fact that this clinic employs all bi/multilingual staff and provides many bi/multilingual materials for patients is quite commendable and radical given that it is situated in the ideologically monolingual United States. In our experience collecting data in this clinic, we observed medical professionals who were dedicated to serving language minoritized Spanish-speaking patients in Spanish, which should be applauded. Generally, we saw health care providers who cared deeply about their patients and strove to give them the best care possible, which why they consented to our study being conducted there. As with any practice, particularly one as little studied as language concordant clinical consultations with language minoritized patients, linguistic analysis can provide insights to improve the practice. In this section, we provide such insights aligned with each excerpt and based linguistic analysis.

5.1 Excerpt 1

In Vickers et al. (2013), we named Carrie's action in excerpt 1, interacting with the computer, "bureaucratic side talk." Indeed, bureaucratic side talk is quite common in our data as medical providers interact with electronic medical records, government paperwork (see excerpt 2), or other medical providers. It would first be important to provide training on typical discursive moves that health care providers use but that they may not recognize because they take them for granted. So to recognize bureaucratic side talk as a discourse move that is common in their professional practice would then allow them to understand how such a move affects interaction with patients. For training bi/multilingual medical providers, it would be important to consider why bureaucratic side talk often instigates a switch to the majority language and allow the provider to recognize the moment and reflect on it. The recommendation is to make medical providers like Carrie aware and encourage them not to code-switch to English when reviewing electronic medical records (or do so silently) or engaging in any type of bureaucratic side talk. Questions that might stimulate provider discussion and reflection include: What were you trying to accomplish at this moment? How did the interaction impact the patient's participation?

Consequently, if the review of the medical records were in Spanish, the patient and the provider could collaboratively use the information in the medical records to co-construct Rosana's health history narrative instead of Rosana becoming a non-participant when Carrie refers to the medical records. Therefore, training to direct the provider to the impact of code-switching could make a major difference in the quality of the patient narrative elicited.

5.2 Excerpt 2

Even though Dr. Thomas was engaged with an artifact in a rather exclusionary way, Dalia and her husband still attempted to engage with her. Suppose health care professionals have access to audio- or video-recorded appointments for training and language intervention purposes. Particular attention can be directed at patient contributions and how they are acknowledged and ratified. Questions to heighten awareness, promote introspection, and stimulate fruitful discussions might include: What information does the patient contribute to the narrative and why? Are languages present that the patient does not use? If so, what might the impact be on the patients' perceptions of interaction?

Patient contributions to the health history narrative are crucial to the diagnosis. However, providers may inadvertently exclude patients from making contributions, particularly when they switch to English. Indeed, problem-solving in an L2 and using English-language artifacts while thinking aloud in Spanish is a major cognitive load. Providers are often under tight time constraints as other patients await, but one practice might be worthwhile for providers to excuse themselves from the immediate interaction for a couple of minutes to troubleshoot, if necessary, to organize their thoughts around the artifact and return with information that they can report to the patient. Then the provider can actively listen and, in turn, account for the patient response to that information as a contribution to the health history narrative that will ultimately be used to diagnose the patient. In other words, maintaining dyadic interaction with the patient in bi/multilingual health care consultations might be beneficial in obtaining a coherent patient-centered health history. Considering their narrative control, bilingual health care providers can make conscious efforts to put artifacts aside and give the patient the floor to move toward more symmetrical narrative construction.

5.3 Excerpt 3

The case of Luisa is a striking example that compels bilingual health care providers to be cognizant when a third-party family member is present, mainly when the patient is monolingual and the family member bilingual. Therefore, in reviewing recording third-party medical consultations with a critical eye, observers should consider the degree to which the patient is a ratified participant, contributing to and understanding the narrative. What pronouns does the provider use to or about the patient? To whom is their gaze directed? What languages are primarily or minimally used? Is there a sense that language more or less constructs someone as more or less capable of managing their own health care regimen? If transcripts are available, word counts can offer a quantitative look at who controls the discourse.

Meta-language reflections, discussions, and interventions can consider how such social dynamics impact the provider-patient rapport and can strip agency from the patient in managing their own narrative and follow-up. In her account, Luisa indexed her ability to act on her perception of a particular regimen that she received, so it stands to reason that she could do so more appropriately when she has a more active, ratified role in her own appointment. In Vickers and Goble (2018), we discussed the affordances of an egalitarian medical provider communication styles such as Carrie's for patient care, but this style may be limited when a bilingual third-party co-constructs English as the normative language and usurps the patient's autonomy in the process in an otherwise Spanish-language medical consultation that could potentially build patient autonomy. We view consciousness-raising as the first step. Practitioners should then overtly acknowledge the implications of third-party interactions before entering the consultation room and consider whether an explicit preference to use the patient's primary language is appropriate.

6 Conclusions

In this paper, we have presented three excerpts involving bi/multilingual medical providers interacting with monolingual patients in medical consultations that are "language concordant" in the minoritized language that the patient uses. These excerpts clearly show micro-interactional moments that become problematic as the bi/multilingual providers switch to English, a language their patients do not use. Mozzon-McPherson's (2013) research methods that doubled as professional development for language learning advisors point to the affordances of establishing a meta-language learning community to understand the implications of language use in a professional practice by working with naturally occurring discourse data. Accordingly, we recommend a discourse-based framework for training bi/multilingual health care providers.

In excerpts 1 and 2, we identified cases of bureaucratic side talk involving documents in both Spanish and English that instigated a switch to English. Discourse-based health care provider training would necessitate recording either role-play scenarios or real-life consultations and attending to instances of bureaucratic side talk. With transcribed and/or audio-recorded data, turning health care providers' attention to bureaucratic side talk and then indicating that such moves tend to result in code-switching to English would raise awareness of how such moves affect patient care outcomes.

As our data shows, code-switches that occur during moments of bureaucratic side talk can place patients in a position in which they become completely detached from their own narratives. The bureaucratic documents become third interactants that patients must be able to access to construct a complete and accurate health history narrative as possible. As Vickers et al. (2012) demonstrated, when health care providers interject too much during the health history narrative, it can affect the quality of the diagnosis. Discourse-based health care provider training would allow bi/multilingual health care providers to reflect on the implications of their own micro-interactional discursive moves.

In Excerpt 3, the presence of a bi/multilingual third-party family member impacts the patient's ability to convey and control the health history narrative. Whether through recorded role-play or recorded authentic medical consultations, raising awareness of the impact of the bi/multilingual third-party family member is crucial. In our data, the presence of a bi/multilingual third-party family member takes the floor away from the patient as the health care provider and family member co-construct the health history in a language the patient cannot understand. Discourse-based health care provider training could allow bi/multilingual health care providers to see how code-switching instigated by a bi/multilingual third-party family member affects the patient's ability to actively co-construct the narrative and to reflect on such moments.

Whether in the case of bureaucratic side talk or bi/multilingual third-party family members, training should include not only indications of the problem but also strategies to overcome the problem. Future research that investigates such strategies would allow a better understanding of how to modify bi/multilingual health care provider interactions in these critical moments. However, immediately apparent is simply the need to maintain Spanish language interaction throughout the medical consultation. Pointing to discourse data to demonstrate how switches to English affect patients and reflection on these moments with other practitioners might allow providers to devise strategies of their own.

Pointing out issues does not need to be a lengthy or involved process. Recording medical provider interactions with the trainer in the room would allow the trainer to indicate issues to be attended to during the role-play (Atkins 2019) or real-time consultation (O'Grady 2016) and then play these scenes for the provider. The trainer could then point out examples of problematic moments to make the provider aware in one or two training sessions.

Following Mozzon-McPherson (2013), training could involve a learning community of bi/multilingual health care providers who, in conjunction with the trainer, could spend time describing, reflecting on, and meeting to debrief on their own and each other's language use in providing health care. With the issues in mind that we have presented in this chapter, participants in the learning community can work to identify problematic moments and contemplate how macro-societal ideologies may influence their discursive moves in the consultation.

Such a preintervention training method (Robinson and Heritage 2014) could allow a researcher to develop strategies for bi/multilingual health care providers to use in their clinical interactions. The research could then move to an intervention stage (Robinson and Heritage 2014) to determine if such strategies result in less code-switching and better patient control over the health history narrative. We propose that such intervention research would lead to discourse competence among bi/multilingual health care providers who serve minoritized-language patients.

References

Antaki, Charles. 2011. *Applied conversation analysis: Intervention and change in institutional talk*. London: Palgrave Macmillan.

Atkins, Sarah. 2019. Assessing health professionals' communication through role-play: An interactional analysis of simulated versus actual general practice consultations. *Discourse Studies* 21 (2). 109–134.

Auer, Peter. 1998. *Code-switching in conversation: Language, interaction and identity*. London: Routledge.

Auer, Peter. 2005. A postscript: Code-switching and social identity. *Journal of Pragmatics* 37 (3). 403–410. https://doi.org/10.1016/j.pragma.2004.10.010

Anderson, Laurie M., Susan C. Scrimshaw, Mindy T. Fullilove, Jonathan E. Fielding & Jacques Normand. 2003. Culturally competent healthcare systems. A systematic review. *American Journal of Preventative Medicine* 24 (3 Suppl). 68–79. doi:10.1016/s0749-3797(02)00657-8.

Anderson, Nancy Lois Ruth, Evelyn Ruiz Calvillo & Marie Ngetiko Fongwa. 2007. Community-based approaches to strengthen cultural competency in nursing education and practice. *Journal of Transcultural Nursing* 18 (49). 49S–59S. DOI: 10.1177/1043659606295567

Aranguri, Cesar, Brad Davidson & Robert Ramirez. 2006. Patterns of communication through interpreters: A detailed sociolinguistic analysis. *Journal of General Internal Medicine* 21. 623–629. doi: 10.1111/j.1525-1497.2006.00451.x

Bauman, Richard & Charles L. Briggs. 1990. Poetics and performances as critical perspectives on language and social life. *Annual Review of Anthropology* 19 (1). 59–88. https://doi.org/10.1146/annurev.an.19.100190.000423

Barnes, Rebecca K. 2019. Conversation analysis of communication in medical care: Description and beyond. *Research on Language and Social Interaction* 52 (3). 300–315.

Berkowitz Bobbie & Marilyn McCubbin. 2005. Advancement of health disparities research: A conceptual approach. *Nursing Outlook* 53 (3). 153–159. https://doi.org/10.1016/j.outlook.2005.03.008

Betancourt, Joseph R. 2006. Cultural competency: Providing quality care to diverse populations. *The Consultant Pharmacist* 21 (12). 988–995. DOI: 10.4140/tcp.n.2006.988

Bisset, Mariana & Barbara Gödeke. 2015. Integrated learner support through language advising: Initial experiences and considerations at Padova University Language Centre. *Language Learning in Higher Education* 5 (2). 423–440. DOI: 10.1515/cercles-2015-0020

Brach, Cindy & Irene Fraser. 2000. Can cultural competency reduce racial and ethnic health disparities? A review and conceptual model. *Medical Care Research and Review* 57 (Supplement 1). 181–217. DOI: 10.1177/1077558700057001S09.

Candlin, Sally & Peter Roger. 2013. *Communication and professional relationships in healthcare practice*. London: Equinox.

Carson, Luke & Jo Mynard. 2012. Introduction. In Jo Mynard & Luke Carson (eds.), *Advising in language learning: Dialogue, tools and context*, 3–25. New York: Pearson.

Carter-Pokras, Olivia, Marla J. F. O'Neill, Vasana Cheanvechai, Mikhail Menis, Tao Fan & Angelo Solera. 2004. Providing linguistically appropriate services to persons with limited English proficiency: A needs and resources investigation. *The American Journal of Managed Care* 10 (SP). 29SP–36SP.

Casey, Michelle M., Lynn A. Blewett & Kathleen T. Call. 2004. Providing health care to Latino immigrants: Community-based efforts in the rural Midwest. *American Journal of Public Health* 94 (10). 1709–1711. DOI: 10.2105/ajph.94.10.1709

Cashman, Holly. R. 2005. Identities at play: Language preference and group membership in bilingual talk in interaction. *Journal of Pragmatics* 37 (3). 301–315. https://doi.org/10.1016/j.pragma.2004.10.004

Castro, Eduardo. 2018. Complex adaptative systems, language advising, and motivation: A longitudinal case study with a Brazilian student of English. *System* 74. 138–148. https://doi.org/10.1016/j.system.2018.03.004

Castro, Eduardo. 2019. Motivational dynamics in language advising sessions: A case study. *Studies in Self-Access Journal* 10 (1). 5–20. http://sisaljournal.org/archives/mar19/castro

Ciekanski, Maud. 2007. Fostering learner autonomy: Power and reciprocity in the relationship between language learner and language learning adviser. *Cambridge Journal of Education* 37 (1). 111–127. https://doi.org/10.1080/03057640601179442

Clarridge, Katherine E., Ernest A. Fischer, Andrea R. Quintana & James M. Wagner. 2008. Should all U.S. physicians speak Spanish? *Virtual Mentor* 10 (4). 211–216. DOI: 10.1001/virtualmentor.2008.10.4.medu1-0804.

Chapman, Rachel R. & Jean R. Berggren. 2005. Radical contextualization: Contributions to an anthropology of racial/ethnic health disparities. *Health* 9 (2). 145–167. DOI: 10.1177/1363459305050583

Crabbe, David, Alison Hoffman & Sara Cotterall. 2001. Examining the discourse of learner advisory sessions. *AILA Review* 15. 2–15.

Egede, Leonard E. 2006. Race, ethnicity, culture, and disparities in health care. *Journal of General Internal Medicine* 21 (6). 667–669. DOI: 10.1111/j.1525-1497.2006.0512.x

Edelson, Dana P. & Cynthia M. LaFond. 2013. Deconstructing Debriefing for Simulation-Based Education. *JAMA Pediatrics* 167(6). 586–587. https://doi.org/10.1001/jamapediatrics.2013.325.

Edwards Karethy. 2003. Increasing cultural competence and decreasing disparities in health. *Journal of Cultural Diversity* 10 (4). 111–112.

Erdmann, J. A. 2008. *Medical interpreter neutrality: Few voices outside of the examining room. A literature review and recommendation for further research on improving linguistic access in health care settings* (nd). University of Minnesota, School of Public Health & HACER: Hispanic Advocacy and Community Empowerment through Research.

Fiscella, Kevin, Peter Franks, Mark P. Doescher & Barry G. Saver. 2002. Disparities in health care by race, ethnicity, and language among the insured: Findings from a national sample. *Medical Care* 40 (1). 52–59. DOI: 10.1097/00005650-200201000-00007.

Flores, H. 2005. Workforce diversity: Addressing health status disparities and the distribution of physician services in California. Statement before the Senate Health Committee on University of California Admissions and Shortages in the Health Care Workforce.

Flores, Glenn, Milagros Abreu & Sandra C. Tomany-Korman. 2005. Limited English proficiency, primary language at home, and disparities in children's health care: How language barriers are measured matters. *Public Health Report* 120 (4). 418–430. DOI: 10.1177/003335490512000409

Gafaranga, Joseph. 2005. Demythologising language alternation studies: Conversational structure vs. social structure in bilingual conversation. *Journal of Pragmatics* 37 (3). 281–300. https://doi.org/10.1016/j.pragma.2004.10.002

Goble, Ryan & Caroline H. Vickers. 2016. 'Shift' 'n 'control': The computer as a third interactant in Spanish-language medical consultations. *Communication & Medicine* 12 (2–3). 171–185. DOI: 10.1558/cam.30177

Goffman, Erving. 1981. *Forms of talk*. Philadelphia: University of Pennsylvania Press.

Greatbatch, David. 1988. A turn-taking system for British news interviews. *Language in Society* 17 (3). 401–430. DOI: 10.1017/S0047404500012963

Green, Alexander. R., Quyen Ngo-Metzger, Anna T. R. Legedza, Michael P. Massagli, Russell S. Phillips & Lisa I. Iezzoni. 2005. Interpreter services, language concordance, and health care quality experiences of Asian Americans with limited English proficiency. *Journal of General Internal Medicine*, 20 (11). 1050–1056. DOI: 10.1111/j.1525-1497.2005.0223.x

Hill, Jane H. 1998. Language, race, and white public space. *American Anthropologist* 100 (3). 680–689. doi:10.1525/aa.1998.100.3.680

Hobgood, Cherri, Susan Sawning, Josie Bowen & Katherine Savage. 2006. Teaching culturally appropriate care: A review of educational models and methods. *Academic Emergency Medicine* 13 (12). 1288–1295. DOI: 10.1197/j.aem.2006.07.031

Holmes, Seth M. 2006. An ethnographic study of the social context of migrant health in the United States. *PLoS Medicine* 3 (10). e448. https://doi.org/10.1371/journal.pmed.0030448

Hutchby, Ian. 1996. Power in discourse: The case of arguments on a British talk radio show. *Discourse & Society* 7 (4). 481–497. https://doi.org/10.1177/0957926596007004003

Hutchby, Ian & Michelle O'Reilly. 2010. Children's participation and the familial moral order in family therapy. *Discourse Studies* 12 (1). 49–64.

Jacobs, Elizabeth A., Lisa C. Diamond & Lisa Stevak. 2010. The importance of teaching clinicians when and how to work with interpreters. *Patient Education & Counseling* 78 (2). 149–153. DOI: 10.1016/j.pec.2009.12.001

Jacoby, Sally, Elinor Ochs. 1995. Co-construction: An introduction. *Research on Language and Social Interaction* 28 (3). 171–183.

Keifenheim, Katharina. E. Martin Teufel, Julianne Ip, Natalie Speiser, Elisabeth J. Leehr, Stephan Zipfel & Anne Herrmann-Werner. 2015. Teaching history taking to medical students: A systematic review. *BMC Medical Education* 15. 159. https://doi.org/10.1186/s12909-015-0443-x

Leahy, Margaret M. & Irenee P. Walsh. 2008. Talk in interaction in the speech – language pathology clinic: Bringing theory to practice through discourse. *Topics in Language Disorders* 28 (3). 229–241.

Leyva, Melissa, Iman Sharif & Philip O. Ozuah. 2005. Health literacy among Spanish-speaking Latino parents with limited English proficiency. *Ambulatory Pediatrics* 5 (1). 56–59. DOI: 10.1367/A04-093R.1

Martinez, Glenn. 2008. Language-in-healthcare policy, interaction patterns, and unequal care on the U.S.-Mexico border. *Language Policy* 7 (4). 345–363. doi:10.1007/s10993-008-9110-y

Morales, Leo S., William E., Cunningham, Julie A. Brown, Honghu Liu & Ron D. Hays. 1999. Are Latinos less satisfied with communication by health care providers? *Journal of General Internal Medicine* 14 (7). 409–417.

Morrison, Brian R. & Diego Navarro. 2012. Shifting roles: From language teachers to learning advisors. *System* 40 (3). 349–359. DOI: 10.1016/j.system.2012.07.004

Mozzon-McPherson, Marina. 2007. Supporting independent learning environments: An analysis of structures and roles of language learning advisers. *System* 35. 66–92. https://doi.org/10.1016/j.system.2006.10.008

Mozzon-McPherson, Marina. 2012. The skills of counselling in advising: Language as a pedagogic tool. In Jo Mynard & Luke Carson (eds.), *Advising in language learning: Dialogue, tools and context*, 43–64. New York: Pearson Education.

Mozzon-McPherson, Marina. 2013. Defining the field: The use of discourse analysis as a reflective tool in the professional development of language learning advisers as practitioners and researchers. *The Language Learning Journal* 41 (2). 219–230.

Mozzon-McPherson, Marina. 2015. Supporting independent learning environments: An analysis of structures and roles of language learning advisers. *System* 35. 66–92. DOI: 10.1016/j.system.2006.10.008

Mishler, Elliot. G. 1984. *The discourse of medicine: The dialectics of medical interviews*. New Jersey: Ablex Publishing Corporation.

Ngo-Metzger, Quyen. Dara H. Sorkin, Russell S. Phillips, Sheldon Greenfield, Michael P. Massagli, Brian Clarridge & Sherrie H. Kaplan. 2007. Providing high-quality care for limited English proficient patients: The importance of language concordance and interpreter use. *Journal of General Internal Medicine* 22 (Suppl 2). 324–330. DOI: 10.1007/s11606-007-0340-z

O'Grady, Catherine. 2016. Clinical communication training for the general practice of medicine – A case for including discourse analytical findings from real-world practice. *Journal of Applied Linguistics and Professional Practice* 13 (1–3). 254–275. https://doi.org/10.1558/japl.31860

Pamies, Rubens J. & Phyllis A. Nsiah-Kumi. 2006. Multicultural medicine and ensuring good health for all. *Ethnic Disparities* 16 (2 Suppl 3). S3-14–20.

Pemberton, Richard, Sarah Toogood, Susanna Ho & Jacqueline Lam. 2001. Approaches to advising for self-directed language learning. *AILA Review* 15. 16–25.

Peräkylä, Anssi & Sanna Vehviläinen. 2003. Conversation analysis and the professional stocks of interactional knowledge. *Discourse & Society* 14 (6). 727–750. DOI: 10.1177/09579265030146003

Peterson, M. C., J. H. Holbrook, D. Von Hales, N. L. Smith & L. V. Staker. 1992. Contributions of the history, physical examination, and laboratory investigation in making medical diagnoses. *Western Journal of Medicine* 156 (2). 163–165.

Philips, Susan U. 2000. *The organization of ideological diversity in discourse*. Unpublished Manuscript.

Philips, Susan. U. 2005. Language and social inequality. In Alessandro Duranti (ed.), *A companion to linguistic anthropology*, 474–495. Victoria, Australia: Blackwell Publishing Ltd.

Pope Charlene. 2005. Addressing limited English proficiency and disparities for Hispanic postpartum women. *Journal of Obstetrics and Gynecology Neonatal Nursing* 34 (4). 512–520. DOI: 10.1177/0884217505278295.

Ramirez, Raul. 2006. Reducing health care disparities: breaking the language barrier is critical first step. *Journal of the Arkansas Medical Society* 103 (1). 8–9.

Robinson, Jeffrey D. & John Heritage. 2014. Intervening with conversation analysis: The case of medicine. *Research on Language and Social Interaction* 47 (3). 201–218.

Rosa, Ute W. 2006. Impact of cultural competence on medical care: Where are we today? *Clinics in Chest Medicine* 27 (3). 395–399. DOI: 10.1016/j.ccm.2006.04.011

Rust, George, Kofi Kondwani, Ruben Martinez, Roberto Dansie, Winston Wong, Yvonne Fry-Johnson, Rocio Del Milagro Woody, Elvan J. Daniels, Janice Herbert-Carter, Laura

Aponte & Harry Strothers. 2006. A crash-course in cultural competence. *Ethnic Disparities* 16 (2 Suppl 3). S3–29–36.

Sarangi, Srikant. 2001. Editorial: On demarcating the space between 'lay expertise' and 'expert laity'. *Text & Talk* 21 (1–2). 3–11. https://doi.org/10.1515/text.1.21.1-2.3

Selig, Suzanne, Elizabeth Tropiano & Ella Greene-Motion. 2006. Teaching cultural competence to reduce health disparities. *Health Promotion Practice* 7 (3). 247S–255S. DOI: 10.1177/1524839906288697

Schegloff, Emanuel A. 2007. *Sequence organization in interaction. A primer in conversation analysis.* Cambridge, United Kingdom: Cambridge University Press.

Schenker, Yael, Andrew J. Karter, Dean Schillinger, E. Margaret Warton, Nancy E. Adler, Howard H. Moffet, Ameena T. Ahmed & Alicia Fernandez. 2010. The impact of limited English proficiency and physician language concordance on reports of clinical interactions among patients with diabetes: The DISTANCE study. *Patient Education & Counseling* 81 (2). 222–228. DOI: 10.1016/j.pec.2010.02.005

Somnath, Saha. 2006. The relevance of cultural distance between patients and physicians to racial disparities in health care. *Journal of General Internal Medicine* 21 (2). 203–205. DOI: 10.1111/j.1525-1497.2006.0345.x

Tassinari, Maria G. 2016. Emotions and feelings in language advising discourse. In Christina Gkonou, Dietmar Tatzl & Sarah Mercer (eds.), *New directions in language learning psychology*, 71–96. Graz, Australia: Springer.

Taylor, Stephanie L. & Nicole Lurie. 2004. The role of culturally competent communication in reducing ethnic and racial healthcare disparities. *American Journal of Managed Care* 10 (SP1–SP4).

Timmins, Caraway L. 2002. The impact of language barriers on the health care of Latinos in the United States: A review of the literature and guidelines for practice. *Journal of Midwifery & Women's Health* 47 (2). 80–96. DOI:10.1016/s1526-9523(02)00218-0.

United States Department of Health and Human Services, Office of Minority Health. 2001. *National standards for culturally and linguistically appropriate services in health care CLAS, final report.* Washington, D.C.

Vega, William A. 2005. Higher stakes ahead for cultural competence. *General Hospital Psychiatry* 27 (6). 446–450. DOI: 10.1016/j.genhosppsych.2005.06.007

Vickers, Caroline H. 2020. Occasioned membership categorization in a transnational medical consultation: Interaction, marginalization, and health disparities. *Journal of Sociolinguistics* 24. 574–592. DOI: 10.1111/josl.12441

Vickers, Caroline H., Ryan Goble & Christopher Lindfelt. 2012. Narrative co-construction in the medical consultation: How agency and control affect the diagnosis. *Communication & Medicine* 9 (2). 159–171.

Vickers, Caroline H., Sharon K. Deckert & Ryan Goble. 2014. Constructing language normativity through the animation of stance in Spanish-language medical consultations. *Health Communication* 29 (7). 707–716. https://doi.org/10.1080/10410236.2013.778224

Vickers, Caroline H. & Ryan Goble. 2011. Well, now, okey dokey: English discourse markers in Spanish-Language medical consultations. *The Canadian Modern Language Review* 67 (4). 536–567. doi:10.3138/cmlr.67.4.536

Vickers, Caroline H. & Ryan Goble. 2018. Politeness and prosody in the co-construction of medical provider persona styles and patient relationships. *Journal of Applied Linguistics and Professional Practice* 11 (2). 202–226. https://doi.org/10.1558/japl.24177

Vickers, Caroline H., Ryan Goble & Sharon K. Deckert. 2015. Third party interaction in the medical context: Code-switching and control. *Journal of Pragmatics* 84. 154–171. https://doi.org/10.1016/j.pragma.2015.05.009

Vickers, Caroline H., Ryan Goble & Christopher Lindfelt. 2012. Narrative co-construction in the medical consultation: How agency and control affect the diagnosis. *Communication & Medicine* 9 (2). 159–171.

Watkins, Satoko. 2015. Enhanced awareness and its translation into action: A case study of one learner's self-directed language learning experience. *Language Learning in Higher Education* 5 (2) 441–464. DOI 10.1515/cercles-2015-0021

Weech-Maldonado, Robert, Leo S. Morales, Marc Elliott, Karen Spritzer, Grant Marshall & Ron D. Hays. 2003. Race/ethnicity, language, and patients' assessments of care in Medicaid managed care. *Health Services Research* 38 (3), 789–808. DOI: 10.1111/1475-6773.00147

Wilson, Elisabeth, Alice Hm Chen, Kevin Grumbach, Frances Wang & Alicia Fernandez. 2005. Effects of limited English proficiency and physician language on health care comprehension. *Journal of General Internal Medicine* 20 (9). 800–806. DOI: 10.1111/j.1525-1497.2005.0174.x

Wilson-Stronks, Amy, Karen K. Lee, Karen, Christina L. Cordero, April L. Kopp & Erica Galvez. 2008. *One size does not fit all: Meeting the health care needs of diverse populations.* The Joint Commission; 2008.

Wynia, Matthew. K. 2006. Balancing evidence-based medicine and cultural competence in the quest to end healthcare disparities. *Medscape General Medicine.* 8 (2), 22.

Zambrana, Ruth. E., Christine Molnar, Helen Baras Munoz & Debbie Salas Lopez. 2004. Cultural competency as it intersects with racial/ethnic, linguistic, and class disparities in managed healthcare organizations. *American Journal of Managed Care* 10. SP37–44.

Zhang, Wei. 2005. Code-choice in bidialectal interaction: The choice between Putonghua and Cantonese in a radio phone-in program in Shenzhen. *Journal of Pragmatics* 37 (3), 355–374. https://doi.org/10.1016/j.pragma.2004.10.007

Zsembik, Barbara A. & Dana Fennell. 2005. Ethnic variation in health and the determinants of health among Latinos. *Social Science & Medicine* 61 (1). 53–63. DOI: 10.1016/j.socscimed.2004.11.040

Section 2: **Applied linguistics, translation, and health**

Boyd H. Davis, Ching-Yi Kuo, Margaret Maclagan
Chapter 3
Children learning about dementia in Taiwan: Using gist translations to clarify adult opinions

1 Introduction

As the global aging population increases, so does the increase in projections of dementia. The United Nations (www.un.org) projects that one out of every six persons will be 65 or older by 2050. By that same date, the World Health Organization (www.who.int) expects the number of people with dementia to triple. Knowledge of and understanding about dementia vary in different countries and cultures. Studies of the impact of disseminating knowledge about dementia typically focus on adults or on adolescents. Little is known regarding the effects of increasing dementia knowledge in pre-adolescent children in Asian countries or its impact on combating the stigma of dementia still prevalent in many societies.

This chapter explores adult reactions in interviews in a small, exploratory study of elementary-school Taiwanese children formally learning about dementia in their classrooms. We begin with features of the context that provides the rationale for our focus. The context explains several critical features in the discourse offered by adult participants who consented to an interview, and suggests wider sociocultural issues to which the study points. Next, we briefly display the results from the two exploratory surveys given to the elementary-school children and move to look at 29 adult interviews from the perspective of interpersonal pragmatics (Locher 2013).

Interviews were conducted in the Taiwanese variety of Mandarin Chinese by the second author who speaks both Mandarin and English. Because neither the first nor the third author is competent in Mandarin, we used post-edited automatic machine translations of the adult interviews. Such translations enable the researcher to understand the gist of the interviews but not nuances of expression, or shades of meaning arising from the way the ideas were phrased and presented

---

Boyd H. Davis, Linguistics, University of North Carolina Charlotte, United States of America
Ching-Yi Kuo, Geriatric counsellor, Tainan
Margaret Maclagan, School of Psychology, Speech and Hearing, University of Canterbury, New Zealand

https://doi.org/10.1515/9783110744804-004

verbally and nonverbally by the interviewees. This gisting forms a second, underlying context of technological adaptation. We briefly discuss issues inherent in using machine translations and finally analyze the gists of the conversational interviews from the adults who were connected to the children's schools in various roles.

2 Context

2.1 Demographics

The twenty-first century has seen Taiwan's constantly increasing industrialization and profitability which, combined with population shifts in both location and density, have contributed to major social changes, including demographic shifts affecting aged care. Economic growth began in the twentieth century in the 1960s, reforms in the health system were underway in the 1980s and studies of the various dementias had already begun to appear in the late 1980s and early 1990s. Healthcare has been a priority for the government: between 2003 and 2008, Taiwan's government presented twelve plans for healthcare and long-term care, leading eventually to the Ministry of Health's 2017 *Act for Long-Term Care 2.0* updated in 2018 and currently offering three tiers of care (https://www.mohw.gov.tw/cp-4344-46546-2.html).

Demographic statistics, as interpreted by researchers of sociocultural trends, underlie many efforts for the development of care for Taiwan's ageing population. The annual Survey of Social Development Trends, sponsored by Academia Sinica, Taiwan's national research academy, makes its data available to researchers and to collaborating data archives in the social sciences. For example, the 2002 survey noted a decrease from 1998 in those families including grandparents (https://eng.stat.gov.tw/ct.asp?xItem=9368&ctNode=1644&mp=5). Keyed to information in the 2011 Survey, Poston and Zhang stated that in 2000, a senior citizen was supported by a little over 8 people, but given the dropping birthrate, their available support would drop to 2.11 people by 2060 (2014: 276). Taiwan's population is aging rapidly. The aging share of the population is currently a little over 16 per cent and is expected to be as much as 40 per cent in another twenty years (https://statistica.com), while the birthrate in 2021 is reported as the lowest in the world (https://www.taiwannews.com.tw/en/news/4180941). Currently, 78.5% of Taiwan's population is urban and the average age for first-time mothers is now 31, as shown in figures released by the Ministry of the Interior in 2020.

2.2 Present issues

Two immediate effects of this demographic shift will be key to understanding future care for the ageing in Taiwan and particularly for those ageing with dementia or disabilities. The first effect is economic: it is created by the rise in projections for dementia care, the falling birthrate and the changing family structure, often assumed to be the result of urbanization, together with a concomitant increase in one-parent households (see Hsueh 2014: 199). These factors have led to the new Dementia Care 2.0 (Ministry of Health and Welfare, Taiwan 2018) which in turn entails a needed expansion for education about dementia and in the caregiving workforce. Dementia Care 2.0 states 'Education and training should be available to the professionals as well as the public.... Besides training for the professionals, dementia awareness campaigns should be provided to police officers, village chiefs, **elementary school students** and the public' [emphasis ours] (Ministry of Health and Welfare, Taiwan 2018: 30). The second effect may be termed sociocultural, as it is reflected in how current assumptions about civic and familial virtue, or filial piety, are affected.

Hiring immigrant care workers has been one attempted solution for older people needing long term care: Wang asserts that by 2010, with other family members often working outside the home, immigrant workers were caring for 60 per cent of the seniors in Taiwan (2010: 766–67). Wang and Chen (2017: 122) state that by 2016, 15% of families with older persons needing care were using day care services or daily home care migrant workers, and 25% of the families had hired a worker to live in the home. An analyst for Taiwan *Business Topics* asserted that by 2018, the National Immigration Agency reported that there were over 250,000 foreign caregivers (Ferry 2018). Reporting in 2020 for *News Lens*, another business news publication, Fahey explained that the part of the Taiwanese population available to work was projected to drop to under 50% by 2065, adding, "Simply put, there will not be enough young people working and paying taxes to support a large population of retired people" (2020: 3). And, as reviewed by Chen and Fu (2020) and summarized by Wu et al. in 2021, new payment policies for the home care system, "intended to be a supplementary system grounded in the traditional Confucian care model" (Yeh 2020: 85) whereby adult children are expected to care for their aging parents, have resulted in changes both in home care services and in the number of persons receiving them.

Lan Pei Cha, perhaps still best known for her explosive 2006 *Global Cinderellas: Migrant Domestics and Newly Rich Employers in Taiwan*, had earlier called attention in 2002 to the language issues implicit in the establishment and maintenance of class boundaries for foreign domestic workers. Such issues are expanded in interactions between foreign care workers who speak neither Mandarin nor Taiwanese, who may lack training as culturally competent care workers (Davis and

Smith 2013) and who have been hired to care for older Taiwanese with disabilities and dementias. Munkejord et al. (2021: 2) note that by 2020, there were more than 260,000 registered live-in migrant caregivers. As reported by Yang (2020), Chen Cheng Fen, 2020 President of the Taiwan Association for Family Caregivers, has found that 96.9 per cent of migrant domestic caregivers face major problems with language barriers, training in caregiver skills, and instruction in food preparation. The Association had previously begun work with these problems by, for example, mounting 38 videos for Vietnamese caregivers on YouTube (外籍勞工照護技巧## 2017).

The "traditional Confucian care model" referenced above refers to the cultural construct of *filial piety*, in which the oldest surviving son (although more commonly his wife) cares for the parents who had cared for him. That sentence is a greatly oversimplified description of a major tenet of thought about civic and individual virtue which has been both familial and sociopolitical in its influence for at least two thousand years. One question before many countries throughout the world is this: with the increasing number of aging people and the declining birthrate, will families "be expected to provide both childcare and aged care?" (Ping and Chun 2019: 1914) Such a question has immediate force in Taiwan, as its birthrate is now the lowest in the world (*Taiwan News* 2021–04–19). Payette and Chien assert that Taiwan's expansion of its long-term care system has shifted "elder care responsibilities from the traditional familial care model to a more socialized one" (2020: 228). However, as Farrell and Yi note (2019: 1893) ". . . in a changing society like Taiwan, neither traditional nor modern norms and roles provide adequate guidelines for interaction in families. Both traditional and modern norms receive varying degrees of support and resistance from family members, and often they conflict with one another."

The emphasis on traditional cultural norms can be seen in the 2017 speech to the Ministry of Education by Sophie Chang, Chair of the Taiwan Semiconductor Manufacturing Company's Charity for "the trigger of revival of filial piety" (https://esg.tsmc.com/csr/en/update/socialParticipation/content/charity_2/). Since then, the TSMC charity has established a website in a well-regarded high school, given prizes, and worked with the Ministry to list filial piety as one of the core values in guidelines for schools to facilitate moral culture (https://english.moe.gov.tw/cp-116-24161-390e9-1.html).

2.3 Relationships of children giving care to older persons with dementia

Assumptions about some features of filial piety and changes in family structure are often embedded in sociocultural discussions of children's relationships with older persons or even as their caregivers. Such discussions entail identifying whether the child is living in a three-generation home or the older person is living outside the child's home, either alone or in a care facility. For example, Assaf et al. (2016: 327) report that in the US in 2005 there were roughly 1.3 million young caregivers providing help to seniors or persons with disabilities, adding that this could make the caregivers vulnerable to later stress. According to the ongoing survey by the National Alliance for Caregiving and the American Association of Retired Persons (AARP), the number of children offering caregiving in the US had increased by 2020. The AARP estimate 3.4 million (or more) children below 18 are providing care to adults, with more non-Whites than Whites providing this care.

Based on a long-term study of Chinese older adults in the Chicago area of the US, those whose families expected filial piety from younger family members were "vulnerable" to stress as they aged (Dong and Zhang 2016). This is partially explained by a conference abstract by Xu, Li and Zhang (2016), published by the Gerontological Society of America, and keyed to 500 interviews with persons in Xu et al.'s study. They found that 43.8% of the respondents explained that older and younger citizens now held differing views of filial piety. Hall and Sikes have published a series of studies about young people living in families with dementia, particularly if the person with dementia is a parent. They report a sizeable number of grieving and even hostile reactions from the younger persons (Hall and Sikes 2017, Sikes and Hall 2018). Such reactions were echoed in questionnaires from a little over 900 British adolescents in Farina et al. (2020) who explained the young people learned about dementia from the media or on the internet, rather than in school.

2.4 Previous work in Taiwan to investigate children's attitudes toward and understanding of dementia

In the mid to late 1990s, a small team of Taiwanese researchers in neurology, whose studies focused on brain disorders, began a lifetime's publishing on dementia which continues today. In early articles from studies often led by Dr. Jong Ling Fuh, they looked at screening tools (Fuh et al. 1995) and caregiver depression (Fuh et al. 1999), behavioral disorders (Fuh et al. 2001), agitation (Fuh et al. 2002), differing features among types of dementia including Alzheimer's dementia (Fuh, Wang and Cumkings 2005), and community understanding of how dementia – called senile dementia throughout the community – might be seen by children and adolescents (Fuh, Wang and Juang 2005). Fuh had begun community surveys as part of a larger team which had surveyed 5297 persons in Taiwan to begin to identify dementia prevalence (Liu et al. 1995). They report that at that time, there were few if any nursing homes as Chinese elders lived with their families who protected them. The elders also had a shorter life span than seniors in the West.

Fuh, Wang and Juang (2005) conducted a 10-question survey, with 5515 students out of 5825 returning the questionnaire. The students, all aged 10–15, attended one of seven schools. The Attitude Toward Dementia Questionnaire created by the authors had 5 yes-no questions and 5 Likert-scale type questions, as displayed in their Table (Fuh, Wang and Juang 2005: 140). Their 5 Yes/No questions included the following: have you heard about senile dementia? 93% responded yes. Will you worry about your parents/grandparents getting it? 70 % yes. The Likert scale was used to respond to whether it was normal to get dementia when one grew old: 44.8% disagreed and 22.4% strongly disagreed; there were similar percentages for whether it was incurable and 'embarrassing'; however, 86% thought dementia was preventable.

Younger students thought dementia was a normal part of aging, a hereditary kind of psychosis, and probably contagious; they would feel "embarrassed" to bring home a friend (Fuh, Wang and Juang 2005: 140). Older students knew more about dementia and were more likely to believe it was preventable. The study's authors called for dementia education since none was available in schools, and few teachers had responded to the questionnaire.

3 Present work in Taiwan to investigate children's attitudes toward and understanding of dementia

3.1 Background and methods

In 2020, Kuo, a geriatric counselor and former elementary school teacher who had completed preliminary PhD studies abroad, initiated an attitudinal study with 299 students in grades three through six in eight small schools in Southern Taiwan. The students were aged from 8 to 11. The schools had been recently incorporated into two sizeable cities and are considered suburban rather than rural. An ethics review was conducted, and approval was given by the National Cheng Kung University in Tainan, Taiwan. The study was sponsored by Kaohsiung Women's Work Association, a non-profit organization including outreach to the aged in Kaohsiung. Schools were contacted for permission through Kuo's relatives and a local politician who was a family friend. In each school, the principal read the proposal and authorized Kuo to administer two short, pencil-paper surveys to school-selected classes of students before and after she delivered a Power Point presentation to them about dementia. Parents in each selected class filled out a consent form allowing their children to take part. There was also a consent form for the children, and since they are considered vulnerable, consented children also gave verbal assent to being recorded at the start of each child interview. The original proposal included a second post-test with the surveys two weeks later, but that was not fully possible with several of the schools. Accordingly, our report does not include data for schools whose students could not take the second post-test. Following the first post-test, focused conversations were held with 19 students and 29 adults in various roles connected to the schools.

The study was designed to elicit what students in grades three through six might know in advance about dementia and what they might gain from the presentation. It was also designed to ascertain what empathy they might have in advance towards people with dementia or what they might gain through the presentation. Two surveys were selected, and permission obtained for their translation. The first survey was *KIDS*, the acronym for the *Kids Insight into Dementia Survey* (Baker 2018a; Overgaauw et al. 2017; see Baker et al. 2018b for a review of its psychometric properties). This Australian study was designed "as a tool to measure children's insight into dementia, and to evaluate dementia education initiatives targeting the youth" (Baker et al. 2018a: 953). The tool includes a brief scenario about a 75-year-old woman with dementia and uses a 5-point Likert scale designed to measure in fourteen questions if and how strongly the respondent aligns with assigning personhood to a person with dementia, stigmatizes the person, or understands/has knowledge about several aspects of the condition. The second survey, *EmQue-CA*, or Empathy Questionnaire for Children and Adolescents, presents respondents with a series of statements and asks them to rate each statement as not true – somewhat true – or true (Overgaauw et al. 2017: 3). Statements fall into three areas: affective empathy, such as when you feel happy or sad keyed to another's feelings; cognitive empathy or understanding why someone acts or feels the way they do; and intention to offer comfort. Different versions of the EmQue-CA contain different numbers of items; the version used in the present study contained 18 statements.

After greeting students, the two surveys were administered. The educational component was a roughly 40-minute, thirteen-slide Power Point presentation, emphasizing medical information. Its contents were: Introduction [with video a "Grandpa forgot about me"]; Differences between dementia and aging; The story of dementia; Drawings of brain with and without dementia; Brain Sickness; Dementia Diagnosis; Early Symptoms [with video b]; Treatment [video c]; and Closing video "I'm Still Me" [video d]. The links to the four short videos in Mandarin can be found here:

(a) https://www.youtube.com/watch?v=xF4PPM8yDSw Taiwan Alzheimer's Disease Association 2012, 4.37 minutes;
(b) https://www.youtube.com/watch?v=HtPl-TgTmdw 2018 Understanding Dementia in 1 Minute-Episode 2. 1.29 minutes;
(c) https://www.youtube.com/watch?v=mqSLXFfY_Jw 2020 Wise Series [video channel], 1.38 minutes; and
(d) https://www.youtube.com/watch?v=9fJOOmlRQtI 2020, 4.45 minutes, reposted from shuj.shu.edu.tw/blog/2020/05/25.

Next, the two surveys were re-administered, after which volunteering consented students and adults participated in dementia-focused, semi-structured interviews (Smith 1995) lasting between six and twenty minutes about dementia (students) or teaching about dementia (adults) which Kuo recorded (see Table 1). The second post-test of the two surveys was administered in 6 of the 8 schools after two weeks. The adults represented a range of roles: principals, teachers, school nurses, volunteer moms (a third of whom were foreign brides) and a crossing guard. The results from the KIDS survey presented here are preliminary; any further analysis will be carried out by the second author, Kuo.

Table 1: Questions and prompts for semi-structured interviews.

Questions for children representing grades 3–6	Q1: Who in your family has dementia?
	Q2: Who told you/when and how did you learn about it?
	Q3: Describe what the person with dementia does.
Conversational prompts for adults representing varied school-related roles	Q1: What do you think, from the school's standpoint, of seeing students learning about dementia?
	Q2: How do you think parents will react to this information? Will they be OK with children learning about dementia?
	Q3: How do we prepare these children to face the coming of a super-high aged society?

The semi-structured interviews, recorded on an Android cellphone, were transcribed using *Transcribear* (transcribear.com) with follow-up review of each transcript against the sound file by a native speaker of Mandarin. To assist analysis by the English-speaking collaborators on the project, whose spoken/written Mandarin was insufficient and because no professionally trained Chinese translator was available, each interview was translated using two automatic machine translation programs. These were DeepL (www.deepl.com), a machine translation program launched in 2017 and Google Translate (translate.google.com), originally launched in 2006: see Croes (2019) for a useful comparison of the two, and our discussion below. The second author, a native speaker of Mandarin, who has studied at the graduate level in the US, reviewed all the English translations for topical accuracy. The English-speaking collaborators harmonized the versions through post-editing (see Figure 3, below for an example). For adults, the subject of the present discussion by the English-speaking collaborators, the gisted translation of questions and responses was analyzed qualitatively using thematic analysis (Braun and Clarke 2006; Kiger and Varpio 2020). The initial harmonized versions of the Google and DeepL transcripts were produced by the third author. The first and third authors separately read both versions of each of the transcripts through several times and the post-editing process continued until both authors were satisfied with the final harmonized version. Any disagreements were discussed and settled to the satisfaction of all authors. We discuss issues involved with the use of machine translation and gisted interviews below.

3.2 Findings: How the children responded to each survey

3.2.1 Responses to KIDS survey

This survey was administered once before and twice after the brief educational intervention to see if the children changed how they assigned personhood to a person with dementia, stigmatized the person, or understood/had knowledge about several aspects of the condition. Although 301 children completed parts of the tests, only 276 completed the pre-test and both post-tests. Data was removed from the analysis if the child failed to answer more than 3 out of the 14 questions.

The three sections of the KIDS survey had different numbers of questions. The section on *personhood* included questions like 'I would be happy to be friends with a person with dementia' (Baker et al. 2018a: 957). There were 5 questions in this section. The section on *stigma* contained 6 questions that covered possible negative reactions to meeting or spending time with someone with dementia. The section on *knowledge* contained 3 questions that covered basic aspects of dementia and its care. Children responded to the questionnaire by marking a 5-point scale with 'agree a lot' at one end and 'disagree a lot' at the other end: the higher the score the more positive the child's attitude to a person with dementia (Baker et al. 2018a: 954). An option 'don't know/unsure' was included at the mid-point on the scale to lower the likelihood that children who did not know about dementia would make random guesses (Baker et al. 2018a). If a child 'agreed a lot' with all questions the maximum possible score would be 70.

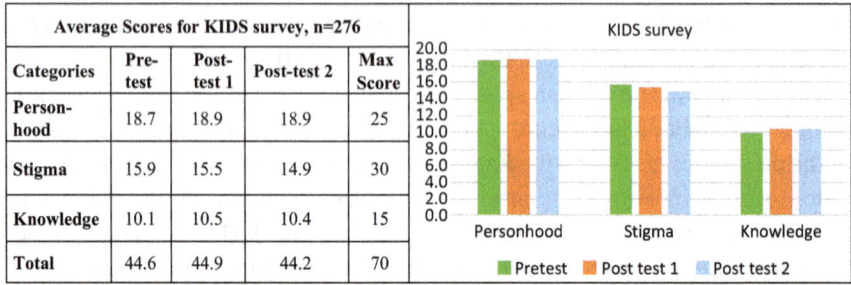

Figure 1: Average scores for KIDS surveys from 276 children.

Figure 1 shows that the Power Point presentation on dementia had little effect on the attitudes measured by the KIDS survey. There were initially very small improvements in two of the categories assessed by the KIDS. After the presentation, in the first post-test, children were slightly more willing to assign personhood to the person with dementia and their knowledge about dementia improved. However, the extent to which they felt dementia attracted Stigma dropped minutely and dropped slightly further in the second post-test. The results for the children's willingness to assign personhood and their knowledge about dementia remained just above initial levels, but the improvements were so small they would not be meaningful in the real world.

3.2.2 Responses to the EmQue-CA survey

This survey was also administered once before and twice after the brief educational intervention to see if the children changed their empathy toward or shared feelings with the person who might have the condition, their knowledge of dementia, or their intention to offer some comfort to the person. The UK version of the EmQue-CA used in this study (https://www.focusonemotions.nl/empathy-questionnaire) contained 18 questions divided into three sections: *affective empathy*, *cognitive empathy* and *intention to comfort*. Seven questions assessed the children's affective empathy, 5 assessed their cognitive empathy and 6 assessed their intention to comfort. In this initial analysis, statements that were coded as not true received one point, those that were somewhat true received 2 points and those that were true received three points. The maximum possible score if a child marked all 18 statements as true was 54. Although 301 children completed parts of the tests, only 272 completed the pre-test and both post-tests. Data was removed from the analysis if the child failed to answer more than 3 questions.

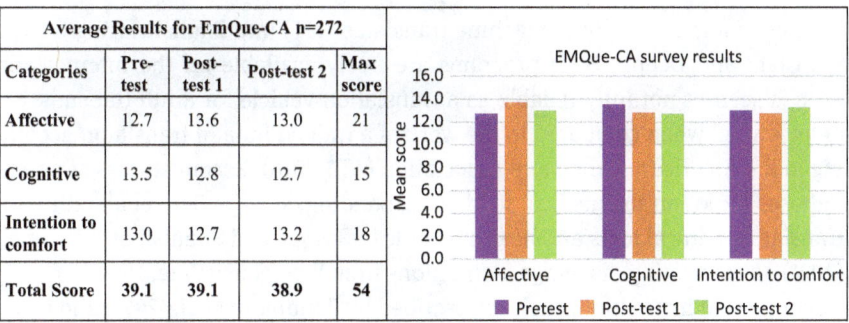

Average Results for EmQue-CA n=272				
Categories	Pre-test	Post-test 1	Post-test 2	Max score
Affective	12.7	13.6	13.0	21
Cognitive	13.5	12.8	12.7	15
Intention to comfort	13.0	12.7	13.2	18
Total Score	39.1	39.1	38.9	54

Figure 2: Average results for EmQue-CA surveys from 273 children.

Figure 2 tells a similar story to Figure 1. The children's scores for affective empathy on the EmQue-CA rose minutely after the Power Point presentation, while the children's cognitive knowledge and the intention to comfort dropped fractionally. By the time of the second post-test, their affective empathy was still slightly above the initial level and their intention to comfort had risen so it also was slightly above the initial levels. Their cognitive understanding showed a further minute decrease. However, as with the results from the KIDS, both the gains and the subsequent losses are too small to be meaningful. We assume that since the original surveys are designed to be administered to children, the cognitive abilities of children in Taiwan would not be below those of the children from Europe, North and South America, Africa, Asia and Australia on whom the survey was validated (Overgaauw et al. 2017: 4). Such details should be included in proposed analysis (by Kuo) of the children's interviews. Since the English-speaking authors have not worked directly with Taiwanese grade-schoolers, they chose instead to work exclusively with interviews of adults, and to report only the outcome of the adult surveys.

4 Findings: The use of automatic machine translation (MT)

In choosing to work with the adult interviews as automatically translated, we knew we would be missing some of the Taiwanese sociocultural and sociopragmatic interpersonal context that could surface, for example, in the length of question-prompts or responses, the choices of one or another lexical item, or in their syntactically and culturally cued arrangement of topic elements within utterances.

Because the first and third authors are not competent in Chinese, our analysis can only go so far, as we can only read and post-edit these interviews that have been automatically or machine translated (MT) into English, using Google Translate and DeepL. Both programs are freely available on the Internet and each is seen as not fully reliable as a translation vehicle for a full transmission of 'meaning' when compared to the work of a trained human translator, according to the American Translators Association (ATA 2018). Recent studies of potential uses for MT in the medical field are expanding, such as Soto et al. (2019) on translating clinical texts and health records in Basque and Spanish or Taira et al. (2021) on translating discharge instructions from Emergency Care. However, physician-patient interaction, such as described by Randhawa et al. (2013) and Davis et al. (2019) on discharge instructions is seen as needing supplemental work from professional human translators.

In tracing the relevant history of the development of such translation programs, particularly to keep up with rapid developments in science and technology since the early 1930s, Hutchins (2010) comments that by the time of the first MT conference held at MIT in 1952, scientists assumed that "full automation of good quality translation was a virtual impossibility, and that human intervention either before or after computer processes (known from the beginning as pre- and post-editing respectively) would be essential; some hoped this would be only an interim measure, but most expected that it would always be needed" (Hutchins 2010: 2).

Research in cognitive linguistics, artificial intelligence and especially the development of very large corpora in multiple languages has reinvigorated the field: of current interest is the appropriation for human translators of tools such as Interactive Neural Machine Translation which is a way "to incrementally feed output to translators from neural networks trained on parallel corpora. . . . The translator generates the translation, starts writing, and the NMT system suggests the next fragment" (ATA 2019: 6; see, for example https://microsoft.github.io/inmt/). To oversimplify, both this technique and MT plus post-editing work well within most of the Western Indo-European languages, such as English-Spanish/Spanish-English (see Cabrera 2017), but as both Turner at al. (2019) and Jia, Carl and Wang explain, English-Chinese pose "great challenges" (2019: 10). And there is more than one way to handle machine translation: Forcada et al. (2018: 192) explain "Machine translation (MT) applications fall in two main groups: assimilation or **gisting**, and dissemination. Assimilation refers to the use of the raw MT output to make sense of foreign texts. Dissemination refers to the use of the MT output as a draft translation that can be post-edited into a publishable translation." (**Emphasis** ours.)

Using House's revised model (House 2015: 65) for comparing a translation with the original text, we can, in our post-edited machine translations, identify the genre (oral interviews), and the field (the elementary education curriculum) and some degree of social interaction. However, we can only infer tenor, or participant relationship, author's provenance and stance, social role relationship, or social attitude. Mode is even more complicated in that we may know the medium to be oral exchange primarily in Mandarin, but we cannot be assured of our analysis of participation. Studies report that in Chinese workplace discourse (Wang 2019: 341) "small talk" is expected as part of developing rapport and establishing positioning in social interactions. And as we demonstrate below, it is used to varying degrees with persons having different relationships to their school and to the interviewer. However, we do not have access by ear or eye to knowing if there are specific Chinese terms of address that were used to signal the interviewer's social equality or superiority of status vis à vis the interviewee, which honorifics might have been used to suggest status of the recipient or which instances of local variation might have signalled something about their relationship.

We were primarily conscious that, in this initial analysis, we needed to be content to work with the gist of what was said, as obtained through machine translation, since we did not know Mandarin well enough to pre-edit the interviews for translation. To illustrate the complexities inherent in any automatic machine translation, we show in Figure 3 the first section of an interview with a teacher, translated automatically by DeepL, and by Google. In order to arrive at the final version we analyzed, we used a two-step process: first we harmonized the DeepL and Google versions and then smoothed the result so that we arrived at the final 'lightly post-edited' version (Shih 2018: 512) which we used for our own gisting. Translation researchers and teachers offer many suggestions on how best to handle post-editing when pre-editing is not possible (see, for example, Koponen et al. 2021). In our own post-editing we followed several of the rules listed in Shih (2018: 512–513). In particular we used the following:

- Use of upper case for the first letter of proper nouns or specialized terms
- Correction of grammatical disagreements (e.g., singular/plurals) and semantic errors
- Change in the word sequence; for example, moving a prepositional phrase from the post-noun position to the pre-noun position
- Restoration of omitted articles
- Use of active voice
- Addition of some words for fluency
- Alteration of incorrect punctuation

We underline some of the main differences between the machine translated versions and our final version in Figure 3. We emphasize again, that it would have been impossible for the current analysis to have been carried out by the first and third authors without using post-edited gisted machine translation.

The well-known translator, Juliane House (2014: 1) explains two key features in what she sees as the multidisciplinary and intercultural act of translation

Voice 14 DeepL	Voice 14 Google Translate	Voice 14 'harmonized'/lightly post-edited
Researcher: I am Guo Jingyi. Thank you for accepting this interview. Can you tell us a little bit about yourself, including your teaching experience, your teaching field, and for you, why you are always on the teaching field? **Interviewee:** hi, my name is Kang Chui-hua, and I have been serving the children for 28 years. <u>The reason why I do not want to retire</u> is because this job is very attractive to me, because I can still see the smiles of many <u>lovely</u> children every day, and the "good morning' every day is also a great help. That's why I feel that I don't want to leave <u>the field of education.</u> And I also work as a counselor, and I get a great sense of achievement from my counselling work. For me, teaching is not a good job, but it's a beautiful thing. For example, when I counselled a child, I could tell from the bottom of my heart that the child had grown or changed.	**Teacher:** Hello, teacher. This is Guo Jingyi. Thank you for accepting our interview. Could you please introduce yourself to the teacher, including your teaching experience and teaching site. For you, why have you always supported the teaching site? **Interviewee:** Hello, my name is Kang <u>Cuihua</u>. I have been serving for 28 years, and the reason I have been reluctant to quit is because this ministry is very attractive to me, because I can still see the smiles of many cute children every day. Then, <u>"Teacher is morning"</u> every day, which is actually a great help. That's why I felt that I would not want to leave the <u>current education scene.</u> Then, <u>I also take part in the counseling work</u>, and the sense of accomplishment I get from the counseling work is quite big. <u>So for me, actually speaking of poor teaching work has its beauty</u>. Like the last time I counseled a child, I can feel from my heart that the child has grown or changed, not that the salary you can compare.	**Teacher:** Hello, teacher. This is Kuo Ching Yi. Thank you for accepting our interview. Can you please tell us a bit about yourself, including your teaching experience and teaching field. For you, why have you always been in the teaching field? **Interviewee:** Hello, my name is Kang Chui-hua. I have been serving the children for 28 years. And the reason I don't want to retire is because this job is very attractive to me, because I can see the smiles of many lovely children every day. Then, "Good morning, Teacher" every day, is also a great help. That's why I feel that I don't want to leave the field of education. Also, I work as a counselor, and I get a great sense of achievement from my counseling work. So for me, teaching isn't just a good job, it's a beautiful thing. Like the last time I counseled a child, I could feel from the bottom of my heart that the child had grown or changed. You can't just compare the salary.

Figure 3: The first section of an interview with a teacher, translated automatically by DeepL, and by Google, and the lightly post-edited version which used for gisting in this chapter. Underlining indicates some of the main differences between the versions.

My feeling like this. Will I still be doing this job? I don't dare to guarantee that I will be able to continue, because we have a mother who is mentally retarded, and she may take up a lot of my thoughts. Before that, I applied for day care, but I felt that the government was not cool enough to set up day care. The government doesn't seem to be aware of this, so when I tried to help my mom apply for daycare, I was told no matter how many places I tried, they all turned me down because they were full. For an elderly person who has just lost his or her mind, if day care is available, he or she can go back to the family of origin at night and interact with the family, which may alleviate his or her dementia.	My feeling is this. Will I continue to hold this job? I don't dare to vouch for it, because there is a demented mother in our family, and I can share a lot of my thoughts there. Fortunately, there are nursing centers that can be entrusted, but I still think it's not enough. I hope my mother lives in Beside me. Before that, I applied for day care, and I think the government still has too few cool points on day care. My mother lives in Yancheng District, Kaohsiung City. There are mostly elderly people in Yancheng District. The government doesn't seem to see this. When I want to help my mother apply for daycare, I have refused as many as I encountered. Because it's full. For an elderly person who has just demented, if he can go to day care, return to his native family at night, and possibly interact with his family, his dementia may slow down	My concern is this. Will I continue to hold this job? I don't dare guarantee it, because we have a mother with dementia, and she takes up a lot of my time. Fortunately, there are nursing centers that can be trusted, but I still think it's not enough. I hope my mother lives in, beside me. Before that, I applied for day care, but I felt the government wasn't aware enough to set up day care. My mother lives in Yancheng District, Kaohsiung City. There are mostly elderly people in Yancheng District. The government doesn't seem to be aware of this. When I tried to help my mother apply for daycare, no matter how many places I tried, they all turned me down because they were full. For an elderly person who is getting dementia, if they can go to day care, and go back to their family at night, and possibly interact with the family, the dementia may slow down.

Figure 3 (continued)

"the source text with its linguistic-stylistic-aesthetic features that belong to the norms of usage holding in the source lingua-cultural community [and] the linguistic-stylistic-aesthetic norms of the target language." Her explanation makes an investigation of one or both sets of norms mandatory; such investigation frequently leads to further exploration via pragmatics. It is no surprise, then, to see the appearance of a recent Routledge handbook in its series on Translating and Interpreting: Tipton and Desilla's 2019 collection of 22 chapters for *The Routledge Handbook of Translation and Pragmatics*. The Introduction identifies several "features of linguistic pragmatics and their treatment in intercultural and interlingual communication" (p. 1), including the emphasis from Verschueren (2017) on the significant differences in language use between Western and "non-Western" cultures and societies (p. 2). In a subsequent chapter, corpus linguist Bernd Meyer reminds us that the qualitative approaches are more frequent in pragmatic studies which "deal with language use in different social contexts and the ways in which language is shaped by, and used to shape, the organisation of social life" (p. 76). We find this description congruent with that of Locher (2013: 176) as she explains relational work in interpersonal pragmatics, a perspective which helps to interpret the interpersonal relationships in the interviews with the Taiwanese adults connected to the schools: relationships are "dynamic constructs that emerge through interaction in situated contexts, relative to situated norms."

Each of the interviews is between the second author and a member of the school administration, or a teacher or nurse, or with volunteer classroom mothers. She must develop a relationship of some kind with each of these previously unknown people as she goes along in order to establish enough trust and reciprocity to request and record something of their opinions. In that sense, these interviews, collected in Mandarin, take on a ritual aspect framed by the interviewer's self-introductions (see Kádár and House 2020: 143: "'Ritual frame' refers to a cluster of standard situations in which rights and obligations prevail, and one is expected to follow these rights and obligations to maintain one's sacred face (Goffman 1967)").

These are face-to-face interviews with conversational tone, usually between two persons. The adults interviewed fell into three groups: people whose social status as administrators would be seen as higher than the interviewer (principals and directors), classroom teachers and school nurses whose status could be considered equal to the interviewer since she was also a teacher; and classroom mothers who could see themselves as of lower social status than the interviewer. The social relationships were indicated by the length of the leadups to the various questions. The second author typically used lengthy leadups with the principals and directors, slightly shorter leadups to nurses and teachers and brief leadups to classroom mothers. The interviews incorporated questions soliciting opinions about educational and cultural approaches to the elementary school curriculum and whether it would be appropriate to introduce dementia education into this curriculum.

The length of the introductory leadup allows the interviewer to announce the forthcoming questions concerning dementia education in a way that validates the interviewer's right to request information in this local situation, often by affiliation with the shared field of education, and offer some praise to the interviewee. The interviewer asked the interviewees to introduce themselves and this allowed her to build on the interviewees' own words in the introductions to the questions. The leadups have several functions. They are a low-key compliment to the worth of the interviewee, which suggests the interviewer has paid full attention to the interviewee, thereby underscoring her worth as an interviewer. They also establish the interviewer's expectation of a commitment from the interviewee to provide some answers in response. Figure 4 shows the way the interviewer approached one of the directors. Bold text indicates how the interviewer used the Director's own words in her introductions to the questions.

I: Director X, thank you for accepting our interview. Before answering these three interview questions, can I first ask you, Director, to introduce some of your own educational experience and how long you have been teaching?

[Biographical overview from Director]

I: Director, **you just mentioned that you have been teaching for 29 years**. You have been in the education scene for so long and **I admire your teaching experience very much.** You said that you entered this job after graduating from university 29 years ago, and so **what are your observations on the changes in the whole society and changes in education**?

[Discussion by Director on social change and parental expectations of education]

I: [after *5 uninterrupted utterances repeating and elaborating* on the Director's discussion of parents]. **What do you think parents would think** about their children coming to receive education on issues related to the elderly, or education about dementia?

Figure 4: Introduction to the first question, from Interview 25. I: is the interviewer.

5 Discussion: Inferences from responses to the gists of the questions in the adult interviews

5.1 Question 1

Question 1 asked if the respondent approved of teaching about dementia in elementary schools. Twenty-six of the 29 adult respondents said yes; three had some reservations or concerns, and no-one disapproved. People with different school-related roles presented slightly different reasons for endorsing the idea or suggestions for its implementation. The twelve volunteer classroom mothers and grandmothers tended to present personal reminiscences about dementia in the family or neighborhood and to encourage school-sponsored interaction with grandparents. They were also concerned with children's family experiences which could affect potential readiness for the information. In the extracts, three dots indicate that material (typically, affirmations and repetitions of key words by the interviewer) has been omitted and a dash indicates a pause (often as interviewees reformulates their responses). As Classroom Mother 75 put it,

(1) *I would suggest a gradual approach, because I feel that children nowadays are relatively unfamiliar with the environment of three generations and four generations living under one roof, because we are all now in small family systems.*

School nurses focused on the hows and the whys for dementia education in the schools: Nurse 21 felt "they will be less likely to fear it" and Nurse 35 said it would be needed because of the increase in older people. Nurses 36 and 52 felt that the content of the presentation should be adjusted to the age of the students. As Nurse 52 said,

(2) *The first grade may be too young, they will be more confused about the situation. Middle grades can be slow, that is, your content should be simple and easy to understand.*

Not surprisingly, the five school administrators (principals and directors) focused on how best to insert additional teaching materials into an already busy curriculum. Four of them were solidly committed to the idea, and one had reservations. Administrator 18 talked about how technology and popular media could help:

(3) *I think it's quite good to do some supplementary work, or even provide some cartoons or online animated learning. That's a good approach. . . . I want to include it in the formal curriculum, but kids only have 8 hours in school and it's getting shorter and shorter.*

Administrator 11 offered several ideas for how dementia education at the elementary level might be implemented and explained why s/he thought dementia education was needed. In addition to embedding dementia education within the curriculum for family education, Administrator 11 wanted the curriculum adapted to grade levels and if possible, for it to involve experiential learning.

(4) *I think that in the future, similar courses can also be done online in flexible courses. Another thing is that I think it's positive for the students to receive such a message and to understand the related knowledge. Because they can observe and pay attention to the people around them who have similar symptoms or are at risk of developing them, and then can provide them with accurate information so that they can go to the doctor early. . . . I think this course will more or less help students learn how to interact with their elders. . . . I think this part of dementia can also be integrated into the topic of our family education, because family education is also very important for students.*

5.2 Question 2

Looking at interpersonal relationships within Taiwanese society, even within the confines of gisted translation, explains some issues with asking and answering the second author's Question 2: "How do you think parents will react to this information? Will they be OK with children learning about dementia?" Asking such a direct question in Mandarin could be pragmatically risky in terms of (im) politeness (see Matsumoto 1988 for a description of the pragmatics of similar situations in Japan). However, from an emerging third wave perspective, work in the area of pragmatics has been overly based on the work of Brown and Levinson (1987) who come from what is seen as an exclusively Western, individualistic and Anglo-centric perspective. Jia and Yang (2021: 1) explain that recent work in pragmatics "emancipates" Chinese research "and instead, constructs theories of (im) politeness based on Chinese socio-cultural values." Hints of those values surface in responses to Question 2. As a certified elementary teacher, Kuo could establish social relationships similar to those of an extended family with the principals, the directors, the nurses and the teachers. In their interviews, she can ask them a direct question and she can expect a direct answer without harming the temporary social relationships that they have established. And that is what happens. Two principals and a grandfather now serving as a volunteer crossing guard identify scenarios for problems with obtaining full parental assent, and only one interviewee, a volunteer classroom mother, does not answer the question in any way. Out of the 29 interviewees, 28 responded: in general, they thought parents could be persuaded to accept dementia education despite potential complications.

It is not surprising to obtain direct responses in the gisted translations from the principals and directors. Their business is to know what parents might think about changes to the curriculum and how best to adjust education about dementia to specific age groups and into which area of the curriculum dementia education might best fit. Given that Kuo had done graduate work, they could be direct and professional in their analyses. As Principal 18 commented,

(5) *I believe that most parents are positive, but there are – some parents are more likely to say that this will – will bring them bad luck, there will be quite a few with this, this kind of logic.*

Three of the four nurses had teaching experience, so they are also knowledgeable about the curriculum and probable parent opinions, as are the teachers. This is not the case with the interviews with the volunteer classroom mothers. Kuo is not a mother so she cannot claim that to use in building a social relationship. The topic is difficult to handle with the classroom volunteer mothers: they cannot be expected to know what parents at the school might think and will be reluctant to speak for parents other than in their own families. They may not wish to explain that they are not interested in or knowledgeable about dementia, knowing she has just given a presentation on it in 'their' school. Accordingly, her interview must be more conversational and must be more indirect so that she can establish a more intimate social relationship so that everyone can enjoy good interpersonal interaction. The mothers who are foreign brides are more direct and more straightforward in offering critical comments about the school and about Taiwanese education.

For example, Volunteer Father 63 said

(6) *I always told the teacher that you have to cooperate with the parents and communicate – parents and teachers have to cooperate with each other.*

And Volunteer Classroom Mother 75 who was a foreign bride said

(7) *The first response could be that it is too early, because it will be too difficult for the child . . . I think this is necessary.*

Re-evaluations of Brown and Levinson's model of politeness (1987), especially by European and Chinese researchers in pragmatics "have resulted in significant paradigm shifts towards relation-based theories of pragmatics and social interaction over the last two decades" (Ye 2019: 1; cf Kádár 2019; Kádár and Haugh 2013; Hanks, Ide and Katagiri 2009) in order to look at the 'society of intimates' in Chinese social interaction, and the establishment of interdependence in Japanese interaction (Matsumoto 1988). The interpersonal interactions concerning Question 2 underscore the importance of looking at features of interpersonal work – a shift in cultural pragmatics – even when such features may be blurred by translation technology. For example, four of the classroom mothers are international brides who offer stronger views about filial piety than the other classroom mothers. They are asked about these views and about teaching children in what appears to be a slightly different way from interactions with the Taiwanese mothers. That is, the temporary relationship between the interviewer and these women is defined primarily by their not being Taiwanese, and the interpersonal relationship is established differently as the interviewer in her leadup offers nothing to hold in common with the interviewee.

The leadup consists of a couple of sentences such as this with volunteer Classroom Mother 33:

(8) *I: The main purpose of this interview is to understand, that is, if we tell you from the standpoint of an educator today, we want to teach children about things related to the elderly, such as dementia. What is your opinion?*

Once the foreign mother reveals how long she has been in Taiwan, and volunteers their home country's name, the interviewer may expand the purpose with a little small talk.

(9) *I: Then you say you are from Vietnam, then I want to know what you would think if your friend in Taiwan said that she heard the teacher tell her that they want to teach your children something related to your elders, specifically dementia which is a disease of the brain. Would you want your children to receive such an education? (Classroom Mother 32).*

There does not seem to be the same degree of concern for the social status of the interviewee as signaled by the length of the leadup to the questioning, and the questioning itself is keyed to the interviewee's otherness and possible lack of understanding of Taiwanese elementary curriculum. The foreign brides may not be expected to establish a temporary intimacy in their interaction. These abbreviated leadups could be viewed from a Western perspective as being less polite than the longer leadups to the Taiwanese classroom mothers. However, following the lead of current third wave pragmatics researchers on relationships and interpersonal interaction in Chinese, such as Gu (1990; cf. Kádár 2018) we would be reluctant to claim that one or another feature we discuss here is a solid example of (im)politeness in workplace discourse focused on the possibility of children learning about dementia in schools.

5.3 Question 3 – and its link to a larger and political issue

Question 3 asked "How do we now prepare children for entering a super-aged society?" To understand the content of the responses, we must turn to studies in gerontology and economics. Interpersonal interaction clearly differed between school personnel and volunteer mothers. Principals, directors, and nurses responded to this topic with an orientation to how they could make students – and parents – aware of the topic through the curriculum and try to "improve" the situation. For example, Principal 11 focused on the need for experiential learning:

(10) *if you have the opportunity, take them to a nearby nursing home to interact with these elderly people. I think this kind of experiential learning will impress them.*

and Principal 19 recommended intergenerational education:

(11) *An ideal school of the future, because of the declining birthrate and the transformation of schools, I think young and old should learn this matter together. . . . the more seniors you have, the less children you have – the fewer children so grandpa and grandma bring their children to class, while the dad and mom go to work, right, then children go to the elementary school, and then that grandpa and grandma go to the senior center.*

Nurses were even more straightforward in emphasizing needs for self-reliance. From Nurse 21:

(12) *Taiwan is now an elderly society, and it will be a great burden for young people to take care of the elderly in the future . . . . I think the people's future now is probably fewer children, and then more elderly and so from now on, the young can't rely on future care by their children. I think the basic point is you have to be able to support yourselves.*

Nurse 52 shared her emotion:

(13) *when we are old, we really have to rely on ourselves. . . . I'm very scared. I don't dare to expect them [to look after me when I am old]. I can only rely on myself. When I see them like that, I don't dare to expect them. I often cry and cry.*

However, the clearest differentiation between the kinds of interpersonal interactions with the interviewer was between school staff and mothers, in their choice of whether to respond to comments about the 2000-year-old emphasis on filial piety. Kuo introduced this construct from a "we both believe in this" stance, as in: "*because we are still in the Asian traditional Confucian filial piety culture.*" She reinforced the topic from this perspective more than once in all but two of the interviews. One administrator did not reply to any comments about filial piety; the other four objected in various ways to its use as a framework for teaching about aging or dementia, thinking dementia education would be best accepted in the framework for family education.

Half of the school nurses, such as Nurse 21, commented that "I think this concept is gradually changing;" the others were "I am 100% dedicated to that" (Nurse 35). Like nurses, teachers were split in their opinions: Teacher 15 was direct and introduced a more political issue which is unusual in interpersonal interaction for a school interview:

(14) *even if it's not under the framework of the Confucian tradition of filial piety, and the final decision is to send them to care, then you must have sufficient financial security and you must be prepared. What's even more difficult is that there is no way to guarantee their safety . . . . Then you see that this issue [filial piety] involves gender equality. Why does the daughter-in-law have to resign and stay at home to take care of the person?*

The opposite opinion can be represented by Teacher 34 who said: "*I hope to really implement it in every child's life*" or Volunteer Classroom Mother 62 who said "*You are very afraid of letting your children know how much money you have. If your children are filial to you, then you are blessed.*"

6 Conclusion

In this chapter, we have started to explore dementia knowledge among elementary school children, focusing on a sample of children in Taiwan together with adults' attitudes towards explicit teaching about dementia within the school curriculum. Because of the projected increase in the number of people living with dementia, knowledge about the disease is becoming increasingly important for people throughout the world. When surveys are carried out, they usually focus on adults or adolescents, though Fuh, Liu and Jiang (2005) did include children as young as 10. The present study lowers the age to 8. The results show that a single Power Point presentation about dementia was not sufficient to make lasting changes to children's attitudes towards people with dementia as measured by the EmQue-CA survey or their knowledge about dementia as measured by the KIDS survey. The adults interviewed included school directors, principals, teachers and nurses as well as parents and grandparents. Most supported the inclusion of education about dementia at school though some were concerned about how it would fit into the already crowded curriculum. No one opposed the idea. Again, all but one of the interviewees thought parents would find such material acceptable. A final question asked how children could be prepared for living in Taiwan's super-aged society. This received mixed responses. Most of the adults thought that parents could no longer rely on traditional Confucian values of filial piety to ensure that they were later cared for by their children. This point was made particularly strongly by the foreign brides who were born in Vietnam and came to Taiwan later in life. They considered that Vietnam's culture adhered much more to traditional values than did Taiwan's. They attributed the difference to the economic differences between the two societies. Several of the adults interviewed emphasized the importance of people needing to be able to look after themselves as they aged.

In order to carry out the analysis of the interviews which were in Taiwanese Mandarin Chinese, the first and third authors (who do not speak or read Mandarin) relied on automatic Machine Translations of the interviews. We used two different translation softwares, DeepL and Google Translate, and post-edited the resulting outputs. In effect, the resulting translations provided the gists of the interviews. This process meant that some of the details (such as specific word choice or use of honorifics: see Gu 1990) was not available for analysis from an interpersonal pragmatics perspective. This analysis has, however, demonstrated that, despite their limitations, such translations, particularly when pre- or post-edited, allow worthwhile analyses of interpersonal and sociocultural issues.

Providing care for the aged, and more specifically for those with dementia, is by no means a simple issue anywhere, and answers dare not be simplistic. This exploratory study has attempted to illustrate a part of the complexity of aging care in what is rapidly becoming the country with the largest aged population. As with the educational presentation, the issues will need to be presented multiple times and adjusted to multiple populations.

References

Assaf, Raymen Rammy, Jennifer Auf der Springe, Connie Siskowski, David A. Ludwig, M. Sunil Mathew & Julia Belkowitz. 2016. Participation rates and perceptions of caregiving youth providing home health care. *Journal of Community Health* 41(2). 326–333. doi: 10.1007/s10900-015-0100-7.

ATA (American Translators Association) 2018. Position paper. Machine translation: A clear approach to a complex topic. *Advocacy & Outreach* (https://www.atanet.org/category/advocacy-outreach/) 2018. 1–10. (accessed 28 August, 2021.)

ATA (American Translators Association) 2019. Using Neural Machine Translation Beyond Post-Editing. *ATA Chronicle, Tools and Technology* (https://www.atanet.org/author/ata-chronicle/). https://www.ata-chronicle.online/highlights/using-neural-machine-translation-beyond-post-editing/ (accessed 30 August, 2021.)

Baker, Jess R., Lee-Fay Low, Belinda Goodenough, Yun-Hee Jeon, Ruby S.M. Tsang, Christine Bryden & Karen Hutchinson. 2018a. *The Kids Insight Into Dementia Survey (KIDS)*: Development and preliminary psychometric properties. *Aging and Mental Health* 22(8). 953–959. doi: https://doi.org/10.1080/13607863.2017.1320703

Baker, Jess R., Belinda Goodenough, Yun-Hee Jeon, Christine Bryden, Karen Hutchinson & Lee-Fay Low. 2018b. The Kids4Dementia education program is effective in improving children's attitudes towards dementia. *Dementia* 18(3). 1777–1789. https://doi.org/10.1177/1471301217731385

Braun, Virginia & Victoria Clarke. 2006. Using thematic analysis in psychology. *Qualitative Research in Psychology* 3(2). 77–101. DOI: 10.1191/1478088706qp063oa

Brown, Penelope & Stephen C. Levinson. 1987. *Politeness: Some universals in language usage*. Cambridge: Cambridge University Press.

Cabrera, Tamara. 2017. The translation and interpreting industry in the United States. *Informes del Observatorio / Observatorio Reports*. 028–02/2017EN ISSN: 2373–874X (online) DOI: 10.15427/OR028-02/2017EN (accessed 28 August, 2021.)

Chen Cheng-Fen & Tsung-hsi Fu. 2020. Policies and transformation of long-term care system in Taiwan. *Annals of Geriatric Medicine and Research* 24(3).187–194. doi: 10.4235/agmr.20.0038

Croes, Li-Ann. 2019. La traducción automática: Una comparación entre las traducciones de Google Translate y DeepL del español al holandés. Universidad de Utrecht: Trabajo Fin de Máster.

Davis, Seethalakshmi H., Julia Rosenberg, Jenny Nguyen, Manuel Jimenez, K. Casey Lion, Gabriela Jenicik, Harry Dallmann & Katherine Yun. 2019. Translating discharge instructions for Limited English-Proficient families: strategies and barriers. *Hospital Pediatrics* 9(10). 779–787. doi: 10.1542/hpeds.2019-0055

Davis, Boyd & Mary Smith. 2013. Cultural challenges in supervision and training in dementia care for direct care workers. *J Continuing Education for Nurses* 44(1). 22–30. doi: 10.3928/00220124-20121101-54.

Dong, XinQi & Manrui Zhang. 2016. The association between filial piety and perceived stress among Chinese older adults in Greater Chicago area. *Journal of Geriatrics and Palliative Care* 4(1). DOI: 10.13188/2373-1133.1000015

Fahey, Michael 2020, June 16. Taiwan's plan to attract foreign talent. *News Lens* [thenewslens.com], Opinion. (accessed 28 August, 2021.)

Farina, Nicolas, Laura J. Hughes, Ellen Jones, Sahdia Parveen, Alys W. Griffith, Kathleen Galvin & Sube Banerjee. 2020. The effect of a dementia awareness class on changing dementia attitudes in adolescents. *BMC Geriatrics* 20(1). 188. https://doi.org/10.1186/s12877-020-01589-6

Farrell, Michael P. & Chin-Chun Yi. 2019. Sociological perspectives on contemporary Taiwanese families. *Journal of Family Issues* 40(14). 1887–1895. https://doi.org/10.1177/0192513X19863195

Ferry, Timothy. 2018. Taiwan Has 250,000 Foreign 'Angels of Mercy' Caring for Its Elderly. Taiwan Business Topics. https://topics.amcham.com.tw/2018/10/foreign-caregivers-fill-the-gap/ (accessed 28 August, 2021.)

Forcada, Mikel L., Carolina Scarton, Lucia Specia, Barry Haddow & Alexandra Birch. 2018. Exploring gap filling as a cheaper alternative to reading comprehension questionnaires when evaluating machine translation for gisting. arXiv preprint arXiv:1809.00315

Fuh J. L., E. L. Teng, K. N. Lin, E. B. Larson, S. J. Wang, C. Y. Liu, P. Chou B. I. Kuo & H. C. Liu. 1995. The Informant Questionnaire on Cognitive Decline in the Elderly (IQCODE) as a screening tool for dementia for a predominantly illiterate Chinese population. *Neurology* 45(1). 92–96. doi: 10.1212/wnl.45.1.92.

Fuh, J. L., S. J. Wang, H. C. Liu, C. Y. Liu & H. C. Wang. 1999. Predictors of depression among Chinese family caregivers of Alzheimer patients. *Alzheimer disease and associated disorders* 13(3). 171–17. doi: 10.1097/00002093-199907000-00010.

Fuh, J. L., C. Y. Liu, M.S. Mega, S. J. Wang & J. L. Cumming. 2001. Behavioral disorders and caregivers' reaction Taiwanese patients with Alzheimer's disease. *International Psychogeriatrics* 13(1). 121–128. doi: 10.1017/s1041610201007517.

Fuh, J. L., M. S. Mega, G. Binetti, S. J. Wang, E. Magni & J. L. Cummings J. 2002. A transcultural study of agitation in dementia. *Journal of Geriatric Psychiatry and Neurology* 15. 171–174. doi: 10.1177/089198870201500308.

Fuh, J. L., S. J. Wang & J. L. Cummings. 2005. Neuropsychiatric profiles in patients with Alzheimer's disease and vascular dementia. *Journal of Neurology, Neurosurgery & Psychiatry* 76(10). 1337–1341. doi: 10.1136/jnnp.2004.056408.

Fuh, J. L., S. J. Wang & K. Juang. 2005. Understanding of senile dementia by children and adolescents: Why grandma can't remember me? *Acta Neurologica Taiwanica* 14(3). 138–142.

Goffman, Erving 1967. *Interaction ritual: Essays in face-to-face behavior*. London: Routledge.

Gu, Yueguo. 1990. Politeness phenomena in modern Chinese. *Journal of Pragmatics* 14(2). 237–257.

Hall, Mel & Pat Sikes. 2017. "It would be easier if she'd died": Young people with parents with dementia articulating inadmissible stories. *Qualitative Health Research* 27(8). 1203–1214. doi: 10.1177/1049732317697079.

Hanks, William, Sachiko Ide & Yasuhiro Katagiri. 2009. Towards an emancipatory pragmatics. *Journal of Pragmatics* 41(1). 1–9. DOI:10.1016/j.pragma.2008.02.014

House, Juliane (ed.). 2014. *Translation: A multidisciplinary approach*. London: Palgrave Macmillan.

House, Juliane .2015. *Translation quality assessment past and present*. London: Routledge.

Hsueh, Cherng-Tay. 2014. Diversity among families in contemporary Taiwan: Old trunks or new twogs? In Dudley L. Poston, Wen S. Yang & Demetrea Farris (eds.). 2014. *The family and social change in Chinese societies*. Springer; The Springer Series on Demographic Methods and Population Analysis. DOI:10.1007/978-94-007-7445-2_12

Hutchins, W. John. 2010. Machine translation: A concise history. *Journal of Translation Studies* 13: 29–70.

Jia, Yanfang, Michael Carl & Xiangling Wang. 2019. How does the post-editing of neural machine translation compare with from-scratch translation? *The Journal of Specialized Translation* 31: 60–86.

Jia, Mian & Guoping Yang. 2021. Emancipating Chinese (im)politeness research: Looking back and looking forward. *Lingua* 251.10328. https://doi.org/10.1016/j.lingua.2020.103028

Kádár, Dániel & Michael Haugh. M 2013. *Understanding politeness*. Cambridge: Cambridge University Press.
Kádár, Dániel. 2018. Politeness and impoliteness in Chinese discourse. In Chris Shei (ed.), *The Routledge handbook of Chinese discourse analysis*. 203–215. London: Routledge.
Kádár, Dániel. 2019. Introduction: Advancing linguistic politeness theory by using Chinese data. *Acta Linguistica Academica* 66(2). 149–164. DOI: 10.1556/2062.2019.66.2.1
Kádár, Dániel & Juliane House. 2020. Ritual frames: A contrastive pragmatic approach. *Pragmatics* 30(1). 142–168. https://doi.org/10.1075/prag.19018.kad
Kiger M, Varpio L 2020. Thematic analysis of qualitative data: AMEE guide no. 13. *Medical Teacher* 42(8). 846–854. doi: 10.1080/0142159X.2020.1755030.
Koponen, Maarit, Brian Mossop, Isabelle S. Robert, Giovanna Scocchera, (eds.) 2021. *Translation revision and post-editing: Industry practices and cognitive processes*. London & New York: Routledge.
Lan, Pei Chia 2002. Subcontracting filial piety: Elder care in ethnic Chinese immigrant families in California. *Journal of Family Issues* 23(7). 812–835. https://doi.org/10.1177/019251302236596
Lan, Pei Chia 2006. *Global Cinderellas: Migrant domestics and newly rich employers in Taiwan*. Durham: Duke University Press.
Lin, Ju-Ping & Chin-Chun Yi. 2019. Dilemmas of an aging society: Family and state responsibilities for intergenerational care in Taiwan. *Journal of Family Issues* 40(14). 1912–1936. https://doi.org/10.1177/0192513X19863204
Liu, H. C., K. N. Lin, E. L. Teng, S. J. Wang, J. L. Fuh, N. W. Guo, P. Chou, H. H. Hu & B. N. Chiang. 1995. Prevalence and subtypes of dementia in Taiwan: a community survey of 5297 individuals. *Journal of the American Geriatric Society* 43(2). 144–149. doi: 10.1111/j.1532-5415.1995.tb06379.x.
Locher, Miriam. 2013. Relational work and interpersonal pragmatics. *Journal of Pragmatics* 58. 145–149. http://doi.org/10.1016/j.pragma.2013.09.014
Matsumoto, Yoshiko. 1988. Reexamination of the universality of face: Politeness phenomena in Japanese. *Journal of Pragmatics* 12. 403–426. http://dx.doi.org/10.1016/0378-2166(88)90003-3
Ministry of Health and Welfare, Taiwan. 2018. Dementia prevention and care policy and action plan 2.0; 2018–2025 https://www.mohw.gov.tw/dl-51182-b894344f-f241-4f7b-adc2-e3a6644d9fb1.html, accessed 10 April, 2022.
Munkejord, Mal Camilla, Tove M. Ness & I-An W. S. Gao. 2021. "This life is normal for me": A study of everyday life experiences and coping strategies of live-in carers in Taiwan. *Journal of Gerontological Social Work*, 64 (5) https://doi.org/10.1080/01634372.2021.1917032
Overgauuw, Sandy, Carolien Rieffe, Evelien Broekhof, Eveline A. Crone & Berna Güroğlu. 2017. Assessing empathy across childhood and adolescence: validation of the *Empathy Questionnaire for Children and Adolescents (EmQue-CA)*. *Frontiers in Psychology* 8 Article 870. https://doi.org/10.3389/fpsyg.2017.00870
Meyer, Bernd. 2019. Corpus-based studies on interpreting and pragmatics. In Rebecca Tipton R & Louisa Desilla, (eds.) 2019. *The Routledge Handbook of Translation and Pragmatics*, 75–92. London: Routledge.
Payette, Alex & Yi-Chun Chien. 2020. Culture or context? Comparing recent trajectories of elder care development in China and Taiwan. *Asian Journal of Social Science* 48(3–4). 227–249.
Poston, Dudley L. & Li Zhang. L 2014. Taiwan's demographic destiny: Marriage market and aged dependency implications for the twenty-first century. In Dudley L. Poston, Wen Shan Yang &

D. Nicole Farris. 2014. *The family and social change in Chinese societies*, 265–280. Springer; The Springer Series on Demographic Methods and Population Analysis. https://doi.org/10.1007/978-94-007-7445-2_16

Randhawa, Gurdeeshpal, Mariella Ferreyra, Rukhsana Ahmen, Omar Ezzat & Kevin Pottie. 2013. Using machine translation in clinical practice. *Canadian Family Physician* 59(4). 382–3.

Shih, Chung-ling. 2016. Can machine translation declare a new realm of service? Online folktales as a case study. *Theory and Practice in Language Studies* 6(2). 252–259. DOI:10.17507/TPLS.0602.05

Shih, Chung-ling. 2018. Machine translation and its effective application. In Chris Shei & Zhao-Ming Gao. 2018. *The Routledge handbook of Chinese translation*, 506–521. London: Routledge.

Sikes, Pat & Mel Hall. 2018. "It was then that I thought 'whaat? This is not my Dad": The implications of the 'still the same person' narrative for children and young people who have dementia. *Dementia* 17(2). 180–198. doi: 10.1177/1471301216637204

Smith, Jonathan A. 1995. Semi structured interviewing and qualitative analysis. In: Jonathan A. Smith, Rom Harre & Luk Van Langenhove. (eds.) *Rethinking Methods in Psychology*. 9–26. Sage Publications.

Soto, Xabier, Olatz Perez-de-Viñaspre, Gorka Labaka & Maite Oronoz. 2019. Neural machine translation of clinical texts between long distance languages. *Journal of the American Medical Informatics Association* 26(12). 1478–1487. doi: 10.1093/jamia/ocz110

Taira Breena, Vanessa Kreger, Aristides Orue & Lisa C. Diamond. 2021. A pragmatic assessment of Google Translate for emergency department instructions. *Journal of General Internal Medicine*. doi: 10.1007/s11606-021-06666-z

Tipton Rebecca. 2019. Introduction. In Rebecca Tipton & Louisa Desilla, (eds.), *The Routledge Handbook of Translation and Pragmatics* 1–9. London: Routledge.

Tipton Rebecca & Louisa Desilla, (eds.) 2019. *The Routledge Handbook of Translation and Pragmatics*. London: Routledge.

Turner, Anne M., Yong K. Choi, Kristin Dew, Ming-Tse Tsai, Alyssa L. Bosold, Shuyang Wu, Donahue Smith & Hendrika Meischke. 2019. Evaluating the Usefulness of Translation Technologies for Emergency Response Communication: A Scenario-Based Study. *JMIR Public Health Surveillance*. 2019 Jan 28;5(1):e11171. doi: 10.2196/11171.

Verschueren, Jef. 2017. Continental European Perspective View, in Yan Huang, ed., *The Oxford Handbook of Pragmatics* 1–22. Oxford: Oxford University Press.

Wang, Frank. 2010. 'From undutiful daughter-in-law to cold-blood migrant household worker', in Kirsten Scheiwe and Johanna Krawietz, (eds.). *Transnationale Sorgearbeit: Rechtliche Rahmenbedingungen und gesellschaftliche Praxis*, 9–28. Weisbaden Germany: VS Verlag, Springer Fachmedien.

Wang, Vincent. 2019. Chinese workplace discourse: Politeness strategies and power dynamics. In Chris Shei, (ed). *The Routledge handbook of Chinese discourse analysis*, 339–351. London: Routledge.

Wang, Frank T. Y. & Chen-Fen Chen. 2017. The Taiwan Association for Family Caregivers: transformation in the long-term care debate for carers, *International Journal of Care and Caring* 1(1). 121–26. DOI:10.1332/239788217X14866308260586.

Wu, Shih-Cyuan, Mei-Chi Peng, Jui-Yuan Hsueh J, Tung-Liang Chiang, Yu-Kang Tu, Yu-Chi Tung & Ya-Mei Chen. 2021. Impact of a new home care payment mechanism on growth of the home care workforce in Taiwan. *The Gerontologist* 61(4). 505–516. doi: 10.1093/geront/gnab010.

Xu Y., G. Li, Y. Zhang. 2016. Filial piety beyond the nuclear family: a qualitative analysis. *The Gerontologist*, 56, (Suppl_3). 107. https://doi.org/10.1093/geront/gnw162.414

Yang, Mien-chieh. 2020, July 13. Immigrant Workers: Taipei launches training program for migrant caregivers *Taipei Times*. (accessed August 29, 2021.)

Ye, Zhengdao. 2019. The politeness bias and the society of strangers. *Language Sciences* 76: 101183. https://doi.org/10.1016/j.langsci.2018.06.009

Yeh, Ming-Jui. 2020. Political and cultural foundations of long-term care reform comment on "Financing Long-term Care: Lessons from Japan." *International Journal of Health and Policy Management* 9(2). 83–86. Doi: 10.15171/ijhpm.2019.90

Robert W. Schrauf
Chapter 4
Research translation as situated practice

1 Introduction

In this chapter, I take a reflective look at what health applied linguists *do* when they do translation. In short, I conceptualize *research translation* as a cumulative process over a series of data analytic situated practices, each with its own purposes and task-specific context, issuing in formal translated data displays and associated commentary for publication. In describing this process, I trace how constitutive moments of deep *intra*lingual engagement with the indexicalities of the source language and sustained *inter*lingual moments of translanguaging and acts of formal translation cumulatively shape up linguistically and culturally equivalent metapragmatic re-presentations of source language material in the target language.

The health applied linguists that I have in mind are the readers of this book: scholars and social scientists whose multilingual capacities are well-developed, who work professionally across more than one language and/or who work extensively in multilingual teams, and who publish their (translated) data in linguistics and/or health literature or in conference presentations, and so on. Further, I assume that the unique focus that the applied linguist brings to health topics – his or her multidisciplinary contribution – has to do with *language*, perhaps as itself the object of study (as for instance, in clinical linguistics), but more broadly, language as a form of social action related to health issues. Thus, his or her *professional vision* (Goodwin, 1994) derives from the conceptual frameworks and associated toolkits of our discipline (e.g., discourse analysis, conversation analysis, semiotics, sociolinguistics, systemic functional grammar, sociocultural theory, pragmatics).

Finally, I assume that, for health applied linguists, it is not only language per se that matters, but specific languag*es*, namely *source languages*, perhaps not as the medium of a unique worldview or alternate ontology (see the edited collection of Severi & Hanks 2015), but certainly as patterned and systematic, locally embed-

---

Acknowledgements: The preparation and writing of this chapter were completed under the auspices of the funded project "Resilience and Helpseeking in Health and Illness by and for the Elderly" (R21MD013701) of the National Institute on Minority Health and Health Disparities of the National Institutes of Health; Patria López de Victoria, Principal Investigator; Robert W. Schrauf, Co-Principal Investigator.

Robert W. Schrauf, Pennsylvania State University

ded, indexically rich, and resonantly familiar sets of communicative resources for social life and self-interpretation. I mention this latter because there is arguably a contrary pull in the culture of biomedicine toward, on the one hand, its own universality (independent of linguistic difference) because it is rooted in the universals of life science (but see Lock & Nguyen 2010), and, on the other hand, a view that a *good-enough* translation will more than suffice. Regarding this latter: it is probably the case that the majority of medical translations *are* in fact good enough (and thankfully routine), but health applied linguists don't set out to do good-enough translations. On the contrary, alive to how people put their *worlds into words* (Strauss & Feiz 2014), applied linguists seek to faithfully convey meanings from a source language text into a target language text while enlivening the contextual worlds of those source performances for target language readers. (Predictably, some of these worlds appear just as mundane in translation as they appear in the source language, but achieving that effect is good translation).

1.1 Organization of the chapter

The chapter is organized as follows (with major concepts in bold print). The first section is a discussion of **translation** itself, beginning with some key formulations from Jakobson ([1959] 2012) and the work of Silverstein on the role of **indexicality** in translation (2003b). In this section, I also adopt Hank's (2015) notion that the inherent reflexivity of language grounds translation proper, and I use that dynamic throughout the chapter to show how applied linguists engage in translation over the duration of their research projects. In the second section, I review the notion of **situated activity** to characterize the purpose-and-context driven features of research projects, activities, and tasks, and I zero in on the many successive **project worlds** that applied linguists construct as the macro-contexts of doing translation. The third section of the paper explores the linkages between translation and specific stages of research: **transcription, coding, analysis and re-transcription**, and the development of **translated data displays**. In the discussion section, I reflect on research translation as a key contribution by applied linguists to health-related social science.

2 Translation

2.1 Intralingual translation

Jakobson famously distinguished *intralingual* translation from *interlingual* translation ([1959] 2012). *Intra*lingual translation, on the one hand, is essentially the ubiquitous "rewording" (p. 127) constantly exercised by speakers within their own language and extends to a whole range of reflexive uses of language-about-language, as for example: definition, typification, paraphrasing, and represented speech (Agha 2007; Lucy 1993). On the other hand, *inter*lingual translation or translation proper is "an interpretation of verbal signs by means of some other language" (Jakobson [1959] 2012: 127), from one natural language to another natural language.

Both clinical medicine and social science research are saturated by *intra*lingual translation. In medicine, an extensive range of healthcare professionals – physician specialists, family physicians, registered nurses, LPNs, dentists, social workers, occupational therapists, and paramedics – are constantly involved in rewording, glossing, and paraphrasing a clinical argot "down" to patients and then back "up" the professional hierarchy (i.e., from the language of medicine to the language of the life-world and then back to the language of medicine).

There is a similar trajectory of intralingual translation in the world of qualitative social science research, starting from data collected from participants in lay language (recorded interviews and events, ethnographic notes, archival documents; ultimately, texts) and up into the professional terminology of qualitative analysis and research (e.g. coding, in vivo coding, annotating, memoing) spoken by PI's, Co-PI's, project managers, research assistants, Internal Review Board officials, conflict-of-interest officers, conference organizers, journal editors, manuscript reviewers, and sometimes back down to the public.

Hanks (2015) has argued that *inter*lingual translation (translation proper) depends on *intra*lingual translation (e.g., the form of linguistic reflexivity just reviewed) because the former is grounded in the resources available in the latter: "In order for a semiotic system to serve as a medium of translation, it must be functionally capable of self-interpretation through metalanguage. As a shorthand, we can say that cross-linguistic translation presupposes intralinguistic translation" (p. 22-23). This is exactly the dynamic that I wish to exploit in this chapter. That is, when a health applied linguist engages in a multilingual research project, he or she moves stepwise and recursively through the following stages of intense intralingual translation: conventionalized transcription from oral/aural to written/read formats → sustained translanguaging associated with coding and data analysis → highly concentrated spates of *intra*lingual re-transcription → careful and sometimes creative *inter*lingual translation proper.

2.2 Interlingual translation

What is translation proper? Jakobson ([1959] 2012) refers to it as a kind of *reported speech*: "the translator records and transmits a message received from another source. Thus, translation involves two equivalent messages in two different codes" (p. 233). Although he does not pursue the comparison in the 1959 chapter, Jakobson's analogy to reported speech has rather intriguing parallels. In their seminal paper on reported speech, Clark and Gerrig (1990) argued that quoting someone was a kind of *demonstration*, and that "demonstrations work by enabling others to experience what it is like to perceive the things depicted" (p. 765). Reported speech is thus a performance that invites the hearer to re-experience something of the original. Nevertheless, Clark and Gerrig note that such demonstrations are analogical representations and inherently (strategically) selective. Thus, reported speech is almost never a verbatim rendition; speakers rarely attempt a complete and comprehensive performance of the paralinguistic and non-linguistic aspects of the original performance. Rather, reported speech is speech performatively re-crafted to achieve a particular effect for a particular purpose in a particular context.

Hence to some extent, the translation ≈ reported speech analogy (Jakobson ([1959] 2012) limps: *unlike* speakers doing reported speech, translators must strain toward the highest fidelity possible in their crafting target productions. Nevertheless, *like* reported speech, translations are meant to be inserted in some new context: shaped for some new audience (who may be culturally naïve vis-a-vis the original context) precisely to achieve some specific purpose. Indeed, as we shall see in the case of research, a translated data segment often takes on a life of its own – a sort of second life – in a world of professional linguistics, clinical medicine, or public health. Given the view that translations are demonstrations – inherently performative in some sense – and that they share important links to their original contexts while taking on links to new contexts, we turn to the *how* of translation.

How do translators translate? Silverstein (2003b) describes three approaches (or perhaps better *processes*) which in practice are densely intertwined. These are: the *grammar-and-lexicon* approach; the *transductive* (indexical) approach, and the *transformation* approach.

2.2.1 Grammar-and-lexicon approach

This approach captures the prototypical sense of translation in which meanings from one natural language are re-worded into another natural language (where "re-wording" comes directly from Jakobson and is meant quite literally). That is, the translator considers words, phrases, and expressions in the language of the source text, attending assiduously to their grammatical categories and denotational meaning. In Silverstein's words: he or she seeks "at least one closest-possible lexical gloss in a target language modulo the grammatical-categorial system (including lexical-semantic categories with distributional correlates) of the two respective languages into which the words and expressions of the denotational text (source and target) are involved" (Silverstein 2003b: 77). That is, the researcher works with *object languages* – source and target natural languages – within an overarching framework of a scientific *metalanguage* (i.e., grammatical categories), that systematizes the selection of formal and functional equivalents (Hanks & Severi 2015). Again, however, at this *grammar-and-lexicon* level, the translator focuses on equivalence as achievable in putatively comparable, Saussurean lexico-grammatic systems (i.e., the source and target languages).

2.2.2 Transduction

In a second approach, *transduction* or indexical translation, the translator focuses on matching the indexical function and force of language-in-use, from text-in-co(n)text in the source language to text-in-co(n)text in the target language. Thus, by their specific selections of morphosyntactic and lexical forms in a source language, language-users invoke, make strategically relevant, or *index* nuanced cultural meanings and social distinctions for just this occasion of language-use (Silverstein 1976) – this conversation, this presentation, this pamphlet, this website – *and* simultaneously position themselves and others as legitimate (or practiced or novice or unlicensed) language-users and members of specific social strata (Silverstein 2003a, 2004). Silverstein refers to the process of translating these indexical invocations from source to target languages as *transduction*: "a process of reorganizing the source semiotic organization (here, in the original problem, denotationally meaningful words and expressions of a source language occurring in co(n)text) by target expressions-in-co(n)text of another language presented through perhaps semiotically diverse modalities differently organized" (2003b p. 83).

In contrast to the grammar-and-lexicon approach of translation, establishing these equivalencies of indexical evocation from source language contexts to target language contexts requires a different kind of expertise than knowledge of the formal, lexical-grammatical metalanguage that (in principle) maps onto both. Working with indexicality demands familiarity with, and (ideally) experience of different sociolinguistic, sociocultural contexts in which the spoken or written text is intricately embedded.

At the source level, these multiply layered contexts include: the situated conversation (or text) itself and the social, institutional, and cultural contexts made selectively and strategically relevant by the interlocutors (or authors) through their linguistic and discursive choices. At the level of the target language, contexts include the language channel of the data presentation (oral and printed) or publication (printed), the professional-institutional culture of the audience or readership (e.g., clinical medicine, public health, and allied health sciences).

The translator's criterion here is *pragmatic appropriacy*. The task is finding linguistic options in the target language that trigger the same contextual linkages, have the same social implications, and carry the same illocutionary force as in the source language – often at fine-grained and exceedingly subtle levels of linguistic detail. Not surprisingly, bilingual and (ideally) bicultural expertise become critically important at this level of translation.

2.2.3 Transformation

Finally, in certain exercises of translation, the re-rendering of lexico-grammatic elements and indexical function-and-force effectively exceed replication of the original text and constitute new meaning(s) in the target culture. We have then a third level of translation: *transformation*. As Silverstein notes: ". . . in transduction, operating in the realm of culture more frankly, there is always the possibility of **transformation** of the [en]textual[ized] source material contextualized in specific ways into configurations of cultural semiosis of a sort substantially or completely different from those that one started with" (2003b: 91). What might transformation into a different cultural semiosis look like? As an example, he offers the translation/transformation of Shakespeare's *Romeo and Juliet* into Bernsteins' *West Side Story*, but unfortunately this is an intralingual transformation.

In sum, in Silverstein's account, the practice of translation proper involves, and perhaps requires, two crucial linguistic operations-cum-criteria: (1) a search for similarly functioning, equivalently meaning-bearing, lexico-grammatic forms in a target language that match those of the source language, and (2) the specific selection those forms (sometimes paraphrases or circumlocutions) which successfully invoke equivalent cultural linkages and social implications as were invoked for original speakers or hearers of the source text.

Attending to indexical invocations in source language texts and seeking for equivalents in the target language (and recognizing that at times the indexical equivalents necessarily exceed the warrants of the source language) demonstrates that the linguistic encounter between source and target language at the very heart of translation is in fact a *cultural encounter*. Interestingly, for the applied linguist-researcher, the months-long alchemy through which this *linguacultural* transformation takes place is the *research project*.

3 Project worlds as the ground of translation

In a typical research career, applied linguists engage in numerous formal research projects, each with its own boundaries, structures, stages, and outcomes. Planful and forward-looking accounts of these projects are found in IRB applications, grant applications, sabbatical proposals, conference abstracts, and publications. Ideally, some selection of these become cumulatively linked into a coherent research program.

Research projects are rarely quick. They require months and sometimes years. Every stage requires troubleshooting, problem-solving, changes of direction, careful and comprehensive notes, curation of records, reading of and reflection on the research literature, conversation with colleagues, trial-and-error in analysis, on-the-fly articulations, and draft reports, summaries, and abstracts. The process is rife with recursivity: research questions are refined and re-articulated; analysis obligates different approaches to data preparation and subsequent re-analysis; conference abstracts suggest whole new research questions; reviewers want to see additional analyses, and so on. Every project involves hours of thought, imaginative energies, painstaking analysis, and days of writing.

All of this constitutes a lived and multi-layered *project world*. Data – those carefully collected and curated traces of life-as-lived by participants – form the foundation of this world. Data are the touchstone. They are the social world that is-what-it-is, though selectively pried from their surrounding context(s) to answer the questions put by the researcher. Whatever the content, the form is linguistic, discursive, and pragmatic.

Work in the project world – the researcher's crafts – involve subtle transformations of data. These transformations are successively refined, meta-pragmatic re-characterizations (the mundane transcription, coding, discursive/narrative/thematic analyses of methods textbooks) which researchers shape into articles, chapters, and books, themselves meta-pragmatic re-characterizations, for readers who live in other professional worlds with other professional interests. These various transformations are each of them unique crafts; each is a situated activity with its own genius or art. Translation is one such situated activity, though, as I will argue in the following paragraphs, good translations are grounded, on the one hand, on the concatenation of carefully practiced transcription, coding, and analysis, and on the other, in the cognitive, psychological, and professional immersion of the researcher in the project world.

When translation takes place varies. Depending on researchers' predilections, circumstances, resources, and goals, translation might take place all at once at the beginning of a project. Thus, some researchers collect audio- or audio-visual data, transcribe the data, and then immediately translate *all* data documents from the source language of participants into a research language (presumably the language of the research team). All project analysis then takes place with translated data. Other researchers engage in formal translation only at the end of the project, when preparing excerpts for publication. Both are real practices, but in the following I reflect on what I expect is the more common process: translation takes place at multiple times throughout a project. Translation is strategically interspersed throughout the project.

4 Translation through multilayered situated practices

A critical concept for framing concatenated research activities is that of *situated practice*. Tracing back to Garfinkel and Sacks' seminal paper (1970; see Lynch, 2019), situated practice refers to the fact that ordinary activities have their own orderliness to which participants orient, and through which participants both produce and interpret their own speech and actions. Key dimensions here are local purposes, fine-grained adaptation of actions-to-immediate tasks, and larger contexts as orienting frames. Thus, we might think of the research project as the macro-context; the standard stages of a project (e.g., design, data collection, analysis) as the meso-layer; and the component research activities within each stage as the micro-layer, with each micro-activity having its own, internally sequenced organization. In effect, situated practices are nested in larger situated practices.

4.1 Transcription

Mondada (2007) strikes precisely these notes in her extended analysis of transcription as a situated practice: "Practices are irremediably indexical (Garfinkel and Sacks, 1970), reflexively tied to the context of their production and to the practical purposes of their accomplishment. Thus, a transcript is an evolving flexible object: it changes as the transcriber engages in listening and looking again at the tape, endlessly checking, revising, reformatting it" (p. 810). She lists the ordered activities surrounding transcription: "data production, digitalization and compression, anonymization, storage and filing, representation and annotation, analysis and so on" (p. 810).

Her reflections draw our attention to the key elements of situated practice: how a *purpose*-driven activity is indexed to layered and multiple *contexts*, within an ordered array of strategically ordered *component activities* (sub-steps), each with its own purposes and contexts, each shaping up the *flexible object* (the transcription) in often recursive and circular fashion. Critically for my purposes, Mondada also thinks about the skills, expertise, and ultimately "professional vision" (Goodwin 1994) that ground the *perceptive practices* of the analyst (Mondada 2007: 811).

In the following paragraphs, I expand on this way of thinking about transcription-as-situated-practice as itself a component element in the larger activity of research translation. I do this primarily by calling attention to the fact that transcription, and the ordered set of activities and contexts in which it takes place, is done *in the source language*.

Data collection results in a corpus of audio- and/or audiovisual files, and these are themselves curated in specific ways (e.g., organized and stored in file folders by themes or by demographics etc.). In most projects, there is a point at which this curated set of a/v files becomes *the* dataset because no additional interviews, recorded events, ethnographic notes, or other documents are added to it. Further, in some projects, researchers transcribe all the a/v files, but in other projects, researchers make selections from the corpus, creating subsets of the data. Choices about what and how much to transcribe are driven by practical questions about the purposes of the research and the targeted content, and the resources (time and money) available for transcription. In effect, researchers divide up the data into "regions," some of which will be mapped in detail, some which are more lightly sketched, and some which remain (frankly) *terra incognita*. Interestingly, the curated corpus of a/v files constitute a slice of the real world, and selective transcription results in a further, strategic slice of that original landscape. In any case, it is still the total data corpora that constitutes the foundational layer of the *project world*, and that world may be subject to years of further transcription, coding, analysis, and publication.

As Mondada points out, transcripts and recordings remain mutually linked: "... transcripts facilitate access to the recordings and highlight detailed features for the analysis; reciprocally, recordings give to transcripts their evidence and substance. They allow and warrant an enriched and contextual interpretation of tiny conventional notations" (2007: 811). This last refers to the conversation analysis of Mondada's own practice, but it is fair to say that applied linguists would generally see the recording-plus-transcript *pair* as the data. I see this latter preference and practice as a definitive characteristic of the applied linguist as social scientist, for whom discourse (talk, text, or both) is quintessentially social action. Every linguistic feature is a choice from among options, and what gets said is inherently linked to how it gets said.

Nevertheless, researchers adopt specific transcription conventions when transcribing, and these conventions are calibrated to specific levels of detail.

Müller (2006) speaks of multilayered transcription to capture these: from simpler orthographic approaches to highly detailed annotations for capturing turn-by-turn multimodal speech (for an overview, see Jenks, 2011). Not uncommonly, early transcriptions in a project are often content driven to facilitate construction of codable indices of topics, speakers. Such transcriptions aim at rendering conversational turns and words spoken, possibly with some minimal attention to longer pauses (captured in parenthesized quantities of seconds), false starts, cut-off speech, and non-verbals (parenthetical inclusion of descriptors: e.g., *laughter, sighs*). Orthographic translations devote less attention to prosody, and standard punctuation is used to signal whether utterances were heard as questions (via question marks) or indicative statements (via periods). Later *re*-transcriptions inevitably involve refinements, corrections, and additional notations, usually driven by more detailed conventions. Transcription is cyclic and increasingly fine-grained.

Transcription is usually intralingual: done from source language a/v files into source language text files, and I will argue that this sustained practice of intralingual meta-pragmatic re-characterization from oral-aural forms to written-read forms is the ideal foundation for faithful indexical, interlingual translation in later stages of the research project. Silverstein's second approach to translation – his *transduction* – involves achieving in the linguistic forms of the target text the same functions and force as are operative in the source forms. Such transduction assumes extensive and intimate familiarity with indexical references in the source language regarding whatever topics are at issue in the research.

We might pause for a moment to consider the kind of linguistic knowledge required to process indexical reference. For a speaker, *doing an indexical reference* implies an act of invocation and an invoked context (e.g., an American who uses the phrase *operating theatre* is likely invoking a British cultural nuance versus the culturally expectable and unmarked *operating room*). We know that speakers invoke contexts via an extensive range of linguistic features (phonological, prosodic, morphosyntactic, lexical, and discursive), and we also know that the range of contexts invoked is correlated with the topic. Thus, the transcriber who is submerged (hour after hour) in the discursive world of the data *and* who must capture the spoken features of talk via fine-grained transcription conventions is forced to cultivate and sharpen an intimate knowledge of source language indexical reference.

In sum, if a major goal of transductive interlingual translation is achieving indexical equivalents in the target language that match the function and force of indexicalities in the source language, then the immersive situated practice of intralingual transcription in the source language provides fertile ground for such translation. In sum, research translation begins with transcription.

4.2 Coding

Coding and the larger analytic techniques that it serves (e.g., content analysis, phenomenology, discourse analysis, narrative analysis) are also situated practices, linked to the layered contexts and purposes of their production. In the following paragraphs, I examine coding as situated steps-and-stages in the gradually emerging process of research translation.

Although coding may seem an atomistic and pedestrian act, it is the foundational practice of qualitative data analysis. To code, we need labels: words or phrases that we use to tag data segments (selected text). We give these code labels longer descriptions; we set criteria for their application; and we attach them to portions of text as useful indices of content. (Indeed, data segments and codes become critically important intermediate analytic objects in the qualitative research process). As codes increase in number, they become a *codebook*, and that collection of codes waxes and wanes as researchers lump some codes (combining code labels that overlap) and split other codes (creating separate but related codes from one overly generalized code). Lumping and splitting involve micro-level metapragmatic discriminations about the content of data segments. Coding is further complexified by the fact that coders often apply several codes to the same data segment. Over time, researchers use the codes themselves to characterize the structure of, and to test relationships within, the project world.

Coding is a quintessential metapragmatic re-characterization of source language talk-and-text, and another form of *intra*linguistic translation. Or so it would seem. In fact, in an interesting twist, coding is also often a first moment of systematic *interlingual translation* because multilingual researchers often work indiscriminately in both the source language of the data and the eventual target language as they engage in the series of situated practices that constitute coding: deriving labels, applying codes, defining codes, articulating criteria for applying the codes, managing the code book, discussing codes, modeling networks of codes, and beginning the process of writing up results. Indeed, it is not uncommon that researchers work in a mélange of languages across all these activities.

As an example, Patria López de Victoria conducted a project about older adults' help seeking in the aftermath of Hurricane Maria in Puerto Rico (see Chapter 7, this volume). Overall, the source language of the study was Spanish: all ethnographic notes were recorded in Spanish; all printed texts and websites were in Spanish; all interviews were conducted in Spanish; and all recorded interviews and events were transcribed in Spanish. However, all team members were Spanish-English bilinguals, and throughout the project, all personnel worked across both languages. As an example, Figure 1 shows an Excel worksheet that represents a portion of the codebook from the project (coded via the QDA program,

Atlas.ti; Muhr 2017). Note that the worksheet is entitled in Spanish, "Subcódigo para identificar eventos de alfabetización en etapa 1 de investigación" (Subcodes to identify literacy events in stage 1 of the investigation). Column A however contains the list of codes in English, while Column B gives descriptions of the codes in Spanish. However, even here there are code switches. For example, in row 2 the words "over the counter" appear in English and in row 6 there is a parenthetical reference to "bedside manner" also in English. Thus, coders in López de Victoria's project applied English language codes to Spanish data segments but elaborated code descriptions in a mix of both Spanish and English.

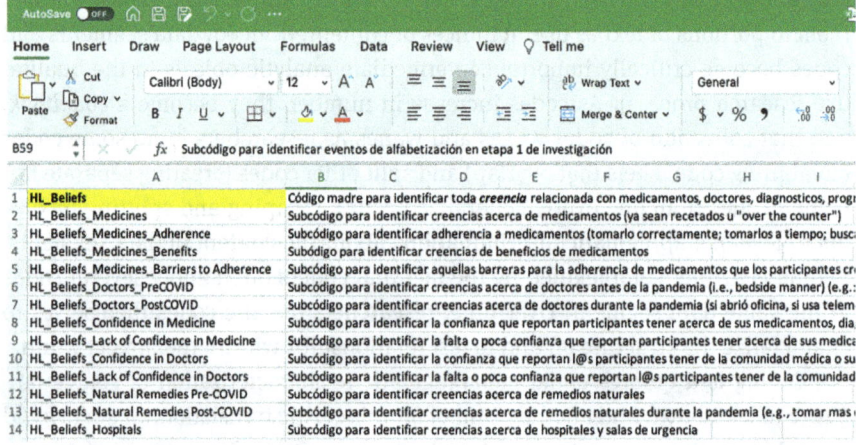

Figure 1: Codebook from The Helpseeking Project (López de Victoria).

It is important to note however, that this pattern of research multilingualism is only one variation. In multilingual projects involving more than two source languages at the data level, all team members may not know all the source languages, but it is almost always the case that they will share at least one common, research language. That is, one language (often English) is used for analysis, presentation, and publication of the results. In such projects then, coding becomes a thoroughly bilingual activity, requiring facility in alternating between languages in two essential channels: *reading and writing* – to do the coding – and *understanding and speaking* – to coordinate, organize, and complete the tasks.

Is this translation? It is arguable that it is not. Rather this facile working in multiple languages is better captured by *translanguaging* which describes how multilingual individuals make flexible use of all the linguistic resources at their disposal to accomplish an immediate communicative task-at-hand. In these moments of selecting material in the transcript and then creating and applying codes in both languages, the applied linguist "dwells in a converged space where diverse semiotic resources subsist and operate in tandem" (Baynham and Lee 2019: 3).

Nevertheless, in interesting ways, translanguaging in this semiotically converged space becomes a powerful resource for research translation. Multilinguals do translanguaging at various levels of awareness. At one end of a hypothetical continuum, two multilinguals in fluid and fast conversation are mostly unaware of their language(s), but there may be flashes of consciousness. Every multilingual momentarily catches himself or herself tripping up over a linguistic choice (though these moments are usually resolved at lightning speed). At the other end of the continuum, interlocutors sometimes explicitly pause at some communicative hiccup and explicitly work to repair it. I'll hazard the guess that neither party would think of himself or herself as translating in such a moment, but of course for such interlocutors, translation is not the point.

For a researcher, however, translation is very much the point since research moves inexorably toward publication and presentation. Moments of tripping up over a linguistic choice or full-stop moments of repair become conscious signals of lexico-grammatic and/or indexical in-equivalence. Critically, these moments also trigger new insights into the cultural differences at the intersection of source and target languages. As Hanks notes for the anthropological translator: ". . . translation so understood is not merely a problem of redescribing a cultural form, but of understanding it in the first place. In other words, it has to do with our ability to gain knowledge of other cultures . . ." (Hanks 2015: 26). Further, insofar as researchers explicitly textualize coding and analysis – typing out code definitions, criteria, summaries of content, and so on – these *translanguaged*, multilingual records are often revisited, modified, corrected, and expanded. Thus, the essentially translanguaged and recursive character of qualitative data analysis raises conscious wonder, questions, doubts, and guesses about linguistic equivalence that will serve formal translation later when the researcher moves meticulously and stepwise toward the formally defined "material outcome that we call a translated text" (Baynham & Lee 2019: 40).

4.3 Analysis and re-transcription

Although coding is the first step in analysis, the transition to deeper analysis occurs with the systematic search for patterns and relationships in the data via constant review of, and reflection on, the codes and involves the following research practices: frequent tacking back and forth between coded data segments; the drafting of models of potential relationships between codes, often visually as concept maps (Wheeldon & Ählberg 2012); continued elaboration of memos, and preliminary articulations (what Latour calls "ad libitum writing trials," Latour 2005: 134–135). Again, where researchers are proficient in the languages of the project, these operations involve constant translanguaging as researchers move up and down through multiple, multilingual layers of transcription, coding, and prior analyses.

It is also common at this stage that researchers engage in re-transcribing portions of data to deepen their insights, test their predictions and hunches, and begin the process of preparing excerpts for publication. Indeed, the cycle of transcription and re-transcription is a key tool in applied linguistic research (Müller 2006; Schrauf 2016, chapter 5). Several steps in the situated practice of re-transcription deserve more detailed comment.

First, the act of selecting data segments for re-transcription involves articulating for oneself some quasi-systematic criteria for doing so. Which segments address which aspects of my research question? Why these segments and not those? Are segments broadly representative, richly descriptive, or intriguingly exceptional? Importantly, because re-transcription is quite time-consuming and labor-intensive, the result of these selections is the creation of yet another subcorpus that gradually accrues canonical status. *This* set of transcribed data segments becomes the pool from which data displays are selected for presentation and publication. Certainly, researchers do in fact continue to revisit the data and test their ideas etc., and therefore the re-transcribed subcorpus is not *the* data. But inertia sets in, and re-transcribed segments themselves trigger new insights, which further cements their canonical status.

A second situated practice in re-transcription concerns the selection and careful application of more detailed transcription conventions. Materially, of course, it is the transcription conventions that mediate the researchers' attention to linguistic, discursive, and interactional forms, and in the re-encounter with the a/v file the transcription conventions tell us what to listen for. At the same time, since it is an activity of *re*-transcription, we usually have before us an already printed, orthographic transcription of what we or another transcriber heard before. Finally, we are conscious at some level of the purposes of our study and its intended audience or readership. All of this to say that the sustained re-encounter with the micro-details of the spoken language dips us back into the source language and dense social reality of the original speech event, while at the same time we are drawing closer and closer to the moments-of-truth in which we will create research *representations* (accurate? faithful? authentic?) of those speech events for public consumption and evaluation.

4.4 Data display in presentation or publication

As analysis moves toward writing, the researcher takes up *translation proper*: Jakobson's interlingual reported speech or Silverstein's lexico-grammatic + transductive operations. The literary object in which this process is crystallized is the *data display* in which selected data segments are transformed into publishable form, embedded at key locations in a manuscript, and integrated into the flow of the results section.

The act of translation itself, including attention to the lexico-grammatic and indexical equivalences, is the final step and culmination of the series of situated activities that precede and prepare this moment (transcription, coding, analysis, re-transcription – as described above). In small projects, researchers may have translated whole transcripts prior to this point, but perhaps more commonly, researchers attend to the translation of the subcorpora of re-transcribed, source language data segments described above. These will be the clearest, simplest, and most rhetorically persuasive bits of evidence around which he or she will weave the results narrative. The immediate context of production of data displays is the researcher's writing the commentary about and around excerpts in the results section of that manuscript. In fact, this surrounding text/commentary is an essential component of the translation. Thus, the following section treats first the data display and second the role and character of the preceding and succeeding commentary.

4.4.1 Translation proper: The excerpt

Before moving on to translation in data displays, it may be helpful to think through the genre of the *excerpt* as the basic data display in qualitative publication. Importantly, excerpts are saturated with indexical associations to both the research process itself as well to the content and context of the data. That is, genre conventions of the published excerpt send powerful semiotic signals about the data collection, the sample, the organization of the data corpus, some of the analytic steps, and the fundamental validity of the research. To set the stage for considering data displays-of-translated-material, in the following example I explore the range of semiotic signals in the standard data display.

The following excerpt comes from a video-recorded session of diagnostic testing (entirely in English) in which a patient is answering questions posed by a behavioral neurologist. As the excerpt begins, the neurologist is asking the patient to recite back to him a name and address given earlier in the testing.

Example 1
Typical Monolingual Data Display (author data)
Excerpt 7 – Delayed Recall (T33)
ITEM #10 – delayed recall
1 DOC: Sir what was that na::me and address
2   that I asked you to remember?
3 (6.1)
4 DOC: Can you remember anything about that sir?
5 PAT: When did you uh give that?
6 (t.4)

Again, standard genre features function as indexical cues for specific details of the research process or research world. The *heading* announces the genre ("Excerpt") which signals the transition from the manuscript narrative to a spate of empirical data. The heading also includes a brief and purposely telegraphic *title* ("Delayed Recall") for easy reference later in the manuscript. The title is followed by a *parenthesized alphanumeric* ("T33") which serves to identify the participant as belonging to a set (the sample) of such participants (the "T's") of whom there appear to be at least thirty-three. The anonymizing alphanumeric also signals that the participant's identity is protected by legal and research protocols. The *line numbers* demarcate each printed line as a potential bit of evidence for reference in the text of the article. The *speaker designations* ("DOC" and "PAT") construct essentialized identities/roles for both interlocutors, and their placement in a special *column* immediately to the right of the line numbers structurally highlights conversational turns. Finally, the *transcription conventions* (i.e., underlines for emphasis; up and down arrows for prosodic shifts; parenthesized pause lengths; colons for elongation, and so on) are instantly readable as belonging to one of the highly developed convention sets available to professional linguists (in this case, Jeffersonian conversation analysis).

Every one of these conventions is optional. That is, there are numerous published data displays in which some of the elements (heading, title, parenthesized identifier, line numbers, speaker designations, and transcription conventions) are not used. Thus, the author may not need to send certain signals. For example, there may be no heading because the excerpt is indented as a block; no title because abbreviated reference back to this excerpt later in the manuscript is unnecessary; no participant identifier because the participant is identified in the preceding narrative text or participants are treated as a homogenous class; no line numbers because it isn't necessary to call attention to specific linguistic features; no turn-taking identifiers because only the participant's words are displayed; no transcription conventions because only the content is important. Thus, from a discourse analytic perspective, the employment of each genre feature is a strategic choice by the author to enhance the reader's ability to link the data to the narrative text or to connect the excerpt back to the larger empirical research from which it comes.

Translated data displays usually appear in published excerpts in one of four typical forms: (a) in side-by-side text blocks, with the source language on one side and the translation on the other, (b) in successive text blocks, with the source language in one block and the translation in the other, (c) in interlinear organization with source language lines followed by translation lines or (d) in an indented block containing only the translation (no source language). In a sense, there is a binary here: options (a)-(c) favor representing the source language and option (d) eliminates it. Let's examine the format of one such data display: option (c).

The following excerpt comes again from López de Victoria's project on help-seeking among Puerto Rican islanders immediately after Hurricane María in September 2017. The participant in the interview is Elsie (E), an older woman who recounts her trip to a community pharmacy in the days after the hurricane (see Chapter 7, this volume).

Example 2
Interlinear Translation of an Excerpt (López de Victoria)
Excerpt 4: I had to pay

54	E:	*Este em- (tsk) y entonce:s este un medicamento no lo tenían disponible*
		Uh mhm (tsk) and then one of the medicines was not available
55		*Me tuve que ir a la farmacia de la comunidad*
		I had to go to the community pharmacy
56	I:	*Okey*
		Okay
57	E:	*.hh y la farmacia de la comunidad no tenía sistema ni nada* ↑
		And the community pharmacy didn't have the billing system or anything

---

What does this arrangement convey? Although I have not reproduced the surrounding commentary from the chapter (but see pp. 172–174, this volume), I note that the data display has a different format from the surrounding text, which works to set it off as a piece of evidence. Many of the same genre features are present here as in the previous example. A heading (*Excerpt 4*) sets the piece off from the preceding text; a title (*I had to pay*) captures the significance of the passage; the lines are numbered, for easy reference in the accompanying text; and speaker roles are marked by capital letters (*E* for Elsie, *I* for the interviewer). Crucially, the Spanish source language is set off in italics, and the interlinear translation is in regular font (which of course matches the rest of the chapter text). Finally, the interlinear pairing sends two subtle signals. First, having the Spanish precede the English signals its priority and leads back to the participant's actual wording.

(Readers who know Spanish can inspect the original and judge for themselves the quality of the translation). Second, connecting the source-target pair to a single line number sends the signal that both lines are equivalent *and* evokes the project world through which the source language text has traveled to this current (translated) setting in the official, representative product: a published chapter.

These choices are trade-offs, of course; not the least of these is that representing the source language text takes up extra space and adds to the word count. Editors can be cautious around these issues, and authors may have to make adjustments: trimming the number of excerpts, displaying less context in the excerpts, lengthening the lines, providing tighter commentary, and so on. Too, there is the question of the journal readership. Readers of linguistics journals take source language representations for granted; readers of medical journals may find source language representations negligible. Nevertheless, interdisciplinary publication, both during manuscript preparation by the team, and during the reading experience by non-linguists, is also an occasion for expanding perspectives. It is also the case that data displays do not stand alone, but are linked to interpretive commentary. This latter is also a site in which authors treat issues of language and culture, and I turn now to this textual framing.

4.4.2 Translation setting: The metapragmatic commentary

Translated data displays are common in many traditions: literary translation (e.g., Proust's *À la recherche du temps perdu* into English as *Remembrance of Things Past* (1982), psychometric translations (e.g., a translation of the *Mini Mental State Examination [MMSE]* into Sinhalese for use in Sri Lanka; de Silva & Gunatilake 2002; see Steis & Schrauf 2009), or institutional translations (e.g., consent forms, discharge instructions). Translated data displays from qualitative social science projects differ from these former traditions in the critical sense that literary, psychometric, or institutional translations are meant to stand alone in their target languages. The activities of reading *Remembrance of Things Past*, taking the MMSE, or signing a consent form should not in principle require accompanying commentary about the source language versions.

By contrast, research translations in qualitative projects always include associated commentary before and after the translated data display. Such commentary usually includes descriptions, explanations, and cultural contextualizations. There are in fact two tasks of contextualization that are indispensably addressed in the surrounding commentary: one has to do with the translation itself – in particular with indexicality. The other has to do with the insertion of the translated data display into its new context: the journal article.

Per Silverstein's (2003b) combined approaches, a good translation necessarily involves *both* the careful mapping of *lexico-grammatic forms* of the source language onto equivalent forms in the target language, largely in the ambit of Saussurean paradigmatic and syntagmatic relations, *and* the transduction of *indexical function and form* from source to target language texts. Again, indexicality is the linguistic invocation of contextual information during ongoing acts-of-communication without detailed explanation or explicit reference. Such information derives from and re-presents dimensions of cultural knowledge, presuppositions, and normativities not immediately apparent in lexico-grammatic equivalents. Crucially, precisely because speakers invoke/conjure/deploy/insinuate such information to fit their strategic purposes, indexical invocation is *performative*. However, as Silverstein notes, "To the degree such complexes of presupposition contribute particularly to the performative efficacy of textual use of words and expressions as social action, they constitute the very limits of normal, denotationally centered approaches to 'translation'" (Silverstein, 2003b: 86). Literary translation, psychometric translation, and institutional translation *must* solve this issue without commentary, but the research translator has the advantage of being able to provide metapragmatic description.

Effectively, the research translator has many more resources at his or her disposal to orient the reader to the finer points of indexical performance in the source language, and to achieve the same indexical force and function in the target language, now not simply through the translated data display, but rather through the pairing of data display with contextual commentary. In this sense, the research translator's craft has everything to do with cultural translation: all of which (again) has been richly prepared by the months-long immersion in the multilingual project world. An interesting effect of the metapragmatic commentary is that it frames the translated data display as an analytic object.

Thus, in reference to the second kind of contextualization mentioned above – the insertion of a data display into the new context of the journal article – the author also re-contextualizes the excerpt in a very different cultural setting: the applied health, clinical, biomedical, or public health context. Obviously, the author/translator will be making links from the data display to the points made in the article, relevant to the research questions, etc.

5 Final reflections

In this chapter, I have re-read the act of research translation as an elongated process that takes place over several months of the researcher's immersion in his or her own research project, and I re-envisioned translation as grounded in, prepared by, and exercised through the standard series of concatenated, situated activities of transcription, coding, analysis and re-transcription, and construction of translated data displays. By way of summarizing how translated data displays (and associated commentary) slowly emerge out of these many steps, we might place the accent on how the applied linguist becomes a translator.

As noted previously, through his or her saturation in the project world, the applied linguist goes through a process not unlike acculturation. Acculturation involves acquiring an experientially fine-tuned knowledge of, and ability to interact socially within, a culture other-than-one's own culture-of-origin. By analogy, the applied linguist's immersion in the project world involves awareness and comprehension of an extensive range of indexicalities in a locally exercised source language, the ability to construct and navigate multiple levels of metapragmatic characterization of that world in both source and target languages; and ultimately facility in translating descriptive statements into professional worlds far-removed from that of the data. In brief, I would characterize research translation as an iterative process of successive intralingual and engagements with source and target languages in specific situated practices:

- Source-language indexical sensitivities are acquired and deepened over long hours of careful transcription (intralingual)
- Practice, refinement, and nuance of interlingual metapragmatic representation comes from *translanguaged* working out a codebook and coding, analytic modeling, and creation/curation of subcorpora associated with specific findings.
- Deepening attunement to source language indexicalities (intralingual) is acquired in re-transcription of excerpts in the data display sub-corpus,
- Authentic representation of the project world for other professionals comes from crafting translated data displays in the target language and linguistic-cultural commentaries that capture the relevant indexical nuances of the source language and culture.

In essence, via his or her construction, revision, and analysis of a particular project world, the applied linguist acquires highly expert, *local* expertise about a particular slice of social life. As a result, he or she then becomes a privileged voice for the re-presentation of that world in the new context of a very different target culture: that of academics. However, because the gold standard of academic production remains the printed article, this voice is primarily exercised in a printed publication, and hence representations of the slices of social life drawn from the source language data are necessarily written/read.

Earlier in this chapter, I distinguished between, on the one hand, literary, psychometric, and institutional translations, and on the other hand, the research translation of scholarship and social science. There I noted that a distinguishing mark of the former was that they necessarily stood on their own as adequate communicative representations of their source language originals (without reference to that source language), whereas the advantage of research translation was the associated commentary. Commentary allows the linguist to provide explanations of indexical reference that the reader needs to grasp the meanings that the source text has in its source-culture context. Thus, at the end of the day, it is the translated data display-*plus*-associated commentary that constitutes the essential and almost only vehicle for communicating source language social life to the professional worlds of other linguists, academic health scholars, and health personnel.

Given that reality, it is important that we think carefully about how these data displays-plus-associated commentary develop, not solely in the moment of translating the excerpt from source to target language, but in the slow, cumulative, thickening development of the applied linguist's linguacultural and research expertise and engagement with the data. This latter is *research translation*: a carefully coordinated series of situated practices, indexically sensitive to the data and the research process itself, and culminating in brief, telegraphic, translated excerpts that, if well framed, give a window onto another social reality, critically linked now to another series of situated practice in clinical, community, and public health. Research translation, I would argue, is a key contribution of applied health linguists to health-related scholarship in the social sciences, especially in the emerging international context of global health. Both our research participants and our research colleagues have justifiably high expectations that we do it well.

References

Agha, Asif. 2007. *Language and social relations*. Cambridge: Cambridge University Press.
Baynham, Mike. & Tong K. Lee. 2019. *Translation and translanguaging*. New York: Routledge.
Clark, Herbert. H. & Richard J. Gerrig, Richard J. 1990. Quotations as demonstrations. *Language*, *66*(4). 764–805.
Garfinkel, Harold & Harvey Sacks. 1970. On formal structures of practical actions. In John C. McKinney & Edward. A. Tiryakian (eds.), *Theoretical Sociology*, 337–366. New York, N.Y.: Appleton-Century-Crofts.
Goodwin, Charles. 1994. Professional vision. *American Anthropologist, 96*(3). 606–633. https://doi.org/10.1525/aa.1994.96.3.02a00100
Hanks, William. F. 2015. The space of translation. In Carlo Severi & William. F. Hanks (eds.), *Translating worlds: The epistemological space of translation*, 21–49. Chicago, IL: Hau Books.

Hanks, William. F. & Carolo Severi. 2015. Translating worlds: The epistemological space of translation. In Carlo Severi & William. F. Hanks (eds.), *Translating worlds: The epistemological space of translation*, 1–49. Chicago, IL: Hau Books.

Jakobson, Roman. 2012. On linguistic aspects of translation. In Lawrence Venuti (ed.), *The translation studies reader* (2nd edition). London: Routledge.

Jenks, Christopher. J. 2011. *Transcribing text and interaction: Issues in the representation of communication data*. Philadelphia: John Benjamins.

Latour, Bruno. 2005. *Reassembling the social: An introduction to actor-network-theory*. Oxford: Oxford University Press.

Lock, Margaret & Vinh-Kim Nguyen. 2010. *An anthropology of biomedicine*. Malden, MA: Wiley-Blackwell.

Lucy, John. A. (ed.). 1993. *Reflexive language: Reported speech and metapragmatics*. New York: Cambridge University Press.

Lynch, Michael. 2019. Garfinkel, Sacks and formal structures: Collaborative origins, divergences and the history of ethnomethodology and conversation analysis. *Human Studies*, 42(2). 183–198. https://doi.org/10.1007/s10746-019-09510-w

Mondada, Lorenza. 2007. Commentary: Transcript variations and the indexicality of transcribing practices. *Discourse Studies*, 9(6). 809–821. https://doi.org/10.1177/1461445607082581

Muhr, Thomas. 2017. *Atlas.ti V8: The knowledge workbench*. Berlin: Scientific Software Development.

Müller, Nicole. 2006. *Multilayered transcription*. San Diego: Plural Publishing.

Nilsson, Elin. 2017. Fishing for answers: Couples living with dementia managing trouble with recollection. *Educational Gerontology*, 43(2). 73–88. https://doi.org/10.1080/03601277.2016.1260911

Proust, Marcel. 1982. *Remembrance of Things Past – Volume 1 – Swann's Way and Within a Budding Grove*. Translated by C.K. Scott Moncrieff and Terence Kilmartin. New York: Vintage – Random House.

Schrauf, Robert. W. 2016. *Mixed methods: Interviews, surveys, and cross-cultural comparisons*. Cambridge and New York: Cambridge University Press.

Schrauf, Robert. W. 2020. Epistemic responsibility – Labored, loosened, and lost: Staging Alzheimer's disease. *Journal of Pragmatics*, 168. 56–68. https://doi.org/10.1016/j.pragma.2020.07.003

Severi, Carlo & William F. Hanks. (eds.). 2015. *Translating worlds: The epistemological space of translation*. Chicago, IL: Hau Books.

Silverstein, Michael. 1976. Shifters, linguistic categories, and cultural description. In Keith. H. Basso & Henry. A. Selby (eds.), *Meaning in anthropology*, 11–56. Albuquerque, New Mexico: University of New Mexico Press.

Silverstein, Michael. 2003a. Indexical order and the dialectics of sociolinguistic life. *Language & Communication*, 23. 193–229.

Silverstein, Michael. 2003b. Translation, transduction, transformation: Skating "glossando" on thin semiotic ice. In Paula. G. Rubel & Abraham Rosman (eds.), *Translating cultures: Perspectives on translation and anthropology*, 75–105. New York: Berg.

Silverstein, Michael. 2004. "Cultural" concepts and the language-culture nexus. *Current Anthropology*, 45(5). 621–645.

Steis, Mindy & Schrauf, Robert. W. 2009. A review of translations and adaptations of the MMSE in languages other than English and Spanish. *Research in Gerontological Nursing*, 2(3). 214–224.

Strauss, Susan & Feiz, Peristou. 2014. *Discourse analysis: Putting our worlds into words*. New York: Routledge/Taylor and Francis Group.
Wheeldon, Johannes & Mauri K. Ählberg. 2012. *Visualizing social science research: Maps, methods, and meaning*. Los Angeles: Sage Publications.
Xiao, Lily. D., Jing Wang, Guo-Ping He, Anita De Bellis, Jenny Verbeeck & Helena Kyriazopoulos. 2014. Family caregiver challenges in dementia care in Australia and China: a critical perspective. *BMC Geriatrics*, *14*, 6. https://doi.org/10.1186/1471-2318-14-6

Section 3: **Applied linguistics and public health**

Peter Joseph Torres
Chapter 5
Modality and interpretative spaces in policies

1 Introduction

Since its inception in the 1960s, language policy and planning (LPP) has continued to evolve. LPP is an applied linguistic research domain focusing on policies regulating language use (Fishman, Ferguson, and Das Gupta 1968). One particular development in the area is the growing presence of scholarship examining health care policies in language policy publications (Schuster, Elroy, and Elmakais 2017; Martinez 2008; Higgins 2010; Ramanathan 2010). Digital advances in data gathering provide an opportunity for applied linguists to integrate collaborative corpus-assisted approaches. These advances aim to explore large-scale discourse data and broaden the scope of LPP research beyond examining language policies towards scholarship analyzing the very language of policies. The goal of the chapter is to outline and apply a systematic, applied linguistics framework – corpus-based discourse analysis (CBDA) – for use in LPP research on health policy. The study presented in this chapter explicates that framework, using CBDA to understand the functions that grammatical features serve in the framing of public health policies.

The first half of this chapter treats LPP and introduces the linguistic theory that grounds my CBDA approach, while the second half reflects on the analysis of a previous study, in which I used CBDA to analyze the roles of modal verbs in framing policies (see Torres 2021 for more detailed discussion). Modality (i.e., verbs like can, will, shall) is a popular choice for framing policies and any other discourses referencing future events because they can communicate attitudes, truths, and stances displaced in space and time (Bhatia, Flowerdew, and Jones 2008; Hacquard 2016; Portner 2009). However, modals can also cause confusion and ambiguity due to their polysemic quality (Asprey 1992; Garzone 2013). American policymakers' excessive use of modals, despite their potential to pose problems for stakeholders tasked with interpreting and carrying out such policies, is a source of curiosity that motivates the investigation presented in the sample study. Specifically, the sample research answers the following research question: *What functions do modal verbs*

Peter Joseph Torres, Miami University, Ohio

https://doi.org/10.1515/9783110744804-006

serve in shaping California opioid policies? Finally, the chapter concludes with a reflection on the potential contributions applied linguists and CBDA could make to advance LPP studies in the context of public health policies.

2 Part I: Linguistic theory

2.1 Situating the study: From language policies to language of policies

Applied linguists interested in policy research face the challenge of situating their work within a field that already considers LPP as one of its well-defined research domains. Language policies, in broad terms, refer to guidelines regulating language use in communities. The first wave of scholarship in the 1960s focused primarily on the codification of national languages, when standardization was regarded as a solution to establishing a unified sense of identity among coexisting communities (Haugen 1959, 1983; Fishman, Ferguson, and Das Gupta 1968). Although not necessarily ill-intentioned, these policies come with top-down solutions that ultimately limited how people think, communicate, and identify themselves (Noss 1967; Das Gupta 1970).

"Critical language policy" emerged in the 1990s, as scholars in the domain began criticizing language policies and their historical and structural mechanisms for causing linguistic inequalities (Fowler 1979). The movement eventually catapulted LPP research towards investigating local policy enactments in areas such as schools and the workplace as researchers began confronting the interpretive nature of policies (Pérez and Nordlander 2004; Levinson, Sutton, and Winstead 2009; Hornberger and Johnson 2007). According to Johnson and Freeman (2010:15), policies can be interpreted and understood in different ways by stakeholders who "appropriate, resist, or change dominant and alternative policy discourses." For instance, Ricento and Hornberger (1996) investigated the role of English instructors as language policy arbiters in the classroom and revealed the discrepancies in the interpretation and enactment of policies. Similarly, Johnson (2012) examined the stakeholders' diverging interpretations of Arizona's language education policy, Proposition 203, to illustrate how interpretation influences stakeholder response. As Hornberger (1998) explained, ignoring the effect of policies discounts the agency of the very people in charge of linguistically interpreting them. Johnson and Freeman (2010) presented the concept of "spaces" within which teachers – the stakeholders in their study – negotiate various possible interpretations of education language policies (see also Menken and Garcia 2010). This concept inspired the notion of "interpretive spaces" introduced later in this chapter.

Incorporating ethnographic and discourse analytic approaches to LPP opened up the domain to the investigation of the language of policies instead of simply "language policies" per se. As Davis (1999) explained, the field has done more than simply establish national languages. In fact, the field has increasingly addressed the language of healthcare policies. Stritikus and Wiese (2006) highlighted health policy interpretation and enactments as a possible direction for future studies in a paper about bilingual education language policies. Moreover, in a special issue of Language Policy, Ramanathan (2010) advocates the importance of addressing 'language' and 'policy' concerns separately instead of as a singular unit in order to address both language and (public) policy concerns around health. Higgins (2010) took up the challenge by examining the language of international public health policies while simultaneously evaluating the linguistic means in which such policies are interpreted in local HIV/AIDS educational sessions in Tanzania. She revealed the tensions between global and local cultural models, demonstrating the need for policymakers, health care practitioners, and applied linguists to collaborate on solutions. Martinez's (2008) ethnography at the U.S.-Mexico border exposed how the language of federal healthcare policies negatively impacts Spanish-speaking patients' health outcomes despite federal policies concerning the provision of interpreter services. Finally, scholars like Ainsworth-Vaughn (1998), Ramanathan (2009), Sarangi and Roberts (2008) have sought to address critical and cultural issues around policies concerning ailments.

2.2 Policies

Applied linguists studying the language of policies also have to navigate through the many different definitions of "policy" from various academic domains. Ball (1990) and Goodnow (2017) define policies as authoritative texts and de facto practices used by governing institutions to reflect social knowledge into plans, procedures, and goals to guide local decision-making. When taken into a linguistic perspective, policies are chunks of language (discourse) made up of lexical and grammatical features that denote a suggestive intent of regulatory measures and courses of action concerning a given issue. By analyzing the emerging patterns present in policies, we can uncover policymakers' hidden ideologies and attitudes towards the issue in question (Gales 2009; see also Stubbs 2001). The language of policies permits the investigation into the current state of the community that implements it (Wodak 2006; Ramanathan and Morgan 2007). After all, the importance of policies relies on the need that calls for it.

There are at least three diverging levels of policies informing health issues in the United States today: federal, state, and local. Each level feeds into and off of another, creating a dynamic intersecting system that informs emerging health issues. Thus, policy scholars must consider these distinctions when deciding which policies to investigate to make connections between the language of policies and local enactments.

According to the Institute of Medicine (1988), the federal government's primary role in healthcare is to fund state health initiatives. Thus, the federal government's influence in implementing change locally is limited because it is not involved in the local realization of the funds. Instead, federal institutions could only draft contracts that obligate states to take action towards a general goal. State governments are responsible for promoting the general welfare of their constituents by establishing state-level healthcare policies for local medical institutions to follow. Furthermore, local institutions such as health centers, clinics, and city hospitals, consider the guidance provided in state policies when drafting the specific mandates or guidance for their workers to follow.

The primary federal units responsible for public health issues in the United States are the Department of Health and Human Services (HHS), Centers for Disease Control and Prevention (CDC), and the Food and Drug Administration (FDA).

2.3 Corpus-based discourse analysis and frameworks

Corpus-based discourse analysis has been widely used in studying public and language policies because it allows for the quantitative and qualitative examination of large data (Flowerdew 2008; Partington 2003, 2008). Corpus Analysis (CA) provides a quantitative textual analysis of specific grammatical features, while Discourse Analysis (DA) allows researchers to interpret the set of possibilities that motivate and explain the patterns that emerged from CA (Baker 2006). Using DA allows policy researchers to make sense of the choices language users make. In the case of the sample study, DA helps shed light on the modal choices of policymakers that could lead to identifying their role in policies. Two relevant frameworks that could assist the analytic process are (1) context models and (2) frames.

2.3.1 Context models

Van Dijk's (1999: 131) context model framework – a schema designed to reduce the complexity of social situations and efficiently contextualize discourse through schematic categories – is an effective guiding principle for the discourse analysis of policies because it efficiently narrows down various contextual features relevant to the analysis. The four contextual categories in Table 1 were conducive to the analytic process in the study cited in this chapter.

Table 1: Four schematic categories accounted for when designing a discourse analysis study of policies.

Category	Policy Information	Purpose (present study)	Use in policy analysis
Time	When was the policy chaptered?	To map the changes in modal usage across time.	Accounting for when policies or amendments were made enables researchers to connect local realities to the changes in the language or framing of policies.
Location	Where is the policy enacted?	To understand the correlation between local events and modal usage.	Choosing a specific area and constituency from which policies are gathered and analyzed keeps the study focused, resulting in key findings that could directly benefit the specific locality.
Participants (Policy stakeholders)	To whom are the policies addressed?	To identify the policy stakeholders (gender-neutral term for actors) who are either limited or empowered by restrictive and permissive modality, respectively.	Identifying the individuals who are expected to address social issues through interpreting language and whether they provide ample representation of the diverse groups in the locality.
Action (Policy action)	What is the policy about?	To reveal the purpose of the proposition that triggered certain modal choices.	Identifying the specific actions state and local leaders are implementing to address concerns.

2.3.2 Frames

Fillmore (1975: 123) describes "frames" as "schemata" that structure one's understanding and interpretation of linguistic expressions and symbolic units such as text. Fillmore (1975) adds that frames are either evoked by the discourse or invoked by the "cognizer" (the receiving end of the discourse). Lastly, Fillmore (1976: 29) describes frames as empty slots within a string of words that could be filled using the information provided by the remainder of the text and applying what one knows about the situation and the world.

(1) "The doctor <u>*may*</u> prescribe me <u>opioids</u> for chronic pain"
                     MODAL   MEDICATION

For example, sentence (a) above has "opioids" occupying the "MEDICATION" frame. For the language user who chose "opioids" out of potential alternatives, the word evokes a frame in which a semantic unit called "opioid" is "a medication prescribed for chronic pain." Similarly, the cognizer could also arrive at their own interpretation of the sentence based on their knowledge of opioids. For example, the receiving end of this sentence may assume that the speaker is suffering from intense pain if they know that an opioid is a controlled substance reserved for relieving intense pain.

The speaker must have implicitly qualified all possible modals to decide on "may" over potential alternatives to occupy the "MODAL" frame. In addition, the knowledge that a language user has on the words "prescription," "chronic pain," "narcotic," "controlled substance," or "painkiller" also affects their level of certainty and, thus, modal choice. Similarly, a cognizer from the 2020s who has knowledge of the opioid crisis may have a different interpretation of the sentence than a cognizer from the 1970s when the public was told that opioids were safe. Simply put, frames allow us to become actively involved in giving meaning to various linguistic texts, such as policies, using our personal knowledge, memories, and experiences at that point in time.

3 Part II: Sample study

3.1 Background: Overview of the opioid crisis

In 2011, the United States Centers for Disease Control and Prevention (CDC) declared prescription drug abuse a national epidemic after deaths from accidental overdose exceeded fatalities from vehicular accidents (Centers for Disease Control and Prevention 2011). This section outlines the landmark policies at both the federal (United States) and state levels (California) to map out the significant shifts in the history and sentiments associated with opioids. As pointed out by Strauss and Corbin (1997), creating a data narrative makes a valuable backdrop against which the discourses under inspection can be grounded.

3.1.1 Phase I: Pain epidemic (1970 to 2003)

In the 1970s, before the opioid crisis, the United States dealt with an entirely different problem – the lack of pain treatment. The solution policymakers across the country came up with was to change the way medical practice addressed pain, from finding its source to directly targeting pain itself (Caudill-Slosberg, Schwartz, and Woloshin 2004). Thus, policies that came out between 1970 to 2003 were less concerned about overprescribing opioids than they are alleviating patients' pain:

1986: The World Health Organization (1986) released the "analgesic/pain ladder," an international guideline which states that if cancer pain relief is not adequate, "another strong opioid drug should be tried."
1990: The state of California passed the Intractable Pain Act, which stated that "no physician shall be punished for prescribing opioids for chronic pain."
1992: The Agency for Health Care Policy and Research (1992) released a guideline for aggressive pain treatment to alleviate post-surgery suffering.
1997: California enacted the Patient's Bill of Rights, officially supporting the use of opioids in treating noncancerous conditions.
1999: The American Pain Society (1999) and the Department of Veteran Affairs (2000) called for pain to be classified as a vital sign.
2000: The California Board of Registered Nursing (2000) required pain as one of the vital signs gathered during clinic intake. Nurses asking patients to rate their pain on a scale of one to ten has become a ritualized component of medical visits. The policy tasked nurses to take action if the patient's pain is beyond their comfort level.

3.1.2 Phase II: Transition (2003 to 2010)

Based on the statistics presented by the CDC and HHS, the US opioid prescription rates increased substantially during this phase, averaging 81.2 prescriptions for every 100 Americans. The policies that were "chaptered" – meaning, approved by policymakers – during this time may have started addressing issues on addiction, but there were also policies that made opioids more accessible in treating any kind of pain.

2004: California released Senate Bill 1838: The Alcohol and Drug Prevention Program, a blanket policy primarily focusing on addictive substances on a larger scale, targeting popular choices such as alcohol and marijuana. While the word narcotic was mentioned briefly, the policy neither mentioned nor addressed opioid addiction. That said, the policy was a declaration of the state's focus on fighting addiction and brought life to rehabilitation programs and centers.
2006: California amended the 1990 Intractable Pain Act: "A physician and surgeon may prescribe, dispense, or administer dangerous drugs or controlled substances for the treatment of pain, including, but not limited to, intractable

pain. No physician shall be subject to disciplinary action for prescribing, **dispensing**, or administering **dangerous drugs or controlled substances**." The insertion of "dangerous drugs" and the coordinating conjunction "or" right beside "controlled substance" twice in the policy imply some degree of equivalency.

3.1.3 Phase III: Opioid Epidemic (2011 to Present)

Ultimately, this era marks the beginning of a more deliberate and aggressive campaign against opioid addiction. The policies that came after 2011 were primarily focused on fighting the epidemic

2011: The CDC used the word "epidemic" to describe the state of opioid misuse in the country after deaths from accidental overdose exceeded fatalities from vehicular accidents (Centers for Disease Control and Prevention 2011).
2013: California turned the law enforcement tool, Controlled Substance Utilization Review and Evaluation System (CURES), into a prescription monitoring system.
2016: President Obama signed the Comprehensive Addiction Recovery Act (CARA), the first major federal legislation on addiction in 40 years and the most comprehensive effort undertaken to address the opioid epidemic.
2017: Physicians were required to consult CURES before prescribing opioids. The transition confirms that the opioid crisis is now predominantly a policy issue instead of a law enforcement concern.

This timeline allows us to understand where the sentiment towards opioids lies at certain points in its history. Clearly, opioids were seen as the solution to the harrowing pain epidemic, only to later become the problem needing to be solved. Figure 1 illustrates the rising opioid-related death rates in California through the three phases.

By paying attention to the emerging patterns in modal usage across the three phases, researchers can evaluate whether correlations exist between modal use and the events happening on the ground.

3.2 Modals

Policy documents are one of the most prominent and consequential outlets by which social issues are discussed (Fairclough 2003). Yet, as discussed earlier, there is a lack of research investigating policymakers' excessive use of modality

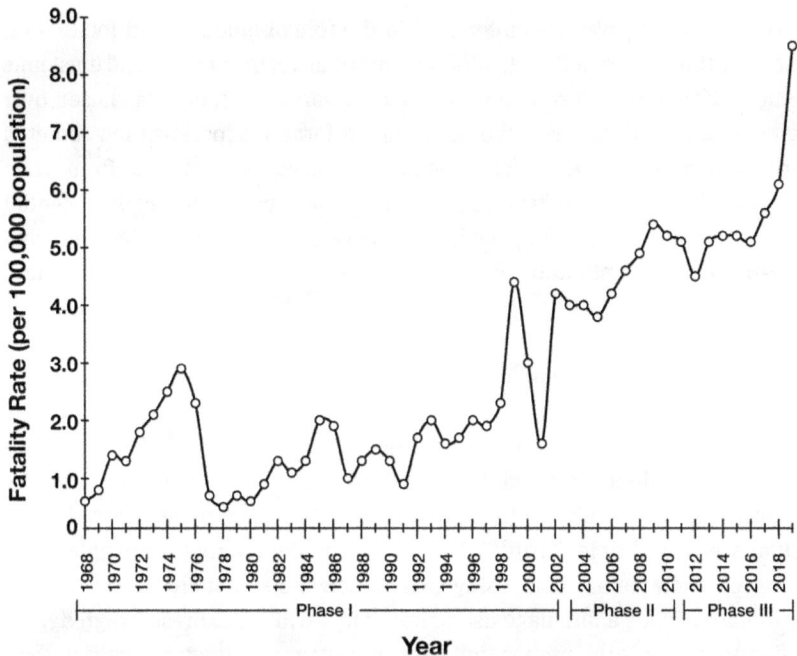

Figure 1: Number of opioid-related Fatalities in California from 1968–2019.[1]

in policies, despite its well-established potential for ambiguity (see Lyons, 1977). This section provides more context on how the polysemic nature of modals could result in varied interpretations of policies.

Modals have been commonly described in linguistics through their deontic (root or intrinsic) and epistemic (extrinsic) interpretations, as summarized in Table 2 (Coates 1983; Saeed 1997; Werth 1999; Kratzer 2012).

Table 2: Deontic and Epistemic Interpretations.

Modal Auxiliary	Deontic (Intrinsic)	Epistemic (Extrinsic)
can, could, may, might	permission, ability	possibility
must, should	obligation	necessity
will, would, shall	volition	prediction

---

[1] Crude rates, or death rates per 100,000 population, are used when age-adjusted rates are not available. Data was gathered from the CDC WONDER database. To generate the report for opioid-related fatalities, the following International Classification of Disease (ICD) codes had to be identified: ICD-8 E853.0 for 1970–1978; ICD-9 E850.0 for 1979–1998; ICD-10 underlying cause-of-death codes: X40–44, X60–64, X85, Y10–Y14 and multiple cause-of-death codes: T40.0- T40.4, and T40.6 for 1999–2018.

Thompson (2001) was also interested in the role of modality but focused on academic writing. He argued that, although informative, the deontic and epistemic distinction offers little information about why a particular modal is chosen over a long list of alternatives. Instead of focusing on form, his investigation centered primarily on the range of rhetorical functions thesis writers aim to perform when using modals. This chapter takes on a parallel approach by examining the potential range of functions performed by modals in the genre of policy drafting, allowing us to deepen our understanding of how language is used in constructing policies.

3.2.1 Modals as a reflection of local realities

In his study of modality within political discourse, Chilton (2004: 57–59) proposed a concept called the "modal axis," which states that people use modality to position themselves relative to their "truth," given the circumstances in that particular space and time. "Truth," here, could be the reality that people deem right or seek to frame as such. Using this model, the statement *"I will visit the doctor tomorrow"* has a language user employing "will" to express a high degree of confidence towards the proposition because visiting the doctor is right in their reality. Therefore, choosing a different modal, such as *may* – as in *"I may visit the doctor tomorrow"* – evokes a meaning that is farther from their truth. With modals as a grammatical feature that expresses force and realities, policymakers' modal choices could indicate their perceptions towards the severity of local issues and the actions they seek to address them. As such, the study presented renders the concepts of "modal axis" and "realities" into a policy perspective to propose that modals mirror the seriousness of local issues.

3.2.2 Modals as permissive and restrictive forces

In their discussion of speech acts and modality, Boyd and Thorne (1969) described modals, particularly those found in imperatives, as illocutionary forces that permit and lay obligations. Talmy's (1988) and Sweetser's (1990) later suggestions are in agreement, referring to modals as forces that "forbid or allow" and "restrict or permit," respectively. More recently, Chilton (2004) uses the terms "command" or "prohibit" to describe the same speech acts and argues that modal interpretation is contingent upon prevailing norms at the time of use. This study recontextualizes all speech acts mentioned into a more policy-oriented perspective; using the word "restrict" to refer to the forces that "forbid" or "prohibit" actions and "permissive" to refer to the forces that "allow" or "let." This study draws on modality's ability to communicate discourses intended to "prohibit" or "permit" particular courses of action to make sense of modality's potential role in policies.

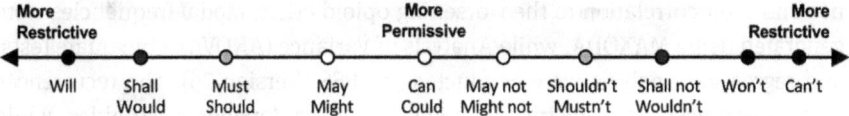

Figure 2: Modals arranged within a "Restrictiveness" and "Permissiveness" scale.[2]

Modals evoking the broadest range of possible interpretations are in the middle, while those intended to be perceived as most confining are found towards both ends. For example, a modal like "may" – with its speech acts that permit or allows – leaves stakeholders with the decision of acting upon a proposition, while modals like "must" carry an obligatory implication restricting stakeholders from certain actions. Thus, modals like "may" and "can" are permissive because they highlight the optionality of policies by allowing stakeholders to negotiate meaning from a broad range of possible interpretations, a quality distinct from restrictive counterparts like "shall" and "will."

In what follows, I discuss how corpus-based discourse analysis allows for both the quantitative and qualitative assessment of policies, helpful in uncovering the role of restrictive modals like "shall" and permissive modals like "may" in policies.

3.3 Methodologies

3.3.1 Creating the corpus

A total of 223 California opioid policies enacted between 1970 and 2019 were gathered from the state's online legislative archive using the following primary keywords: opioids, controlled substance, schedule II, and narcotic. Each result was reviewed so that all of the state's policies concerning opioids were included. The corpus was divided into a subcorpus of original policies and another of amendments to avoid conflating frequencies. In addition, the changes in all preceding and ensuing versions of amendments were carefully compared to account for newly added, deleted, and changed modals.

---

[2] Combines the findings from key pieces of literature – including Boyd and Thorne (1969), Chilton (2004), Saeed (1997), and Werth (1999) – on the restrictiveness and permissiveness of modality.

3.3.2 Quantitative analysis

Through frequency analysis, the study tracked restrictive and permissive modal use and their correlation to the worsening opioid crisis. Modal frequencies were generated using MAXQDA, while Analysis of Variance (ANOVA), chi-square tests, and regression analysis were conducted in SPSS (Version 26). The recurrences of both permissive and restrictive modals were the dependent variables, while "time" and "fatality rates" were the predictors representing the worsening crisis. Instead of the commonly used Euclidean distance, the study detects outliers using Mahalanobis distance because it accounts for variables with different units when analyzing correlation (Divjak and Fieller 2014).

3.3.3 Qualitative analysis

This analysis uses Van Dijk's (1999) context model framework, discussed above, as a starting point for the coding process. Specifically, the study focused on finding what Van Dijk referred to as (1) "participants" or the stakeholders to whom policies are addressed and (2) "actions" or the proposed measures to be enacted by the participants. Coders trained in discourse analysis finalized the specific categories as they emerged from the text – a process called axial coding (Strauss and Corbin 1997). This method allows for data to naturally fit into categories instead of forcing them into pre-determined groups that may not necessarily be accurate representations for the data. Tables 3 and 4 present the policy participants and actions that emerged from the sample study.

Table 3: Stakeholders addressed in California policies.

Policy Stakeholders	Example
1. State departments	Sectors of state government responsible for public health concerns. *i.e., California Department of Health Care Services, California Department of Justice, Drug Enforcement Administration, California Department of Social Services, California Health and Human Services Agency*
2. Health care providers	Medical providers prescribing opioids. *i.e., Physicians, Surgeons, Dentists, Pharmacists, Paramedics, EMT personnel, Nurses, Midwives, Emergency responders, Physician Assistants, Anaesthetists, etc.*

Table 4: Policy actions proposed in California policies.

Policy Action	Example
A. Handling pain	Policies stating who can administer opioids in health centers.
B. Prescribing guidelines	Policies on opioid prescribing, including dosage limitations and procedures for electronic prescriptions.
C. Education requirements	Mandatory certification requirement for physicians to take continuing education on the risks of opioids.
D. Oversight	Policies allowing the regulatory board to suspend licenses.
E. Diversion programs	Policies on establishing and running diversion programs.

Coding was done in tandem, which allowed coders to offer their expertise, discuss differences, and keep each other consistent (see Henry et al. 2020; Hood-Medland et al. 2021). The research is better served when everyone's explanation is heard instead of accepting the code most coders chose, especially in highly specialized discourses such as policies and medical consultations.

Finally, the patterns that emerged from the quantitative findings helped direct the discourse analysis component of this study towards particular modal usage that warrants a more detailed investigation. Specifically, this part of the study zooms in on the amendments in which only modal verbs were changed while the rest of the clause remained constant. As part of discourse analysis, "interpreting" and "explaining" the motivations behind policymakers' decisions to change modals concerning the severity of the crisis in the state sheds light on modality's function in policies.

3.4 Results and Discussions

3.4.1 Modal frequency

A frequency analysis of modal verbs in California opioid policies was conducted using MAXQDA, separating the original policies from their amendments to avoid conflation (Table 5).

Table 5 reveals that "shall" and "may" are the most used modals of California policymakers in framing the state's opioid policies. As presented in Figure 2, "shall" and "may" are found towards the restrictive and permissive sections of the modal scale, respectively. Therefore, the modal frequencies indicate a restrictive-permissive distinction taking place in the framing of policies. Referring back to Fillmore's (1975) frame theory, language users fill empty frames with the help of the information provided by the rest of the text paired with their knowledge of the situation. Language users also qualify the set of potential entries when

Table 5: Modal Frequencies in Original Policies and Amendments.[3]

	Original Policies n=30,013 words				Amendments n=80,095 words		
	Modal	Frequency per 100,000 words	Percentage		Modal	Frequency per 100,000 words	Percentage
1	shall	1586.0	70.8	1	shall	1644.3	74.1
2	may	509.8	22.8	2	may	454.5	20.5
3	can	93.3	4.2	3	will	47.4	2.1
4	will	20.0	0.9	4	would	42.5	1.9
5	would	13.3	0.6	5	can	21.2	1.0
6	could	6.7	0.3	6	should	8.7	0.4
6	should	6.7	0.3	7	must	1.3	0.1
7	might	3.3	0.2	0	could	0.0	0.0
0	must	0.0	0.0	0	might	0.0	0.0

deciding which lexical item best fits the frame. The frequency analysis shows that policymakers satisfy empty modal frames by overwhelmingly using "shall" over any of its restrictive alternatives like "should" or "must" and by repeatedly picking "may" instead of other permissive options such as "can" and "might." Such glaring patterns suggest that policymakers find it most appropriate to frame "restrictive" and "permissive" propositions with "shall" and "may," respectively.

3.4.2 Modal distribution

The study uses "time" and "fatality rates" to represent the worsening crisis as the issue continues to be increasingly fraught (Torres, Henry, and Ramanathan 2020) and opioid-related fatalities continue to rise in California. The ANOVA and regression analysis, with P values ≤ 0.05 considered statistically meaningful, show that time has a significant positive correlation with the frequency of restrictive modals at $p<0.05$ and a non-significant correlation with the increase in permissive modals at $p<0.05$ (Figure 3). Note that each modal would have appeared in a unique policy clause; therefore, the frequency of restrictive or permissive modal is synonymous with the number of restrictive and permissive clauses. The positive correlation is also supported by the gap between the regression coefficients of restrictive ($\beta=.774$) and permissive ($\beta=.159$) clauses, which means

---

[3] Frequency values were calculated using MAXQDA, and Frequencies are relative to every 100,000 words to balance the uneven subcorpus (see Baker 2006). There are a total of 97 original policies and 126 amendments.

restrictive clauses significantly increase five times more than permissive clauses each year.

Similarly, the number of fatal cases has a significant positive correlation with the increase in restrictive modals at p<0.05 and a non-significant correlation with the increase in permissive modals at p<0.05. The results of the outlier test using Mahalanobis distance, with a chi-square ($\chi2$) cut off of p<0.01, revealed one restrictive and two permissive outliers, all of which were insignificant to the results.

In what follows, I focus on amended policies to examine the changes in modal usage between the original and succeeding versions of the same policy.

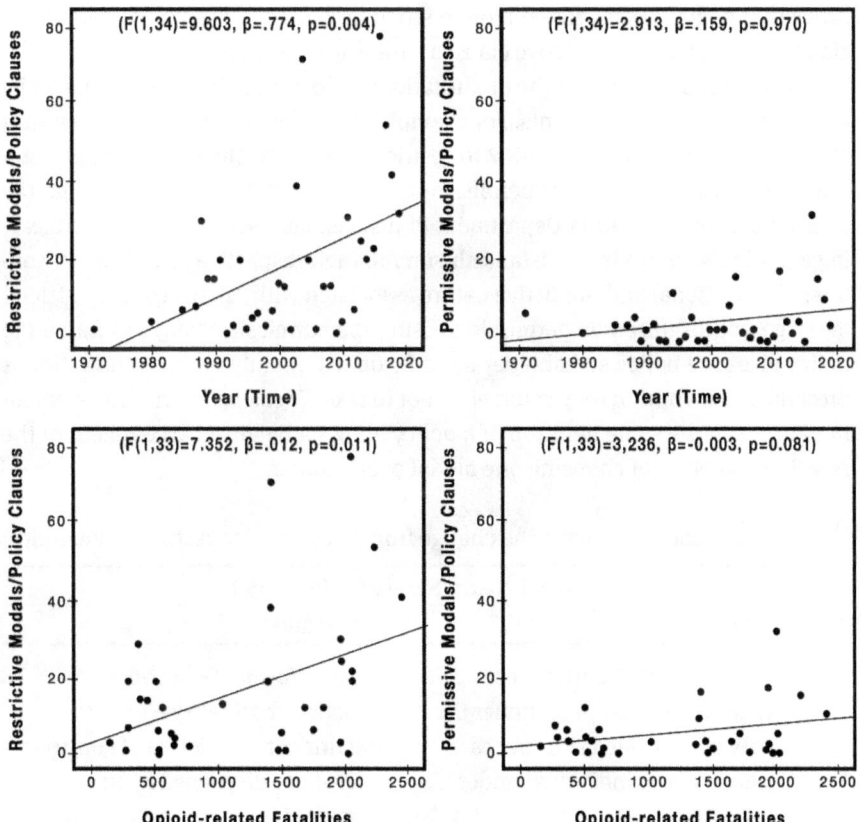

Figure 3: Number of restrictive (left) and permissive (right) modals/clauses across time and fatality rates.

3.4.3 Modal shifts in amendments

Amendments could take the form of adding or deleting provisions as well as reword already existing ones. Thus, these modifications may result in changes in modal frequency. After accounting for all the unique modal changes, amendments can either be a more restrictive or permissive version of the policy. ANOVA and regression analysis revealed a strong association between time and the increase in stricter amendments at $p<0.05$ ($F(1,20)=14.541$, $p=0.01$) and an insignificant association between time and the increase in permissive amendments at $p<0.05$ ($F(1,7)=0.370$, $p=.562$). The standardized regression coefficients for more restrictive ($\beta=.649$) and more permissive ($\beta=-0.224$) amendments similarly prove that policymakers added more restrictive clauses, erased more permissive clauses, or amended permissive clauses with restrictive ones.

Even more striking than the quantitative results are the findings from the discourse analysis of amendments. For example, the following excerpt shows a shift from permissive modality in 2002 to restrictive in 2013. The deontic interpretation associated with "may" is permission. Thus, the 2002 policy denotes that the stakeholder, the California Department of Justice, has the discretion over releasing a patient's controlled substance history to their respective physician. In contrast, the volitional and predictive nature associated with "shall" coveys a stricter message not disguised as permission. Using the permissive "may" to frame the policy gives the policy stakeholder more flexibility, mainly because the action is presented as an option they could elect not to take. Focusing on the only element that differs in the same iteration of a policy allows a balanced assessment of the possible outcomes of choosing one modal over another.

(1) An amendment showing the change from permissive to restrictive modality[4]

Health and Safety Code 11165.1	
2002 [Phase I]	**2013 [Phase III]**
The [California] Department of Justice **may** release to that practitioner the history of controlled substances dispensed to an individual under his or her care ...	The [California] Department of Justice **shall** release to that practitioner the history of controlled substances dispensed to an individual under his or her care ...

---

[4] The statute was clipped for brevity. The rest of the content can be retrieved from the internet through California's legislation website.

Fillmore's (1975) "frames" and Chilton's (2004) "modal axis" frameworks taught us that language users fill empty frames using the best-fit exemplar that adequately represents their reality at that particular point in time. Similarly, discourse analysis assumes that deliberate linguistic events – such as going through the trouble of writing, debating, and voting on "amendment resolutions" only to change a single word – cannot be accidental. Rather, the change must be necessary or meaningful enough for the motivations behind the amendment to make sense. When taken all together, discourse analysis and the frameworks that inform it suggest that the increased use of the restrictive "shall" is indicative of a shift in the policymaker's reality, one that can only be addressed or satisfied if "may" were to be replaced by "shall."

As discussed earlier, policy researchers – such as Levinson, Sutton, and Winstead (2009) and Hornberger and Johnson (2007) – emphasized that policies are meant to be suggestive, and that enactment is dependent on the interpretation and decisions of the arbiters or stakeholders to whom policies are addressed. The following example provides insight as to how modals could highlight or hide the suggestive intent of policies.

(2) An example of modal amendment from permissive to restrictive[5]

Health and Safety Code 11165.5	
2003 [Phase I]	**2011 [Phase III]**
The [California] department of justice **may** revoke its approval of a security printer for a violation of this division [mishandling/unlawful production of prescription slips]	The [California] department of justice **shall** revoke its approval of a security printer for a violation of this division [mishandling/unlawful production of prescription slips]

The difference between the two versions in (2) is that the permissive "may" give the state's justice department more space to negotiate the various interpretations implied by the policy before deciding how they would like to operate. This same space becomes narrower in the 2011 version because "shall" (a) highlights a mandatory rather than suggestive intent, (b) elicits more definitive outcomes, and (c) de-emphasizes or downplays a policy's suggestive and interpretive property.

---

5 Security printers refer to entities that supply printouts of high-value documents such as identifications and prescription slips.

The following excerpt shows an amendment to the other direction, from a policy that started as prohibitive and later amended to be permissive.

(3) An amendment showing the change from restrictive to permissive modality[6]

Business and Professions Code 2746.51	
1991 [Phase I]	**2001 [Phase I]**
Drugs furnished by a certified nurse-midwife **shall not** include controlled substances...	Drugs furnished by a certified nurse-midwife **may** include controlled substances...

Example (3) affirms the role of modality as a reflection of the locality's current state. Policies in the nineties were restrictive of what nurse-midwives can do without an attending physician, including the furnishing of controlled substances, as shown in the example above. With the advancement in workplace training as well as demands to address pain, nurse-midwives were eventually allowed to furnish opioids without supervision, as shown in the 2001 amendment of "shall not" to "may."

The policy went from framing the distribution of opioids as a strongly prohibited action to being at the discretion of nurse-midwives. The modal change grants stakeholders some space to renegotiate whether to enact the policy. Suffice to say, modality can broaden or limit the range of possible actions stakeholders could take.

(4) An amendment showing a change in modality from slightly permissive to restrictive[7]

Business and Professions Code 3502.1	
1994 [Phase I]	**2017 [Phase III]**
A physician assistant **may not** prescribe controlled substances without a physician's order.	A physician assistant **shall not** prescribe controlled substances without a physician's order.

---

6 Opioids are controlled substances. This statute was shortened for brevity; however, the changes do not affect the analysis. The rest of the content can be retrieved from the internet through California's legislation website.

7 The statute was shortened for brevity, and the changes do not affect the analysis. The rest of the content can be retrieved from the internet through California's legislation website.

"May" can convey a broader range of interpretation than "shall" because the modal ambiguously implies consent, leaving stakeholders with the choice to interpret the proposition as an action they "may" or "may not" accomplish. Example (4) offers a different picture because the 1994 version of the policy specifies the "not" instead of only using "may." "May not" is more precise in the sense that it defines part of may's ambiguity. Because the policymakers choose "may not," they are not providing the overt consent that "may" evokes, signaling that the action's completion could violate the proposition. While "may" and "may not" have slight differences, they are still more permissive than "shall" and "shall not." In fact, changing from "may not" to "shall not" in the 2017 amendment suggest that policymakers agree that both differ. The change implies that the restriction "may not" evoked was inadequate at the time. As local policymakers, their knowledge of the severity of the opioid crisis within their constituency makes "shall not" a more fitting choice called for by their immediate environment. The choice of "shall not" is an overt denial of permission that further minimizes what was already a weak semantic expression of possibility evoked by "may not."

These examples offer tangible evidence that appends a policy perspective to Talmy (1988) and Sweetser's (1990) understanding of modality as forces that "stops" or "allows." The analysis in this section opens up the idea of modals as grammatical features that "limit" or "broaden" the interpretive spaces in which policy stakeholders function. Moreover, the specific targeting of modals indicates that policymakers pay attention to modality and see their significance in policy framing relative to the events happening on the ground.

The use of modal verbs indicates the presence of subjects or agents and predicates or actions. The idea that modality denotes restrictions or permissions begs the question of the intended recipients of restrictive policies and the particular actions for which restrictive modality are used. The following section outlines how the sample study answers this question.

3.4.4 Patterns of modal use

Informed by Van Dijk's (1999) context model framework (see Table 1), this section presents the frequency results from the coding process aimed at answering "who and what are these policies for?" Specifically, the policy stakeholders and actions associated with each restrictive and permissive modal were identified to understand the context in which these policies were written and assess whether patterns emerge from them. Table 6 shows the distribution of restrictive and permissive modals across the three phases of the opioid crisis.

Table 6: Distribution of restrictive and permissive policies across the three phases of opioid crisis.

	Restrictive policies		Permissive policies	
	State employees	Health care provider	State employees	Health care provider
Phase I: p=0.003	35%	65%	56%	43%
Phase II: p=0.049	46%	54%	58%	42%
Phase III: p=0.599	59%	41%	61%	38%

A chi-square test revealed that a significant correlation at p<0.05 exists between the stakeholder and the modal used during Phases 1 and 2. The results denote a higher likelihood for stricter opioid policies directed towards health care providers during the first two phases when opioid was known as the effective painkiller that solved the country's pain crisis. The insignificant distribution of restrictive and permissive policies during the third phase means that restrictive policies no longer targeted health care workers as the distribution is defined by chance. The results also suggest that policymakers initially considered opioid-related issues as concerns bound within hospital walls but later changed their perspectives as state department employees become more active participants in the state's opioid narrative.

Table 7: Policy actions and their percentage share of restrictive policies.

Policy Action	Share of restrictive policies (change from previous phase)					
	Phase I	Phase II		Phase III		
A. Handling pain	11.7%	8.1%	(−3.6 %)	4.2%	(−3.9%)
B. Prescribing guidelines	59%	47.6%	(−11.4%)	42.8%	(−4.8%)
C. Education requirements	18.6%	14.0%	(−4.6%)	12.0%	(−2.0%)
D. Oversight	4.8%	4.4%	(−0.4%)	6.6%	(+2.2%)
E. Diversion programs	5.9%	25.8%	(+19.9%)	34.4%	(+8.6%)

Policies framed using restrictive modals hint at the actions policymakers consider to be priorities at that particular time. The findings in Table 7 show the shifting focus of restrictive policies across the three phases. Policy actions concerning (A) handling pain, (B) opioid prescribing guidelines, and (C) learning about opioids had a higher share during Phase I, when the problem in the state was the lack of pain treatment. The share of the same three policy categories dwindled in the succeeding phases, as the state's problem transitioned to the worsening opioid crisis, as shown by the percentage change in parenthesis. Meanwhile, the shares of restrictive policies tackling (D) oversight and (E) diversion showed growth from Phase I to Phase III – when opioid prescription rates and overdoses skyrocketed – validating the claim that the circumstances in which restrictive modality is employed mirror the needs of the community. In this case, actions framed with restrictive modality index high importance.

Of course, the sample study is not without its limitations, including relying on proxies such as time and fatality rates to quantify the worsening crisis. Moreover, the restrictive and permissive framework is not intended to be a definitive categorization of the core roles modal auxiliaries serve in policies, as the corpus is limited to a particular locality, and discourse analysis, while based on overt palpable evidence, is intended to be inferential (Wodak 2004).

3.5 Conclusion of the sample study

The findings suggest two potential functions of modals in policies: (i) to mirror or call attention to the gravity of the issues happening on the ground, and (ii) reconfigure the interpretive spaces in which stakeholders operate. The frequency analysis of the corpus revealed "shall" and "may" as the most occurring modal verbs, suggesting a restrictive-permissive distinction existing in California opioid policies. The quantitative findings further proved that the growing use of restrictive modality has a positive correlation to the worsening crisis. Meanwhile, a close analysis of the amendments in which only modals were changed suggest that policymakers choose between restrictive and permissive modality based on the option they believe best satisfies the pressing concerns of the time. In other words, having permissive and restrictive modals be in complementary distribution is indicative that modal choices carry a particular significance to policymakers. Moreover, having either permissive or restrictive occupy the same frame means the two serve the same discourse functions; that is, both reflect the gravity of local realities and both shape policy interpretation, albeit in different directions. As Thompson (2001: 151) points out, paying attention to modal usage "reveals something of the choices that are available" in expressing meanings and "something of the way written discourse is constructed."

The enactment of policies is the culmination of a complex process that includes parsing modals alongside other grammatical features in the policy. I refer to these agentive spaces, where stakeholders negotiate the meanings they make out of the collective semantic prosody evoked by policies, as "interpretive spaces." An alternative term could have been "implementational spaces," used by Hornberger and Johnson (2007). However, the concept of interpretive spaces accounts for the meaning-making process more than it addresses how actions are accomplished. In this sense, implementational space is the holistic processing of policies, while interpretive is the precursor, if not an aggregate, of a more comprehensive implementational space. In other words, interpretive spaces are concerned with "how policies are understood" while implementational spaces refer to "how one's interpretation is put into action." Paying attention to modality has significant implications for policy implementation. If policymakers adapt the proper modal to align with their desired outcomes, then they can attenuate the extent to which interpretive spaces unfold, which, in turn, influences the implementational spaces where stakeholders enact policies.

Nonetheless, the approach employed in this study saves policymakers and researchers valuable time examining the policies of pertinent local issues. The mining of modals from a complete and well-defined corpus can: (i) provide researchers and policymakers an overview of the general tone of policies, as either restrictive or permissive, (ii) reveal the entities to whom most restrictive and permissive policies are addressed, and (iii) identify the actions policymakers have implemented thus far. These can inform future amendments and policy planning when addressing certain local concerns.

4 Chapter conclusion

This chapter provides a cogent applied linguistic framework for extending LPP research to include scholarship analyzing the language of policies through corpus-based discourse analysis. The sample study shows that the synergy between quantitative and qualitative approaches results in a robust examination of policy discourse, an approach that can be extended further to data of various types and sizes. Finally, this chapter proves that corpus-based discourse analysis carries heuristic value for applied linguists and other researchers who recognize the weight of language choices within societies.

References

Agency for Health Care Policy and Research. 1992. *Acute pain management: operative or medical procedures and trauma*. Rockville, Md.: U.S. Dept. of Health and Human Services, Public Health Service, Agency for Health Care Policy and Research.
Ainsworth-Vaughn, Nancy. 1998. *Claiming power in doctor-patient talk*. New York: Oxford University Press.
American Pain Society. 1999. *Guideline for the management of acute and chronic pain in sickle cell disease*. American Pain Society.
Asprey, Michele M. 1992. Shall must go. *Scribes Journal of Legal Writing* 3. 79–84.
Baker, Paul. 2006. *Using corpora in discourse analysis*. A&C Black.
Ball, Stephen J. 1990. *Politics and policy making in education : explorations in policy sociology*. London; New York: Routledge.
Bhatia, Vijay, John Flowerdew & Rodney H. Jones (eds.). 2008. *Advances in discourse studies*. Routledge.
Boyd, Julian & J. P. Thorne. 1969. The semantics of modal verbs. *Journal of Linguistics* 5(1). 57–74. https://doi.org/10.1017/S002222670000205X.
California Board of Registered Nursing. 2000. *The BRN Report*. California: California Board of Registered Nursing. https://www.rn.ca.gov/pdfs/forms/brn500.pdf (8 April, 2019).
Caudill-Slosberg, Margaret A., Lisa M. Schwartz & Steven Woloshin. 2004. Office visits and analgesic prescriptions for musculoskeletal pain in US: 1980 vs. 2000. *Pain* 109(3). 514–519.
Centers for Disease Control and Prevention. 2011. *Prescription painkiller overdoses at epidemic levels*. Press Release. https://www.cdc.gov/media/releases/2011/p1101_flu_pain_killer_overdose.html (26 April, 2019).
Chilton, Paul A. 2004. *Analysing political discourse: theory and practice*. London; New York: Routledge.
Coates, Jennifer. 1983. The semantics of the modal auxiliaries (Croom Helm Linguistics Series). *London, Sydney & Dover, NH: Croom Helm*.
Das Gupta, Jyotirindra. 1970. *Language Conflict and National Development: Group Politics and National Language Policy in India*. Vol. 5. Univ of California Press.
Davis, Kathryn A. 1999. The sociopolitical dynamics of indigenous language maintenance and loss: A framework for language policy and planning. In Thom Huebner & Kathryn A. Davis (eds.), *Sociopolitical perspectives on language policy and planning in the USA*, 67–97. Amsterdam/Philadelphia: John Benjamins Publishing Company.
Department of Veterans Affairs. 2000. Pain as the 5th vital sign toolkit. *Washington, DC: Department of Veterans Affairs*.
Divjak, Dagmar & Nick Fieller. 2014. Cluster analysis: Finding structure in linguistic data. In Dylan Glynn & Justyna A. Robinson (eds.), *Corpus methods for semantics: Quantitative studies in polysemy and synonymy* (Human Cognitive Processing), vol. 43, 405–441. Amsterdam: John Benjamins Publishing Company. https://doi.org/10.1075/hcp.43.16div. https://benjamins.com/catalog/hcp.43.16div (22 June, 2021).
Fairclough, Norman. 2003. *Analysing discourse: Textual analysis for social research*. Psychology Press.
Fillmore, Charles J. 1975. An alternative to checklist theories of meaning. In *Annual Meeting of the Berkeley Linguistics Society*, vol. 1, 123–131.

Fillmore, Charles J. 1976. Frame semantics and the nature of language. *Annals of the New York Academy of Sciences* 280(1). 20–32.
Fishman, Joshua A., Charles Albert Ferguson & Jyotirindra Das Gupta. 1968. *Language problems of developing nations.* Wiley New York.
Flowerdew, Lynne. 2008. Corpora and context in professional writing. In Vijay Kumar Bhatia, John Flowerdew & Rodney H. Jones (eds.), *Advances in discourse studies*, 115–127. Routledge.
Fowler, Roger (ed.). 1979. *Language and control.* London: Routledge & Kegan Paul.
Gales, Tammy. 2009. 'Diversity' as enacted in US immigration politics and law: a corpus-based approach. *Discourse & Society.* SAGE Publications Ltd 20(2). 223–240. https://doi.org/10.1177/0957926508099003.
Garzone, Giuliana. 2013. Variation in the use of modality in legislative texts: Focus on shall. *Journal of Pragmatics* 57. 68–81. https://doi.org/10.1016/j.pragma.2013.07.008.
Goodnow, Frank J. 2017. *Politics and Administration: A Study in Government.* Routledge.
Hacquard, Valentina. 2016. Modals: meaning categories? In Joanna Błaszczak, Anastasia Giannakidou, Dorota Klimek-Jankowska & Krzysztof Migdalski (eds.), *Mood, aspect, modality revisited: new answers to old questions*, 45–74. Chicago London: The University of Chicago Press.
Haugen, Einar. 1959. Planning for a standard language in modern Norway. *Anthropological linguistics* 8–21.
Haugen, Einar. 1983. The implementation of corpus planning: Theory and practice. *Progress in language planning: International perspectives* 31. 269–290.
Henry, Stephen G., Anne Elizabeth Clark White, Elizabeth M. Magnan, Eve Angeline Hood-Medland, Melissa Gosdin, Richard L. Kravitz, Peter Joseph Torres & Jennifer Gerwing. 2020. Making the most of video recorded clinical encounters: Optimizing impact and productivity through interdisciplinary teamwork. *Patient Education and Counseling* 103(10). 2178–2184. https://doi.org/10.1016/j.pec.2020.06.005.
Higgins, Christina. 2010. Discursive enactments of the World Health Organization's policies: Competing cultural models in Tanzanian HIV/AIDS prevention. *Language Policy* 9(1). 65. https://doi.org/10.1007/s10993-009-9151-x.
Hood-Medland, Eve Angeline, Anne EC White, Richard L. Kravitz & Stephen G. Henry. 2021. Agenda setting and visit openings in primary care visits involving patients taking opioids for chronic pain. *BMC Family Practice.* BioMed Central 22(1). 1–11. https://doi.org/10.1186/s12875-020-01317-4.
Hornberger, Nancy H. 1998. Language policy, language education, language rights: Indigenous, immigrant, and international perspectives. *Language in society* 27(4). 439–458.
Hornberger, Nancy H. & David Cassels Johnson. 2007. Slicing the onion ethnographically: Layers and spaces in multilingual language education policy and practice. *Tesol Quarterly* 41(3). 509–532.
Institute of Medicine. 1988. *The Future of Public Health.* Washington, DC: The National Academies Press. https://doi.org/10.17226/1091. https://www.nap.edu/catalog/1091/the-future-of-public-health.
Johnson, David Cassels & Rebecca Freeman. 2010. Appropriating language policy on the local level: Working the spaces for bilingual education. In *Negotiating language policies in schools*, 27–45. Routledge.
Johnson, Eric J. 2012. Arbitrating repression: language policy and education in Arizona. *Language and Education* 26(1). 53–76. https://doi.org/10.1080/09500782.2011.615936.

Kratzer, Angelika. 2012. *Modals and conditionals: New and revised perspectives*. Vol. 36. Oxford University Press.
Levinson, Bradley AU, Margaret Sutton & Teresa Winstead. 2009. Education policy as a practice of power: Theoretical tools, ethnographic methods, democratic options. *Educational policy*. SAGE Publications Sage CA: Los Angeles, CA 23(6). 767–795.
Lyons, John. 1977. *Semantics (Vol. 2)*. Cambridge [England]; New York: Cambridge University Press.
Martinez, Glenn. 2008. Language-in-healthcare policy, interaction patterns, and unequal care on the US-Mexico border. *Language Policy* 7(4). 345–363.
Menken, Kate & Ofelia García. 2010. *Negotiating language education policies: Educators as policymakers*. Routledge.
Noss, Richard B. 1967. *Language policy and higher education*. Unesco and the International Association of Universities.
Partington, Alan. 2003. *The linguistics of political argument: The spin-doctor and the wolf-pack at the White House*. Routledge.
Partington, Alan. 2008. The armchair and the machine: Corpus-assisted discourse research. *Corpora for university language teachers*. Peter Lang Bern 74. 95–118.
Pérez, Bertha & Amy Nordlander. 2004. Making decisions about literacy instructional practices. *Sociocultural contexts of language and literacy*. Lawrence Erlbaum Associates 2. 277–308.
Portner, Paul. 2009. *Modality*. Vol. 1. Oxford University Press.
Ramanathan, Vaidehi. 2009. *Bodies and language: Health, ailments, disabilities*. Multilingual Matters.
Ramanathan, Vaidehi. 2010. Introduction to thematic issue: language policies and health. *Language Policy* 9(1). 1–7. https://doi.org/10.1007/s10993-009-9154-7.
Ramanathan, Vaidehi & Brian Morgan. 2007. TESOL and policy enactments: Perspectives from practice. *Tesol Quarterly* 41(3). 447–463.
Ricento, Thomas K & Nancy H. Hornberger. 1996. Unpeeling the onion: Language planning and policy and the ELT professional. *Tesol Quarterly* 30(3). 401–427.
Saeed, John I. 1997. *Semantics*. Oxford; Malden, Mass.: Blackwell Publishers.
Sarangi, Srikant & Celia Roberts. 2008. *Talk, work and institutional order: Discourse in medical, mediation and management settings*. Vol. 1. Walter de Gruyter.
Schuster, Michal, Irit Elroy & Ido Elmakais. 2017. We are lost: measuring the accessibility of signage in public general hospitals. *Language Policy* 16(1). 23–38. https://doi.org/10.1007/s10993-015-9400-0.
Strauss, Anselm L. & Juliet M. Corbin (eds.). 1997. *Grounded theory in practice*. Thousand Oaks, Calif.: Sage Publ.
Stritikus, Tom & AnnMarie Wiese. 2006. Reassessing the role of ethnographic methods in education policy research: Implementing bilingual education policy at local levels. *Teachers College Record* 108(6). 1106–1131.
Stubbs, Michael. 2001. *Words and phrases: Corpus studies of lexical semantics*. Blackwell publishers Oxford.
Sweetser, Eve. 1990. *From etymology to pragmatics: metaphorical and cultural aspects of semantic structure*. Cambridge [England]; New York: Cambridge University Press.
Talmy, Leonard. 1988. Force dynamics in language and cognition. *Cognitive science* 12(1). 49–100.

Thompson, Paul. 2001. *A pedagogically-motivated corpus-based examination of PhD theses: macrostructure, citation practices and uses of modal verbs*. Reading, UK: University of Reading.

Torres, Peter Joseph, Stephen G. Henry & Vaidehi Ramanathan. 2020. Let's talk about pain and opioids: Low pitch and creak in medical consultations. *Discourse Studies*. SAGE Publications Sage UK: London, England 22(2). 174–204. https://doi.org/10.1177/1461445619893796.

Torres, Peter Joseph. 2021. "The Role of Modals in Policies: The US Opioid Crisis as a Case Study". *Applied Corpus Linguistics*. https://doi.org/10.1016/j.acorp.2021.100008.

Van Dijk, Teun A. 1999. Context models in discourse processing. *The construction of mental representations during reading* 123–148.

Werth, Paul. 1999. *Text worlds: representing conceptual space in discourse*. Harlow: Longman.

Wodak, Ruth. 2004. Critical Discourse Analysis. In Clive Seale, David Silverman, Jaber F. Gubrium & Giampietro Gobo (eds.), *Qualitative Research Practice: Concise Paperback Edition*, 186–201. SAGE Publications.

Wodak, Ruth. 2006. Linguistic analyses in language policies. In Thomas Ricento (ed.), *An introduction to language policy: Theory and method* (Language and Social Change 1), 170–193. Oxford: Blackwell Publishing.

World Health Organization. 1986. *Cancer Pain Relief*. Geneva: World Health Organization.

Brett A. Diaz
Chapter 6
Discourses at work in elderly, health policy communication: Uncovering aspects of semantic preference and prosody in the rural opioid epidemic

1 Introduction

1.1 The context

In the summers of 2017 and 2018, I conducted initial one-on-one conversations with several directors of rural, older adult health services agencies to learn about the experiences of rural people as they enter the later stages of their lives. However, what began as an ethnographic study about aging in rural contexts quickly turned to the issue of opioids in those contexts. Directors, independently, focused on the ravages of opioids in their population, and the unique challenges they experienced as they pivoted to face an unexpected and rampant health crisis. I would subsequently learn that while overdoses were certainly an issue in their communities overall, from the perspectives of these directors, the sociocultural effects of the opioid epidemic were the major figure of opioids in rural, elderly lives. Crucial to this chapter, the directors underscored that the influence of opioids on their populations remains under-addressed or misunderstood by the current slate of older adult services policies. For instance, older people are common sources of opioids to family because of over-prescription. This issue alone, to say nothing of other phenomena, has deleterious effects on family bonds via drug diversion, and leads to emotional and bodily abuse, neither of which are immediately apparent. These behaviors are in addition to dramatically increased financial exploitation, another more visible issue. Further, current policies did not adequately take into account the modern realities of protective services inves-

---

Acknowledgements: Marika K. Hall for her assistance in semantic prosody analysis, and to the committee members during my dissertation, without whom this chapter would certainly have turned out very differently.

Brett A. Diaz, The Wilson Centre, University of Toronto; Centre for Faculty Development, Unity Health Toronto

https://doi.org/10.1515/9783110744804-007

tigations, such as substantial changes in financial institutions regarding obtaining records, dramatic increases in caseloads, and physical, emotional, and social abuse – all of which present difficulties for the timeframes set out in the protective services code. The misalignment between the current policies and claims by these agents represented evidence of policy implementation breakdown.

The devastation of opioid-related overdoses looms large in public consciousness, and in few places larger than Pennsylvania. According to the National Institute on Drug Abuse (2018), in Pennsylvania in 2016 there were 2,235 opioid-related overdose deaths, or 18.5 deaths per 100,000 persons. The national average was 13.5. Between 2015 and 2016, rural counties saw a 42% increase in overdoses, compared to 34% for urban counties, representing a disproportionate increase of 25% (National Institute on Drug Abuse 2017). Health interventions have focused on Naloxone prescription, resulting in emergency services administering 3,705 doses state wide in 2017, of which only 422 doses were in rural counties (*The Pennsylvania Opioid Data Dashboard*). Making naloxone readily available is an essential tactic in the strategy against the damaging effects of opioids, and cannot be discounted. Yet, rural individuals often face additional challenges in access and social services (e.g., fewer services, greater distances, less reliable roadways). Crucially, for older people there is also loss of physical ability, reduced social visibility, and reliance on kin or close friends for security. Hence, the opioid crisis affects the rural older population in different ways than even young or middle-aged individuals in rural areas, and of course policy should be strategically responsive to the specific needs of different populations. As an example, the Pennsylvania Department of Aging's 2016–2017 report on older adult protective services reported increasing financial exploitation and abuse as key parts of the opioid epidemic. Ideally then, at successive levels of implementation, policy language should convince and motivate administrators of rural, older adult services agencies and their protective services case managers to address specific dimensions of local needs (Majone 1989) – in this case, the ways in which the opioid crisis tears the social fabric of intergenerational relations in rural society, and policy.

Through my conversations with health services agents and an initial review of current policies, it became immediately apparent to me that there was a socially-grounded inconsistency in the implementation pathway. Official policies portrayed aging and older adult health needs in one way, through one channel of *how* and *why policy gets done*. And yet, these agents seemingly represented different positions, or different beliefs, about those same *how* and *why* questions for their populations. This observation led me to the question, how do values, goals, and cultural beliefs interact between rural, older adult health services and official policy documents, as they confront the ravages of the opioid epidemic?

1.2 Health policy implementation

Policy implementation is commonly studied as phenomena of policy transmission and compliance (Alexander 1985; Bauer et al. 2015; Bowen and Zwi 2005; Sallis, Bauman, and Pratt 1998; Watt, Sword, and Krueger 2005). For example, Brownson et al. (1997) define policies as "those laws, regulations, formal and informal rules and understandings that are adopted on a collective basis to guide individual and collective behavior," citing Schmid et al. (1995). They further define interventions as "measures that alter or control . . . the environment" (735). Policies are then objects, and interventions the activities meant to alter an environment to which policy will be applied. A methodological approach informed by this notion would view sites of health services as simple interventional spaces, and the people recipients of a composite item called a policy. This would mean that health policy is not a social-interactional, distributed activity. In the area of health policy implementation (HPI) research, research that focuses directly on the social aspects of implementation is sparse. At least, such research is sparse by comparison to work that takes implementation to be a process by which mandates, documents, and procedures etcetera are transmitted to sites of implementation to be carried out. I understand frameworks of these types as forming "policy as object" models. In this way, researchers frequently treat interventions as packaged activities that conform or do not conform to policy, rather than enacted interventions in collaborative, socially dynamic places.

Many frameworks of policy implementation research nonetheless refer to the impact of individual beliefs, organizational culture, and interpersonal relationships (Damschroder et al. 2009; Sabatier 1988). Yet, in many cases, sources still seem to adhere to a belief in policy as object. In contrast to what could be considered prevailing approaches in scholarship, some authors have found that policy documents, and otherwise static objects, are often ideologically reorganized and repurposed to suit situational needs (Kreindler 2016; Wimmelmann 2019). Perhaps most importantly, those situational needs were defined and chosen by the health policy professionals. To wit, policies are not merely objects, but activities that are shaped and reshaped by the individuals in-context.

1.2.1 Health policy & beliefs

Despite the predominance of linear, policy-as-object models of implementation (Bowen and Zwi 2005), health policies are not merely monolithic textual objects and activity modules distributed by governmental organizations. Rather, they are conceptually diverse operations acted on and enacted by people (Russell et al.

2008; Sabatier 1986). Where policies and service provision meet, people must manage their life experiences, professional expectations, political obligations, and so on, in present social environments. In simple terms, providers have beliefs that undergird their respective decisions.

One framework, the Advocacy Coalition Framework (ACF) introduced by Paul Sabatier (Sabatier 1988; Sabatier and Weible 2007; Weible, Sabatier, and McQueen 2009), positions policies as beliefs held by different actors, coalitions, and their subsystems, in the policy implementation process. Subsystems are defined by their functional dimension or area of concern within coalitions (e.g., older adult health services), and their territorial zone (e.g., rural counties in Pennsylvania). Subsystems include not just organizations, but the people that compose those organizations, such as the directors, caseworkers, and other agents that carry out subsystem activities. Beliefs fall into hierarchically structured categories, descending in scope: (1) core beliefs, (2) core policy beliefs, and (3) secondary beliefs. Core beliefs are deeply held, normative beliefs. Core beliefs are structured by things such as religion, cultural practices etcetera, and undergird the value systems that form coalitions' identities. Core policy beliefs are smaller in scope, and focused on policy preferences and decision-making. Core policy beliefs are generally subsystem-wide, and highly salient. Secondary beliefs are not subsystem-wide and tend to focus on things such as budgetary considerations, staffing decisions, and so on. The three belief types intersect in the implementation process. Normative values influence the ways that agents understand the purposes of their coalitions and subsystems, and thus what the purpose of policies should be. Conversely, policy values shape the applicable form that core values take in the policies, what their goals and ends can feasibly be, and how to achieve them.

1.3 Stance-taking: Capturing the expression of beliefs

Discursive events are often central to the activities that structure human relationships, social roles, and the organizational constraints that guide our everyday lives. Using socioculturally pertinent language is arguably the indispensable means of enacting social relations among the people that constitute organizations (Silverstein 1993: 34). Discourse, as a universal human function for making sense in the world (Ochs 1996; Silverstein 1976), is presumably under way wherever humans engage in social activity. So, wherever people are asked to participate in culturally valorized decision-making processes, we should seek the processes by which those people seem to "construct satisfactory lives and a coherent sense of self" (Ochs 1993: 299). Further, when social contexts ask of them to inhabit competing identities (Silverstein 2004), it is imperative to understand the practices people select to publicly establish their cultural sensibilities in those fluid social moments. HPI is just the sort of high-stakes, possibly conflicted social activity that necessitates such understanding.

1.3.1 Stance-taking, collocation, and semantic preference

The position taken in this chapter is that people have culturally socialized values which are a matter of expression rather than enduring, essential properties. The primary form of expression for these values is taking stances on subjects and objects of discourse. Stance-taking events occur through overt, communicative acts, where communicators stake out positions for subjects, evaluate discursive objects, and align with the prior stances, in a present stance field (Biber and Finegan 1989; Du Bois 2007; Jaffe 2009; Kärkkäinen 2006; Kockelman 2004). Much like the social values that they express, stances are fluid, emerging across time in shifting discursive spaces (Ochs 1996; Sinclair 2004: 49–54).

Stance-taking has been extensively explored in verbal, interactive spaces (see above work by e.g., Du Bois 2007; Jaffe 2009; Kärkkäinen 2006). However, in this chapter, I will deal with stance events at an intertextual level through John M. Sinclair's Extended Lexical Unit (Sinclair 2004; Stubbs 2009), especially (1) collocations, (2) semantic preference, and (3) semantic prosody. Collocations are the consistent, systematic co-occurrence of two or more words (Firth 1957; Sinclair 1991), within a certain span of word sequence, identified usually by statistical means such as mutual information score (MI) within some corpus of language use (Cheng, Greaves, and Warren 2006; Church and Hanks 1990; Stubbs 1995; Xiao and McEnery 2006). As words occur together, they produce meaning that is different than individual words simply adding up in an additive, consecutive manner. That is, collocations form phrases with an internal meaning that may not have anything to do with the individual words. Frequently occurring collocations indicate topics of a corpus, or what that corpus might be about. In signaling this *aboutness*, the topics of stance can be ascertained for further examination. That is, the quantitative and automatic identification of collocations serves as a first step in the analyses of the language use.

Examining the local text in which collocations appear provides insight into the meanings behind collocations as units. The habit of communicators to use collocations with certain subjects in their co-text gives rise to their semantic preference (Bednarek 2008; Stubbs 2009). Certain forms of collocations, with specific words and syntagmatic constructions, will occur in certain semantic fields and subjects of discourse. Thus, the collocation, as a single unit, carries semantic information that can be recovered by examining the language use around it. This requires a mixed form of qualitative analysis based on the quantitatively derived, significant, frequent collocations in a corpus.

A prime example of collocations and semantic preference is *white wine* (Sinclair 2004: 135–136). White, the color, and wine, the alcoholic substance typically made from grapes, have specific meanings unto themselves (a color, an alcoholic substance). Yet *white wine* comes in a range of colors, from a golden hue to light green shades, to sometimes nearly colorless, and more. Therefore, the meaning of white wine cannot, in fact, be confined to white (color) + wine (alcoholic substance) meaning a specific color of wine. Rather white, when followed by wine represents a specie of wine, as a single collocation.

1.3.2 Evaluations, attitudes, and semantic prosody

One of the core aspects of stance-taking is evaluation. Yet, the nature of attitude and evaluation in social activity is also deeply rooted in the study of affect, and emotion (Caffi and Janney 1994; Edwards 1999; Ochs and Schieffelin 1989; Prior 2019). Nonetheless, scholars in language use and discourse analysis have sometimes been hesitant to discuss emotion in social activity, due in large part to a perceived strict separation of cognition from the social (see e.g., Deppermann 2012; Prior 2019, for exploration of the history of this distinction). Yet, Du Bois and Kärkkäinen (2012) and Wetherell (2012) both called for a reorientation to emotion in discourse studies, citing emotion as present in any important, socially expressed event. Accordingly, discourse analysts should be aware of the manifold embodied experiences, social co-constructions, and shared social realities that occur through the feeling, perception, and expression of what can be considered emotional phenomena.

Much work in psychology has been done to investigate emotion. Most relevant to the project at hand, the positive-negative evaluative aspect of emotion has been extensively studied in the form of valence (Barrett 1998, 2006a; Moors 2014; Russell 2003, 2009). Barrett (2006b: 45) has asserted that valence is "an invariant property of emotional life that can be found in virtually every form of emotional responding." Sociocultural norms partly shape core affective dimensions into complex emotional episodes. Complex emotional categories are, in a sense, scripts for understanding the phenomena that are human experience. These scripts implicate language in both internal and external aspects of the process (Barrett, Lindquist, and Gendron 2007; Lindquist 2017), because language is one of the main streams of acquiring cultural knowledge and norms, and thus how one participates in cultural activity (Vygotsky [1962] 1994).

Furthermore, valence has a corollary in Sinclair's semantic prosody, the discourse function of a collocational pattern, or the way that it *colors* the meaning of the local linguistic event as a whole (Hunston 2007; Louw 1993; Sinclair 2000, 2004). Like semantic preference, semantic prosody is established by analyzing frequently occurring collocations in their local textual usage. Two primary treatments of prosody have persisted in the literature. Scholars in one tradition have commonly treated prosody as positive-negative or pleasant-unpleasant evaluations (Bednarek 2008; Partington 2004; Xiao and McEnery 2006). In this account, semantic prosody is a feature of the collocation itself. That is, a collocation and its words are per se pleasant or unpleasant. This mode of seeing semantic prosody fits neatly into an evaluative aspect of discourse. It allows the neat analysis of collocations for evaluative characteristics, and thus a comparison of collocations that are shared between existing texts, interviews, and so on.

In contrast, a more expansive approach to semantic prosody sees it as a semantic *feel* that includes not just the collocation, but patterns in surrounding text and subjects that tend to accompany the collocations (Hunston 2007; Sinclair 2000). In this model, semantic preference is a necessary component in understanding the purpose behind a particular collocation being used. The importance of a collocation is thus not merely its positive or negative character, but the way that it impresses an intention of the writer or speaker into the language use. A collocational form will be used when discussing certain subjects, tending toward pleasant or unpleasant contexts, and so selecting a collocation reflects the surrounding text pattern. Moreover, the specific collocational variant, based on what specific words tend to be present, will influence the tendency of a collocation's meaning within local text. Thus, rather than prosody being a description of a collocation itself, it describes a tendency of collocation in a preferred semantic environment, and thus the attitudinal function of the overall language pattern.

1.4 Summary & specific questions

HPI is ultimately a social activity carried out by people spread across many sites and infrastructural levels. People's normative values, priorities, and organizational norms will have effects on not just what they do, but why and how they accomplish their goals. People communicate their beliefs, such as they are, through the linguistically patterned stances they take. By collecting the claims, statements, and other language use at different discourse levels, the beliefs of different subsystems can be compared to better understand where beliefs are aligned or misaligned during the implementation process.

It bears clarifying that this analysis is comparative, but is firstly about what is present at each subsystem level. The similarities and differences are meant to reveal aspects of meaning related to those that produce it, to understand the borders between the different coalitions they represent. This is why the exact collocations will not necessarily be the same, as they are drawn from specific uses and contexts in which they obtain meaning. In essence, this is a question about the language used for the specific purpose of health policy implementation, in the rural, older adult context of Pennsylvania facing the opioid crisis. The claim that invites comparison is that, from a health policy perspective, the two subsystems (producers of official policy and texts; agents on the ground across Pennsylvania) are intertwined and considered to be part of a single process. Thus, the questions are, how *do* they communicate, and what *do* they mean? Once this can be squared away, only then can we see how that claim holds together.

2 Methodology

To answer my questions, I utilized corpus-assisted discourse analysis (Partington et al. 2013). I collected a multi-modal corpus of text (n = 100; 571,481 words), in the form of official policies, brochures, and outreach materials from older adult health agencies, and talk, in the form of bi-monthly ethnographic interviews (n = 29; 171,492 words) with six director-level agency administrators and five of their protective services case workers. Texts were digitized and changed to plain text format, preserving design or editing conventions (e.g., paragraph, line breaks) where possible. Interviews were audio-video recorded and transcribed verbatim to focus on content rather than structure (e.g., turn-taking). This allowed both subcorpora to be queried and compared in similar fashion.

2.1 Keywords and collocations

I first extracted frequent keywords and collocations from both subcorpora. A keyword or key term has been defined as a term present in a corpus at a frequency that is statistically different from a reference corpus (Gabrielatos and Marchi 2011; Scott 1997). Log-likelihood is a frequently used method of extracting such key terms (Paquot and Bestgen 2009; Pojanapunya and Watson 2018). I then used those keywords as referent words for collocations. I used AntConc (Anthony 2020) to identify and extract keywords and collocations via the following measures:

1. **Keyness:** Log-likelihood (4-term), with a p value < 0.0001 (+Bonferroni), %DIFF for effect size, and selected from the Top 100 keywords
2. **Collocation:** Span of +/- 4 words from the referent word, MI + Log-likelihood score ($p = < .05$) > 3.0, and Frequency > 3 times for Documents, > 2 for Interviews

2.2 Semantic preference

I then qualitatively analyzed a collocation's semantic preference via concordance lines (Sinclair 2004). Because of the highly formulaic and generic format of the policy documents, I only selected candidate collocations that were whole sequences (e.g., *OLDER ADULT PROTECTIVE SERVICES ACT*), collocates shared between the two subcorpora, synonyms, or all of the above, for comparison. Many collocations within a subcorpus have important uses and semantic properties, such as citing major legislation, but are not suitable for comparison between these subcorpora. Yet, there are still many collocations between the two subcorpora that reveal important distinctions between the values and meaning invoked by official policy documents, and the agents implementing those policies.

2.3 Semantic prosody

I then analyzed the semantic prosody of each collocation, again using concordance lines. Two raters first evaluated (negative, positive, neutral) a subset of collocations from each corpus. We calculated inter-rater reliability using Cohen's Kappa (κ) twice, with one round of review and discussion (Loewen and Plonsky, 2015: 90, 93). Our inter-rater reliability was $\kappa = .8$, and $\kappa = .88$, indicating reliable judgments between raters.

During semantic prosody analysis, I constrained maximum samples of collocations so that some very high frequency collocations did not overwhelm the prosody results from other collocations, some of which were mere fractions of more predominant sequences. To do this, I sorted all concordance results by sequence, showing every n^{th} instance to produce up to 100 instances of each collocate. This had the effect of retaining the numerical presence of high frequency collocations, while also including other forms. For collocations with 100 or fewer total lines, I evaluated all collocations. As Louw (1993) demonstrated, subsets of collocations, sorted by n^{th}, deliver insights about collocational behaviors in the sampled language.

To report semantic prosody findings, I will use Xiao and McEnery's (2006) typographic classification system to display and discuss results. All items and neutral uses will be italicized (*neutral*), but items with a negative prosody are also underlined (*bad*), and positive are also **bolded** (***good***). A referent word will be said to have negative, positive, or neutral tendency after accounting the overall ratio of the three evaluations of all collocations, in the form of negative:positive:-neutral. So, if a collocate e.g., *opioid* has a total of 16 negative instances, 6 positive, and 2 neutral, it would have a ratio of 8:3:1, and be considered to have an overall negative prosody in the corpus.

3 Results

I will report on the semantic preference and semantic prosody of three salient keywords and their collocations: *opioid*, *protective*, and *older*. These referent words were selected from the available keywords because (1) they are shared between both subcorpora, and (2) integrally related to the heart of this study, given that the subject is an older adult population, opioids, and protective services provision.

3.1 Opioid

3.1.1 Semantic preference

Opioid as a referent word tends to appear with a rather tight semantic pattern in the corpus overall. Collocates for *opioid* in the Documents subcorpus tend to come in the context of either diagnoses (OPIOID USE DISORDER), overdosing, or impacts of the opioid situation in the U.S. In the Interviews, *opioid* as a collocate follows a similar semantic pattern around use, and the extent of the phenomenon. Interestingly, the interviews include several words which extend the grouping, offering alternative lexemes aligned around the same semantic content: *crisis* but also *issue* and *epidemic*; *use* but also *addiction* and ***abuse***.

    Opioid crisis appears when agencies change their activities, including naming different kinds of exploitation and needs, and changing state level priorities. In the Documents subcorpus, the collocation appears in 14 documents describing the context that leads to policy change, both as a threat and to describe the challenges communities are working to face. In the Interviews, *opioid crisis* is used by 4 directors and 1 protective service worker. The agents also use close synonyms *issue*, *issues*, and *epidemic* in related ways. Each synonym appears with certain boundaries that guide their use. *Epidemic* has a similar sense to *crisis*, showing up when the agents are focused on ways in which opioids are affecting their services, especially appearing with intensifying items such as *afflicted* and *increasing*, and *every aspect of life*.

By extension, *opioid issue*, in the singular form, appears related to the accompanying grammatical article. When *the opioid issue* appears, it is in the context of the health services community attending to or addressing opioids as a health problem. By contrast, *an opioid issue* is more local, and about the people and communities in which it occurs. It could be supposed that *the opioid issue* is representative of a public health subject to be addressed, while *an opioid issue* is something people have, or that particular communities experience. Further exploration of the term in a larger corpus would be needed to discover the durability of the article as the defining semantic feature of *opioid issue*.

Prescription in the Documents subcorpus is used consistently in two ways with *opioid*, either as an adjective modifier, or as a noun modified by *opioid*. Each case has specific meaning associated with its syntagmatic organization. Adjectival *prescription*, appears frequently in descriptions of the *opioid crisis*. The frequency of this grouping shows at least some convention in which the opioid crisis is a prescription opioid crisis. Further, adjectival *prescription* appears with explanations and reports of the problem, for example: *increases in use*, *misuse*, and statistical reports. *Prescription opioids* are a major element to the crisis and, importantly, because it is a specific type of opioid, the documents use its identification to provide solutions. That is, by identifying *prescription opioids* with certain concrete problems, there are public health deliverables available.

When *opioid* modifies *prescription*, it appears consistently in guidelines for medical professionals. This pattern typically coincides with technical explanations of dosage, and prescribing guidance. This pattern is tightly constrained around its semantics not just in this way, but also in that it contributes further to the collocation of *opioid* and *prescription* as being centrally connected to providing concrete information that can lead to public health deliverables. Medical professionals can be given different treatment, dosage, medication guidelines etcetera which target *opioid* use reduction.

It is worth noting that *overdose* collocates with *opioid* in significant frequency in the Documents subcorpus but not in the Interviews. This is a critical distinction between the corpora, because intuitively this *opioid crisis* is about overdosing. Yet the *opioid overdose* problem is cited primarily by official policy, and not by the agents on the ground. This could mean that overdoses are not as visible an issue for the agents, that they do not accompany *opioid* so often as a cause, that *overdoses* are seen as related to some other semantic content, or some combination thereof. Any of these being true, the exclusion of *opioid* and *overdose* as a leading collocation shows that the respective meaning and experiences of *opioid* for these two infrastructural levels is quite different.

Table 1: Semantic prosody of *OPIOID*.

Documents				Interviews			
Collocate	NEG	POS	NEU	Collocate	NEG	POS	NEU
overdose	54	22	12	crisis	12	3	0
use	85	15	0	use	8	1	0
drug	16	23	26	issue	9	0	0
crisis	32	3	1	addiction	8	1	0
prescription	23	4	0	issues	6	1	0
				prescription	4	0	0
				epidemic	4	0	0
				abuse	1	3	0
				think	2	2	0
Total	210	67	39	**Total**	54	11	0

3.1.2 Prosody

As might be expected, *opioid* is negative for both the Documents and the agents' Interviews (Table 1). With the exception of *drug* in the Documents corpus, collocations for *opioid* will nearly always occur in predominantly negative contexts, with an overall ratio of 88:26:13.

Despite *opioid* having a negative character, *drug* modifies its use in several distinct positive and neutral environments, with an overall tendency toward positive or neutral uses. The reason for this is that when *opioid* and *drug* occur together, it is most frequently with **overdose reversal**, especially the sequence *opioid overdose reversal drug*. This sequence appears positive, when it is reported as a solution to the <u>crisis</u>, and neutrally when policies are created policing and regulating the distribution of these *reversal drugs*. When the sequence is *opioid drug*, it tends more toward negative contours describing misuse, over-prescription, and other features or causes of the opioid epidemic. Although there are more collocates that are not, for example, formulaic sequences or parts of larger sequences, in the interviews, there seems to be a much tighter prosody around the word for these agents than in the documents.

3.2 Protective

3.2.1 Preference

Protective provided an interesting case especially around two collocates: *services* and *service*. The usage of *protective* was directly related to the morphological marker for plurality. The plurality of *protective* then led to specialized collocations, and thus different semantic categories for its use.

Protective services (plural) are a designated program, with target populations, criteria for access, and descriptors of what that program is meant to do. *Protective services* predominantly appears in documents to create or regulate programs, and its neutrality comes from this procedural usage. This programmatic usage extends to the agent interviews. *Services* only appears when describing the programs and procedural aspects of carrying out those programs, usually in a decontextualized manner. One important aspect of *protective services* is that it also modifies *staff* and **worker** in both subcorpora, though they did not collocate as closely with *protective* in the Documents. This is one of the few indicators that, even in its programmatic or procedural sense, *services* are sometimes associated with provision by agents and workers, as the ones that will follow the criteria and implement the programs.

Service (singular), in contrast, is something exclusively carried out by agents. In the Documents corpus, *service* is restricted to an adjective for agencies, activities, cases, and clients. The one exception here is that annual reports treat *service* as a noun (e.g., provided service). Yet for the agents, *protective service* operates as a modifier specifying disciplinarity or specialization for workers and cases. They predominantly use *protective service* with **workers**, *staff*, and to a lesser extent, apparent from concordance analysis, *investigators*. Protective *service* **workers** is commonly used in the context of describing the concrete events and procedures of providing service, such as how many workers go, how many are currently employed at the agency, and the effects of current agent counts.

One senses from the subtle differences in semantics here that there is a feeling of ownership or materiality to *protective service* compared to *services*, which are more abstract. While *protective services* are an aspect, or a key program, of older adult services, *protective service* is a category describing people and activities.

Table 2: Semantic prosody of PROTECTIVE.

	Documents				Interviews		
Collocate	NEG	POS	NEU	Collocate	NEG	POS	NEU
services	22	14	64	services	74	17	9
need	76	0	12	service	18	15	2
service	20	2	2	workers	5	16	2
				staff	4	2	1
Total	**118**	**16**	**78**	**Total**	**101**	**50**	**14**

3.2.2 Prosody

Protective is used primarily in negative ways in both subcorpora (Table 2). It could be argued that *protective* is intuitively positive. Protecting others from harm, or against harm, for example, would be thought of as positive. The use of collocations, and the local context in which they occur, reveals that for older adult services, *protective* is often an issue related to negative situations, rather than a sort of intervening, positive influence. There are two specific cases in which this negative prosody does not obtain, *services* which is predominately neutral in the Documents, and with **workers** in the Interviews. Overall, *protective* tends to be negative with a ratio of 219:66:92.

Protective services, used in highly programmatic sense in both corpora, nonetheless shows up differently in each subcorpus. It is used to create programs and services in the Documents corpus, and so ultimately appears frequently in formulaic and neutral contexts, as *adult protective services*. When it appears in this neutral way, it is often decontextualized, relying on prior co-text to establish its need, but its local use is procedural. Occurrences where *services* are negative are more closely bundled with reasons for its creation, and criteria for their use. There is an interesting contrast with the Interviews, because *protective services* is overwhelmingly negative. Though the programmatic semantics of this collocation persists, it is often more closely attached to the environment of abuse or need as an explanation for its existence. Additionally, agents often report dissatisfaction with the state of *protective services*, and a general antipathy or mistrust of *protective services* from their populations.

While in the policy documents, *service* remains overwhelmingly negative, for agents, *protective service* is something associated closely with the agents and **workers**, and thus has a more balanced negative-positive ratio, and is very positive when explicitly referring to *protective service workers*. In that light, there is a very close split between the negative versus positive or neutral usage. Although the contexts in which service workers find themselves are negative, the workers and the work they do are positioned positively. They represent the good reasons and the hard work of rural health service provision. There are distinct indications of, and explicit use of the term "pride" related to *protective service* as both an activity that workers carry out, and meeting the needs of their populations. When the collocation is with *staff*, a synonym with **worker** that is arguably a more abstracted category, there is more negativity associated with *protective*. In most cases this again is related to shortages and fulfillment at the procedural and infrastructural level.

3.3 Older

3.3.1 Preference

Older tends to appear with collocates that involve people for both subcorpora. However, the use of synonyms for people tend to be quite different between them.

In the case of both *individuals* and *adult* in the Documents subcorpus, *older* is always a modifier that sets criteria for services. All instances of *older* with *adult* are a general class of qualified recipients. When the documents invoke this class, it tends to accompany the grounds of inclusion, such as being victims of financial exploitation, or neglect. By extension, this collocation *older adult* also frequently occurs with *report of need*, or its acronym RON, or with *need*. In combination, *older adult* with *need* reinforces the generic subject-class to which policies can be applied, and the specific causes for those services.

Individuals, while still appearing as a class for service provision, tends to appear in a different context. *Older individuals* appears with *income* (specifically *low income*). In contrast with *adult*, which tends to address specific phenomena or causes for services, *individuals* is more associated with the conditions in which those people live. Conditions, as such, are still broadly about the reasons for services being created, but do not usually address things such as exploitation. Rather, they invoke social determinants. It is worth noting that ironically, *individuals* is still not about particular people or concrete examples. In this sense, the plural form is necessary to establish the class or group in need of service, rather than any individual member.

In contrast to the documents, agents' interviews use *older* in both group-type reference and to express unique, concrete experiences that their populations face. On one hand, agents' use of *older* with *adults*, *folks*, *people*, and *population* describe groups to which their services apply. The difference occurs, for example, in that when agents use *older folks*, they are used in active constructions of the experience rather than the passive, and are grammatical subjects as often as objects. This has a strong effect on the perspective one has in understanding perhaps why, or how, services are necessary. This contracts the space between services, and the people and conditions that give rise to them. This contraction, as a semantic feature, reinforces the relationship between the agency and real people that they serve, rather than simple classification.

Table 3: Semantic prosody of *OLDER*.

Documents				Interviews			
Collocate	NEG	POS	NEU	Collocate	NEG	POS	NEU
individuals	57	30	13	adult	75	25	1
adult	97	0	3	adults	65	12	1
adults	53	24	23	folks	31	4	1
income	72	11	2	people	11	5	2
need	78	7	19	think	9	2	0
				person	10	3	0
				population	7	2	0
				help	2	5	0
Total	357	72	60	**Total**	210	58	5

3.3.2 Prosody

Older comes across quite negatively with a ratio of 567:130:65 (Table 3). This overall negativity is greatly related to the propensity of *older* to appear as a characteristic of certain groups that are in <u>need</u>. The only exception is **help** in the Interviews, which is positive except for two instances. **Help** appears in its infinitive verb form in 5 of 7 instances. It is only in its verbal form that **help** is positive. When it appears as a noun, **help** with *older* is in fact negative: people cannot get help, or are in need of help. The noun form of **help** reflects the larger trend in collocations of *older* that some class or category is the target of services or, **help**. Thus, *older* as a modifier functions with predominant negativity as it manages the people, populations, adults, and so on, that have attracted the attention of health policy creators and implementers.

4 Discussion

4.1 Preference

The Documents subcorpus has rather tightly constrained semantic patterns with regard to *opioid*, *protective*, and *older*, likely owing much to the formulaic genre conventions from which many of the documents are drawn. I attempted to avoid some of the pressure exerted by these conventions by sorting and then selecting from a subset of the possible concordance lines, through the methods described above. Still, some over-occurrence must be present. Nonetheless, the findings in this analysis bear fruit in the distinct similarities and differences in which shared collocations do occur between documents, and between documents and agents, and in which synonyms or closely-linked meaning could be established.

Opioids are about the communities and people that agents serve. At a practical level, it could be argued that official health policy documents, which are often meant to serve broader communities and contexts, cannot be about real individuals and specific experiences. Thus, the meaning categories would be formed and constrained by broad groupings and populations, and so depict *opioids*, *protective*, and *older* through those optics. Agents, in contrast, refract their needs for policy provision through the people they meet every day, valenced reports by their agents, and the pressures felt in administering services. Pressures, though, are multi-sited. Administrators talk about what populations need, and they connect the material experiences of abuse and exploitation with opioids. But they are also reflective of agency administration, procedural restriction, and oversight. When administrators face the opioid epidemic, they make sense of policies and what the policies demand of them. Just as well, they face the needs of a vulnerable population that change by day, by call, and by report. In this way, agency directors form a linchpin between the documented policies, case managers, and populations. As a result, agents on the ground frequently share categories or descriptions of their populations with the policies, but attach other synonyms to each category. They have an arguably fuller, or at least more varied, repertoire of ways to talk about the opioid epidemic. As a result, they produce different prosodic dimensions in their interviews, especially in their self-reflective accounts of how they are perceived in the field and the specific, evocative depictions of people in need.

Directors and case managers frequently have disagreements with the policy mandates and decisions they are tasked with. In fact, agents rely comparatively little on referencing the mandates and legal texts that give them authority. Only in the context of *protective* did we see collocations that had distinct, technical use behind them that mirrored the documents. Even in this case, collocates extended to **workers** and *staff*, underscoring the material activities of *protective service*, rather than only the prescribed procedures.

The departure in what *opioids* are about, and by extension the means to address *opioids*, is perhaps best captured in the over-presence of <u>overdose</u> collocations in the Documents, and their relative absence in the Interviews. This is a critical distinction between the corpora, because intuitively this *opioid* <u>crisis</u> is about overdosing. Yet the *opioid* <u>overdose</u> problem is cited primarily by official policy, and not by the agents on the ground. This could mean that <u>overdose</u> is not as visible an issue for the agents, that it does not accompany *opioid* so often as a cause, that overdoses are seen as related to some other semantic content, or some combination thereof. Any of these being true, the exclusion of *opioid* and <u>overdose</u> as a leading collocation shows that the respective meaning *opioid* for these two infrastructural levels can be quite different.

As it impacts implementation, it is clear that there is a need for a fuller vocabulary of sorts than clinical and biomedical intervention, in order to adequately address the needs of the rural, older adult population with regards to *opioids*. If policy mandates can be said to layout the criteria, intentions, and programs for confronting the opioid epidemic, then the language that is used to accomplish that ought to be understood as *saying what it means to say*. This being a reasonable assumption, (1) *opioids* must be considered a social-community issue for elderly folks and their agency directors, with many dimensions of experience rather than only preventing overdose-related deaths; (2) *protective services* and *protective service* are read differently between policy, caseworkers, and the populations that receive that service, and thus impacts construal of being a health services worker, staff, investigator etcetera; (3) *older* as a referent word is somewhat adrift between corpora, where in documents *older* collocations are categorical criteria, and for agents they are touchstones of concrete experiences, and real people that may, or may not, admit to prescribed categories.

4.2 Discussion: Prosody

The semantic prosody of *protective*, together with its collocates, demonstrates the need to look deeper at the situated language use, and the function of affect in discourse that extends beyond single-word connotation. During interviews with agents, there becomes a distinction between the perceptions of the agents and the perceptions of the population. This has some effect on the perspective-taking that occurs. When asked about the procedures of protective service, agents would often produce accounts of their populations being afraid of, or suspicious of, case workers. Yet the agents would often take these accounts as wedge points, where they then outline the approaches they would take, and reasons for being there. These different accounts illustrate yet another infrastructural departure: agents from their population. Agents perceive their roles and activities positively. The population, at least as reported by agents, is more likely to ascribe negative stances toward the agents. Different evaluations in the third person accounts are perceptible in the prosody of *protective* presented above.

The evaluative content of *protective* is framed, first person, by the caseworkers for themselves. It is simultaneously related to prior experiences, as in different evaluations of *protective* by people that are not present. What I mean is that the case workers are pivoting their evaluations (positive, negative) of aspects of *protective* between perspective-taking: theirs compared to their populations. For example, the meaning and so-called aura of *protective* was intimately bound up with (1) whether it appeared with the plural *services* or the singular *service*, and further still (2) how that collocation was linked to *workers* or *staff*, or neither. These different collocations are necessary constituents at the local level, the specific use of them during interaction, but also ties them into larger discourses present in multiple parties, texts, and regimes.

Tying accounts of local experiences and their accompanying prosodies into larger discourses is precisely the crux of attending to organizational beliefs across levels of implementation, such as over subsystems per the ACF. The semantic prosody of a pattern of language use, as the evaluative aspect of discourse, provides insight into the perspectives that agents hold, given their proposed duties and expectations. More importantly, the presence or absence of similar constructions between implementational levels can alert implementation and evaluation researchers to the areas where services are not reflected as perhaps expected. As pointed to by scholars in the prior sections, health policy implementation ought to be conceived of as a social event, impacted by organizational culture, and fashioned by interpersonal relations. To this end, people build up their ways of seeing and talking about service provision, and in turn structure their different core, policy, and secondary beliefs. Consistent linguistic constructions are socially grounded keys to the different areas of service that agents find themselves in, and whom they propose to be stakeholders in those services, while semantic prosodies are one platform on which agents announce their beliefs about those services.

5 Conclusion

This chapter presented several subjects and collocations about health services for older populations that exhibited shifting qualities depending on the variant form or context of use. These semantic shifts showed that the discourse around health policy implementation concerning older adults in rural Pennsylvania is nuanced by situationally negotiated, and sometimes contested, beliefs. Policy beliefs, such as whom policies target, what they are meant to do, and who carries them out, express varying levels of social (mis)alignment between the macro-level of policy mandates, and the micro-interactional stances taken by agency workers. There are portions of official policy reflected in the many perspectives that agents take. At other times, there are gulfs of space between official policies and what agents seem to mean. In response to the original claim laid out in this chapter, that subsystems are part of a single process, comparative findings have revealed that the process is more distributed than linear, and less coherent than officially intended.

Ultimately, the programs created to address different health needs look different to differently positioned stakeholders, whose prominence waxes and wanes in the implementation process. Actors in subsystems distributed across the implementation process perceive health policy needs with unique socioenvironmental influences on their attention, which directly impacts the outcomes in mind, and the language they employ to construct their identities and roles. The findings in this chapter are but one aspect of the overlap in stated policy beliefs, identified through simple keywords or collocations, showing how the meaning behind those beliefs is often subtly misaligned. Thus, the specifics of agent reports on everyday service delivery are just as important as what the relevant mandates might enjoin agents to do. In order to accurately depict the enactment of health policies, implementation researchers must capture the interfaces between the official, textual policies, and the personal beliefs and stances of the people on the ground.

References

Alexander, Ernest R. 1985. From idea to action: Notes for a contingency theory of the policy implementation process. *Administration & Society* 16(4). 403–426.

Anthony, Laurence. 2020. *AntConc*. Tokyo, Japan: Waseda University. http://www.laurenceanthony.net/software.

Barrett, Lisa F. 1998. Discrete emotions or dimensions? The role of valence focus and arousal focus. *Cognition and Emotion* 12(4). 579–599.

Barrett, Lisa F. 2006a. Solving the emotion paradox: Categorization and the experience of emotion. *Personality and Social Psychology Review* 10(1). 20–46. https://doi.org/10.1207/s15327957pspr1001_2.

Barrett, Lisa F. 2006b. Valence is a basic building block of emotional life. *Journal of Research in Personality* (Proceedings of the 2005 Meeting of the Association of Research in Personality) 40(1). 35–55. https://doi.org/10.1016/j.jrp.2005.08.006.

Barrett, Lisa F., Kristen A. Lindquist & Maria Gendron. 2007. Language as context for the perception of emotion. *Trends in Cognitive Sciences* 11(8). 327–332. https://doi.org/10.1016/j.tics.2007.06.003.

Bauer, Mark S., Laura Damschroder, Hildi Hagedorn, Jeffrey Smith & Amy M. Kilbourne. 2015. An introduction to implementation science for the non-specialist. *BMC psychology* 3(32). 1–12. https://doi.org/10.1186/s40359-015-0089-9.

Bednarek, Monika. 2008. Semantic preference and semantic prosody re-examined. *Corpus Linguistics and Linguistic Theory* 4 (2). https://doi.org/10.1515/CLLT.2008.006. http://www.degruyter.com/view/j/cllt.2008.4.issue-2/cllt.2008.006/cllt.2008.006.xml (21 November, 2016).

Biber, Douglas & Edward Finegan. 1989. Styles of stance in English: Lexical and grammatical marking of evidentiality and affect. *Text & Talk*. De Gruyter Mouton 9(1). 93–124. https://doi.org/10.1515/text.1.1989.9.1.93.

Bowen, Shelley & Anthony B. Zwi. 2005. Pathways to "evidence-informed" policy and practice: A framework for action. *PLOS Medicine*. Public Library of Science 2(7). e166. https://doi.org/10.1371/journal.pmed.0020166.

Brownson, Ross C., Craig J. Newschaffer & Farnoush Ali-Abarghoui. 1997. Policy research for disease prevention: challenges and practical recommendations. *American Journal of Public Health* 87(5). 735–739.

Caffi, Claudia & Richard W. Janney. 1994. Toward a pragmatics of emotive communication. *Journal of Pragmatics* 22(3). 325–373. https://doi.org/10.1016/0378-2166(94)90115-5.

Cheng, Winnie, Chris Greaves & Martin Warren. 2006. From n-gram to skipgram to concgram. *International Journal of Corpus Linguistics* 11(4). 411–433. https://doi.org/10.1075/ijcl.11.4.04che.

Church, Kenneth W. & Patrick Hanks. 1990. Word association norms, mutual information, and lexicography. *Computational Linguistics* 16(1). 22–29.

Damschroder, Laura J., David C. Aron, Rosalind E. Keith, Susan R. Kirsh, Jeffery A. Alexander & Julie C. Lowery. 2009. Fostering implementation of health services research findings into practice: a consolidated framework for advancing implementation science. *Implementation Science* 4. 50. https://doi.org/10.1186/1748-5908-4-50.

Deppermann, Arnulf. 2012. How does "cognition" matter to the analysis of talk-in-interaction. *Language Sciences* 34(6). 746–767.

Du Bois, John W. 2007. The stance triangle. In Robert Englebretson (ed.), *Stancetaking in discourse: Subjectivity, evaluation, interaction*, 139–182. Amsterdam/Philadelphia: John Benjamins Publishing Company.

Du Bois, John W. & Elise Kärkkäinen. 2012. Taking a stance on emotion: Affect, sequence, and intersubjectivity in dialogic interaction. *Text & Talk* 32(4). 433–451.

Edwards, Derek. 1999. Emotion discourse. *Culture & Psychology* 5(3). 271–291. https://doi.org/10.1177/1354067X9953001.

Firth, John R. 1957. *Papers in linguistics 1934-1951*. London: Oxford University Press.

Gabrielatos, Costas & Anna Marchi. 2011. Keyness: Matching metrics to definitions. In. https://research.edgehill.ac.uk/en/publications/keyness-matching-metrics-to-definitions-2 (2 June, 2020).

Hunston, Susan. 2007. Semantic prosody revisited. *International Journal of Corpus Linguistics* 12(2). 249–268. https://doi.org/10.1075/ijcl.12.2.09hun.

Jaffe, Alexandra. 2009. Introduction: The sociolinguistics of stance. In Alexandra Jaffe (ed.), *Stance: Sociolinguistic perspectives*, 3–28. United States: Oxford University Press.

Kärkkäinen, Elise. 2006. Stance taking in conversation: From subjectivity to intersubjectivity. *Text & Talk* 26(6). 699–731. https://doi.org/10.1515/TEXT.2006.029.

Kockelman, Paul. 2004. Stance and subjectivity. *Journal of Linguistic Anthropology* 14(2). 127–150.

Kreindler, Sara A. 2016. What if implementation is not the problem? Exploring the missing links between knowledge and action. *International Journal of Health Planning and Management* 31(2). 208–226. https://doi.org/10.1002/hpm.2277.

Lindquist, Kristen A. 2017. The role of language in emotion: existing evidence and future directions. *Current Opinion in Psychology* (Emotion) 17. 135–139. https://doi.org/10.1016/j.copsyc.2017.07.006.

Loewen, Shawn & Luke Plonsky. 2015. *An a–z of applied linguistics research methods*. Macmillan International Higher Education.

Louw, Bill. 1993. Irony in the text or insincerity in the writer? The diagnostic potential of semantic prosodies. In M Baker, G Francis & T Tognini-Bonelli (eds.), *Text and technology: In honor of John Sinclair*, 157–176. Amsterdam: John Benjamins.

Majone, Giandomenico. 1989. *Evidence, Argument, and Persuasion in the Policy Process*. Yale University Press.

Moors, Agnes. 2014. Flavors of appraisal theories of emotion. *Emotion Review* 6(4). 303–307. https://doi.org/10.1177/1754073914534477.

Ochs, Elinor. 1993. Constructing social identity: A language socialization perspective. *Research on Langauge and Social Interaction* 26(3). 287–306.

Ochs, Elinor. 1996. Linguistic resources for socializing humanity. In John J. Gumperz & Stephen Levinson (eds.), *Rethinking linguistic relativity* (Studies in the Social and Cultural Foundations of Language), 407–437. Cambridge: Cambridge University Press.

Ochs, Elinor & Bambi Schieffelin. 1989. Language has a heart. *Text* 9(1). 7–25. https://doi.org/10.1515/text.1.1989.9.1.7.

Paquot, Magali & Yves Bestgen. 2009. Distinctive words in academic writing: A comparison of three statistical tests for keyword extraction. In Andreas H. Jucker, Daniel Schreier & Marianne Hundt (eds.), *Corpora: Pragmatics and discourse* (Language and Computers), vol. 68, 247–269. Brill Rodopi. https://doi.org/10.1163/9789042029101_014. https://brill.com/view/book/edcoll/9789042029101/B9789042029101-s014.xml (24 December, 2020).

Partington, Alan. 2004. Utterly content in each other's company. *International Journal of Corpus Linguistics* 9(1). 131–156.

Partington, Alan, Alison Duguid & Charlotte Taylor. 2013. *Patterns and Meanings in Discourse: Theory and practice in corpus-assisted discourse studies (CADS)*. John Benjamins Publishing.

Pojanapunya, Punjaporn & Todd R. Watson. 2018. Log-likelihood and odds ratio: Keyness statistics for different purposes of keyword analysis. *Corpus Linguistics and Linguistic Theory* 14(1). 133–167. https://doi.org/10.1515/cllt-2015-0030.

Prior, Matthew T. 2019. Elephants in the room: An "affective turn," or just feeling our way? *The Modern Language Journal* 103(2). 516–527. https://doi.org/10.1111/modl.12573.

Russell, James A. 2003. Core affect and the psychological construction of emotion. *Psychological Review* 110(1). 145–172.

Russell, James A. 2009. Emotion, core affect, and psychological construction. *Cognition and Emotion* 23(7). 1259–1283. https://doi.org/10.1080/02699930902809375.

Russell, Jill, Trisha Greenhalgh, Emma Byrne & Janet McDonnell. 2008. Recognizing rhetoric in health care policy analysis. *Journal of Health Services Research & Policy* 13(1). 40–46. https://doi.org/10.1258/jhsrp.2007.006029.

Sabatier, Paul A. 1986. Top-down and bottom-up approaches to implementation research: A critical analysis and suggested synthesis. *Journal of Public Policy* 6(1). 21–48. https://doi.org/10.1017/S0143814X00003846.

Sabatier, Paul A. 1988. An advocacy coalition framework of policy change and the role of policy-oriented learning therein. *Policy sciences* 21(2–3). 129–168.

Sabatier, Paul A. & Christopher M. Weible. 2007. The advocacy coalition framework: Innovations and clarifications. *Theories of the policy process* 2. 189–220.

Sallis, James F., Adrian Bauman & Michael Pratt. 1998. Environmental and policy interventions to promote physical activityaaThis work was prepared for the CIAR Conference on Physical Activity Promotion: An ACSM Specialty Conference. *American Journal of Preventive Medicine* 15(4). 379–397. https://doi.org/10.1016/S0749-3797(98)00076-2.

Schmid, Thomas L., Michael Pratt & Elizabeth Howze. 1995. Policy as intervention: Environmental and policy approaches to the prevention of cardiovascular disease. *American journal of Public Health* 85. 1207–1211.

Scott, Mike. 1997. PC analysis of key words – And key key words. *System* 25(2). 233–245. https://doi.org/10.1016/S0346-251X(97)00011-0.

Silverstein, Michael. 1976. Shifters, linguistic categories, and cultural description. In Keith Basso & Henry A. Selby (eds.), *Meaning in anthropology*, 11–55. Albuquerque: University of New Mexico Press.

Silverstein, Michael. 1993. Metapragmatic discourse and metapragmatic function. In J.A. Lucy (ed.), *Reflexive language*, 3–58. New York: Cambridge University Press.

Silverstein, Michael. 2004. "Cultural" concepts and the language-culture nexus. *Current Anthropology* 45(5). 621–652.

Sinclair, John M. 1991. *Corpus, concordance, collocation*. Oxford University Press.

Sinclair, John M. 2000. Lexical grammar. *Naujoji Metodologija* 24. 191–203.

Sinclair, John M. 2004. *Trust the text: Language, corpus and discourse*. Routledge.

Stubbs, Michael. 1995. Collocations and semantic profiles: On the cause of the trouble with quantitative studies. *Functions of Language* 2(1). 23–55.

Stubbs, Michael. 2009. The search for units of meaning: Sinclair on empirical semantics. *Applied Linguistics* 30(1). 115–137.

Vygotsky, Lev S. 1962. *Thinking and speaking*. (Trans.) Eugenia Hanfmann, Gertrude Vakar & Norris Minnick. The M.I.T. Press.

Watt, Susan, Wendy Sword & Paul Krueger. 2005. Implementation of a health care policy: an analysis of barriers and facilitators to practice change. *BMC health services research* 5. 53. https://doi.org/10.1186/1472-6963-5-53.

Weible, Christopher M., Paul A. Sabatier & Kelly McQueen. 2009. Themes and variations: Taking stock of the Advocacy Coalition Framework. *Policy Studies Journal* 37(1). 121–140. https://doi.org/10.1111/j.1541-0072.2008.00299.x.

Wetherell, Margaret. 2012. *Affect and emotion: A new social science understanding*. Los Angeles: SAGE Publications Ltd.

Wimmelmann, Camilla L. 2019. Local enactments of national health promotion policies: A Danish case. *The international journal of health planning and management* 34(1). e219–e229. https://doi.org/10.1002/hpm.2638.

Xiao, Richard & Tony McEnery. 2006. Collocation, semantic prosody, and near synonymy: A cross-linguistic perspective. *Applied Linguistics* 27(1). 103–129.

2017. *Analysis of overdose deaths in Pennsylvania, 2016*. Philadelphia: U.S. Department of Justice, Philadelphia Division.

2018. *Pennsylvania Opioid Summary*. National Institute on Drug Abuse. https://www.drugabuse.gov/drugs-abuse/opioids/opioid-summaries-by-state/pennsylvania-opioid-summary (17 January, 2019).

The Pennsylvania Opioid Data Dashboard. https://data.pa.gov/stories/s/Pennsylvania-Opioids/9q45-nckt/ (8 January, 2021).

Patria C. López de Victoria Rodríguez,
Elba L. González Márquez, Krystal Colón Rivera

Chapter 7
Responding to crisis, responding to needs: Older adults seeking medical care in the aftermath of storms

1 Introduction

When hurricanes Irma and María swept the island of Puerto Rico in September 2017, they caused major flooding, thousands of landslides, island-wide and months-long power and water outages, and 95.2% of cell phone tower sites to be downed (2017, October 6). Both events, barely two weeks apart, precipitated and made excruciatingly tangible the other crises in Puerto Rico: the $72 billion public debt, the crippling austerity measures that have hobbled public institutions, and an underfunded Medicaid plan for the island, worsened by a drop of nearly 5,000 doctors in the last decade (Bonilla 2020; Bonilla and LeBrón 2019; Mora et al. 2017; Perreira et al. 2017). Older adults – already living through severe cuts to public health infrastructure – were especially threatened by the lack of electricity, water, and everyday resources to deal with their health and multiple chronic illnesses. As a result of severe recovery mismanagement at a local and federal level, older adults' chronic health conditions exacerbated causing thousands to die as they awaited the *long durée* of disaster recovery and reconstruction (Kishore et al. 2018; Santos-Lozada and Howard 2018).

Acknowledgements: We wish to thank the National Institute on Minority Health and Health Disparities of the National Institutes of Health for funding the project "Resilience and Helpseeking in Health and Illness by and for the Elderly" (R21MD013701). We are particularly thankful for the older adults, caregivers, and health care professionals who contributed, consented, and recommended others to participate twice in the interviews held for this project. Data collection (2019–2021) was possible with the assistance of a team of undergraduate research students from UPR Cayey whom we would also like to thank: Adriana Álvarez Rivera, Paola Aguayo Alvarado, Miguel Cardona Rodríguez, Victoria Cotto Rivera, Gabriel Cruz Rodríguez, Valeria de Jesús Benjamín, Gianni Lugo Bermudez, Ashley Ortiz Velez, and Keyla Velez Malave. Lastly, we would like to thank Robert W. Schrauf for suggestions and comments on a previous version of this chapter.

Patria C. López de Victoria Rodríguez, Elba L. González Márquez, University of Puerto Rico at Cayey
Krystal Colón Rivera, University of Puerto Rico Mayagüez

https://doi.org/10.1515/9783110744804-008

This chapter illustrates and discusses helpseeking actions of older adults (60+) in the aftermath of disasters to explore the role of language as a medium for social action and as a response to the lack of government aid at a time of crisis in interviews we – Spanish speakers and residents of Puerto Rico – carried out with the contribution of older adults recruited in a town in the interior of the island. We define helpseeking as the social links that persons make to obtain information about, and access to, social assistance, pharmaceutical remedies, medical equipment, clinical diagnosis, physical or psychological treatment, within the constraints of Medicare and Medicaid or private health insurance and fee-for-service programs. We present collected data which documents and explains health and medical helpseeking among these older residents in the years following Hurricanes Irma and Maria.

This study addresses the helpseeking strategies in health and illness from the patient side (older adults >60 yrs. old) from a discourse-analytic ethnographic lens. While research in applied linguistics and other disciplines, such as medical anthropology and medical sociology, addresses the institutional provision of healthcare, there is less research on the patient "search" side (Ramanathan 2014). The structural damage by Irma and Maria exacerbated an underfunded and under-resourced health system already in crisis, and now four years later, many elderly Puerto Ricans still face overwhelming odds in finding appropriate health care for common, chronic, and acute diseases associated with aging (e.g., diabetes, hypertension, cardiovascular disease, cancer, dementia). Using a discourse-oriented approach to analyzing ethnographic, narrative interview data (De Fina and Georgakopoulou 2011; Riessman 2008; Schrauf 2016; Schrauf et al. 2020; Strauss and Feiz 2013; Strauss et al. 2018), we specifically focus on how older adults talk about how they interfaced with family, friends, neighbors, and/ or health personnel to pursue effective helpseeking in the aftermath of Hurricanes Irma and Maria. We also address areas where effective helpseeking was mobilized but resulted in failure as a result of the underfunded and under-resourced local health system. We aim to show that applied linguistics research – in particular, the microanalytic lens shed on collaborative acts of helpseeking as seen through performativity, indexicality, and talk-in-interaction – has much to contribute to the study of aging, illness, and health in contexts of healthcare and crises.

1.1 Language as social action in health and illness helpseeking interviews

While discourse analysis has much to offer to the understanding of the language of health and illness as refracted through a person's own concerns and accounts of action, the analysis of agency as emerging from discourse can also provide in-depth understanding of people's own conceptualization of causality or responsibility for events (Ahearn 2010). How people talk about their own actions vis-à-vis other's actions and how they attribute responsibility for events in their sociohistorical context can provide insights into the ways in which people operationalize and conceptualize agency in their or others' acts of help seeking. The notion of agency may be best understood as the "the relation between a person and a course of action and its effects" (Enfield 2017: 7). Two key additional definitions of agency are employed in this chapter: those of Alessandro Duranti (2004) and Paul Kockelman (2007). According to Duranti, agency is defined as "the property of those entities (i) that have some degree of control over their own behavior, (ii) whose actions in the world affect other entities (and sometimes their own), and (iii) whose actions are the object of evaluation" (453). Kockelman, on the other hand, defines agency as "the relatively flexible wielding of means toward ends" (375). As such, these definitions suggest that agency is distributed unevenly across networks of persons, organizations, and places and accomplished via language. Along the chain of actors in a helpseeking pathway, individuals have differential flexibility to control place, time, actions, and uptake, and differential levels of accountability for their actions and decisions (Enfield and Kockelman 2017; Kockelman 2007).

Drawing on the notion of agency in language and language in action while using linguistic ethnography as a methodology, we analyze older adults' language use as a form of social action. We study how agency emerges in the specific context of the daily action-steps and decisions made by people at the micro-level of medical helpseeking. We show the kinds of small-scale everyday helpseeking activity older adults carry out in the context of larger, macro-scale events by in-depth analysis of linguistic resources (prosodic, morphosyntactic, lexical, discursive, and pragmatic) that they use to describe, characterize, and interactively manage the search for material resources, the coordination of familial, social, and professional social networks, and their interface with health personnel.

In choosing a discourse analytic tradition of applied linguistic analysis, we also focus on how language is used to talk about and make sense of the social world (Chafe 1994; Ochs and Capps 2009; Potter and Wetherell 1987) in interactions that take place in real-world contexts (in this case life, health, and illness after a major hurricane). Moreover, the discourse analytic perspective applied to the data presented in this chapter not only underscores the importance of linguistic analysis in medical helpseeking talk from an applied linguistic lens but also stresses the central role language has in most aspects of medical encounters (Candlin and Candlin 2003; Sarangi 2012).

1.2 Agency in performativity, indexicality, and talk-in-interaction

To talk about agency in helpseeking in the context of compounded disasters in Puerto Rico is to talk about meaning-making processes which can be distributed in a social, spaciotemporal context. That is, in the context of social science interviews, discourse and discursive practices are semiotic productions that circulate through real-time, event-bound contexts. The task of meaning-making occurs in interaction, co-constructing meaning through linguistic and non-linguistic semiotics. In these discursive occasions, we rely on three key linguistic/ discursive devices: indexicality, performativity, and talk-in-interaction in interviews. Unpacking these structures to analyze different perspectives and distributed agency on helpseeking and sociocultural phenomena in-depth and how these are communicated is the methodological goal of the data presented here.

When we refer to performativity in interaction, we refer to philosopher John Austin's work on speech act theory in pragmatics and the philosophy of language (1962). Austin's work (later expanded upon by Searle 1975; Searle 1976; Searle et al. 1969) shifted the way language was defined: language does not solely name or describe objects in the world, but it acts upon a sociocultural context and co-text and create social facts about social relations (Agha 2007). When we talk, we also do things. If two friends got to talking and one said to the other, "*Qué sed tengo*" (I'm so thirsty), this may have various effects depending on the context. If the same friend visits the other friend in their home, this may be viewed as a request for water, which could result in one giving the other a glass of water. However, if said friends were in a restaurant setting, and one were to utter the same phrase, it may not be a request for action so much as perhaps a critique of the restaurant's poor/slow service or perhaps a suggestion of the food's high salt content. The interpretation of this would be dependent on the turns at talk that came previously and may bring to bear how meaning-making and action in these events are culturally- and contextually bound. The principle of performativity then views language as a social action in interaction, which is also bound to normative sets of practices in a cultural context.

Indexicality or the pointing to or signaling of an object within a given sociocultural context is another way we make meaning in discourse. An index, then, is a sign that points to or signals something contiguous to it in a given context and as such has meaning-making capability when anchored in a context. Canonical structures in language that fall under indexicality are personal pronouns and verb tenses (also known as "shifters") (Silverstein 1976, 2003). Silverstein classifies indexicals as referential or nonreferential. It is the quality of nonreferentiality that makes indexicality particularly powerful in interaction. For instance, indexicals in talk-in-interaction may work in chains or groups in interaction; a given speaker's word choice in a turn at talk may not only unfold notions of register, dialect, and lexical preference, but its prosodic features may reveal a speaker's stance in a context, which in turn indexes aspects of their identity. Indexicality can thus have a number of implications on macro dynamics (i.e., ideologies and views of health in the context of colonialism, classism, racism, debt, decreased medical funding) and micro ones (such as unfolding ideologies in talk-in-interaction), which merits its close analysis.

Talk-in-interaction refers to the turn-by-turn co-construction of meaning within the context of the interview. That is, when we talk in most contexts (and especially within the context of a research interview), we mostly follow a one-at-a-time speaker rule with little or no gap or overlap within turns at talk. While doing so, we may not even notice that we are taking part of a joint action wherein we hold ourselves and other interactants morally accountable for following a series of unspoken rules: taking turns, answering questions, formulating questions, holding others accountable for following the rules, and rebuking others when these are not followed (Sacks et al. 1974; Schegloff 2007). Turn-by-turn dynamics of talk are usually evidenced at the level of an utterance, which can be analyzed for its content (the literal meaning of what was said) and interactional meaning (the contextual meaning). Interactional meaning, unlike the meaning of an utterance content, requires that we pay careful attention to each turn at talk and what came before and after a given utterance. Additional attention must be cast on *how* something was said (i.e., intonational qualities, hesitation, silences, speed, audible sounds) as well as *who* said it (e.g., speaker, attribution of reported speech) (Tracy and Robles 2013).

In applying these different methodological approaches to the data analysis, we hope to show how agency is not only enacted but is rooted and represented through language choices and social practices. Moreover, the cultural logics to which people appeal in order to rationalize their choices, behaviors, and decisions as they seek help (Enfield 2000; Enfield and Sidnell 2017) address the local adoption and strategic deployment of older adults in the aftermath of the storms and other cascading events in the local context.

2 Methods and data: Discourse analysis

The data in this chapter come from a longitudinal study[1] on the psychosocial concept of resilience within the frame of medical helpseeking in the by and for the elderly after the passing of hurricanes Irma and María through Puerto Rico. The data comprise repeated ethnographic interviews with older adults, caregivers, and medical professionals, all which were recruited via purposive referral sampling (Tashakkori et al. 2020; Teddlie and Yu 2007) in six different barrios or districts surrounding the urban center of a municipality in the interior of the island. The research team composed of the authors and 10 undergraduate students from University of Puerto Rico – Cayey conducted in-depth, face-to-face interviews twice in people's homes, healthcare settings, and university offices.

We carried out a total of 64 interviews during 2018–2019 (22 older adults, 19 caregivers, and 23 health care professionals) and re-interviewed 46 persons (17 older adults, 13 caregivers, and 16 healthcare professionals) during Year 2 (2019–2021). We recruited and interviewed four additional medical professionals in Year 2 to substitute those who unable to complete the second interview. All who contributed to the data presented here are Spanish-speakers who resided and/or worked in the interior of the island when hurricanes Irma and Maria struck the island and sought or offered medical or psycho-social aid after the hurricanes and during the pandemic. The data presented here are for some of the older adult interviews carried out in Year 1. Table 1 displays these older adults' basic demographic characteristics (age, gender, education level, years of education, household income), health insurance coverage, reported chronic illnesses, and their self-perceived ratings of current general health outlook, compared health outlook with others of the same age, and health outlook after hurricanes Irma and María.

Data collection is focused on (a) longitudinal, successive accounts of helpseeking by older adults, their caregivers, and medical professionals, and (b) documentation of helpseeking networks (including persons, places, and organizations). Each participant was asked to provide 2–3 accounts of helpseeking in each interview and prompted for details about persons, places, and organizations in their accounts. All study contributors were interviewed twice, with some interviewed in intervals of 9–12 months between interviews and others at a 12–18 month interval given the interruption to data collection in March 2020.

Besides focusing on successive accounts of helpseeking, interviews also consisted of basic demographic questions, general health perceptions as well

---

[1] The study was approved by the Institutional Review Board of the University of Puerto Rico at Cayey.

Table 1: Demographic Characteristics of Subset of Interview Contributors.

Participant pseudonym (age, gender)	Education level/ years	Annual Income (U.S. dollars)	Health insurance	Self-reported chronic illness	Self-reported general health outlook**	Self-reported health compared with others	Self-reported health after hurricanes
Marisol (66, Female)	Higher education (13)	$4,200	Mi Salud*	Breast cancer, depression, hypertension, thyroid disease	Poor	Worse	Worse
El Viejo (73, Male)	Elementary (1.5)	$9,000	Mi Salud	Arthritis, depression	Poor	Better	Worse
Lilian (76, Female)	High School (10)	$9,000	Mi Salud	Arthritis, thyroid disease, depression	Poor	Better	Worse
Elsie (69, Female)	University degree (16)	$43,080	Private	Diabetes, hypertension, thyroid disease, arthritis	Poor	Same	Worse

*Mi Salud was the government-based health insurance. In 2018, a newly elected governor changed the government's public health insurance name as well as some of its regulatory conditions; its recipients were permitted to choose additional coverage from private health organizations managing the government insurance at an additional cost.
**Self-reported health based on Likert-scale rating (1=Excellent, 2=Very Good, 3=Good, 4=Poor, 5=Bad).

as return of basic utility services questions. Finally, older adults and caregivers were also asked questions from the McGill Illness Narrative Interview, Section IV Service and Response to Treatment (Groleau et al. 2006). The length of the transcribed interviews ranged from 45 minutes to 3 hours. These were audio recorded and transcribed verbatim (Hutchby and Wooffitt 1998; Jefferson 2004).

The segments of data that we analyze from the interviews with older adults focus on scripted and unscripted questions related to helpseeking immediately after the hurricanes. As stated previously, the role of language as social action in talking about helpseeking after these major events is the focus of this work. All names presented are pseudonyms, chosen by or assigned to the speakers.

3 Findings and analysis

In the data excerpts presented below, we draw on interviews with older adults seeking medical or social help immediately or shortly after (2–3 weeks) the hurricanes of September 2017. While the focus of the analysis is on each older adult's helpseeking strategies in times of need and/or the obstacles towards healthcare, we also present each case providing a rich, context-based background of the telling including the older adult's self-rated health as well as the health situation or event that triggered the helpseeking. The connections we hope to demonstrate in these excerpts transcend the local environment of each older adult. Transcription conventions are found in the appendix.

3.1 The long delay to medical help and the multiple obstacles to seeking help after the storms

In Excerpt 1, we present a story of health and illness in times of chaos. Marisol is a 66-year-old woman living in one of the oldest and most elderly-populated subdivisions in the urban sector of her town, which was about four months without electricity (although water services were restored within a few days of the events). A recipient of Plan Vital, the government-regulated health care program, Marisol reported living on less than $350 monthly, of which about $100 was taken from her social security check every month to pay for the Medicare Part B provider. She did not drive, but she lived less than five miles from a tertiary healthcare center and from a municipal diagnosis center; the home where she lived – belonging to her mother who lived in the States – was a one-story cement structure surrounded by other one- and two-story homes.

As she talked about her health and illnesses before and after the storms, she reflected on the chaos she lived health-wise. She revealed that she was a breast cancer survivor and had a mastectomy two months prior to September 2017. She felt the confidence to show us the scar that ran down the right side of her chest and commented upon the horrid pain she still experienced each time she touched the wound area. It goes without saying that having had a mastectomy two months prior to the hurricanes was extremely challenging, not only because of the recency of the procedure but because of her severe depression which was diagnosed four years prior to the operation. Given the nightmare of the post-operative recuperation, the extraction of her right breast meant an exacerbation of her already severe mental health diagnosis. Reeling with pain and unable to do the simple activities she did before, she had lost faith in her own body, her self-image, and her relationships with others. Faced with little in the way of a cancer support group, friends, or family for support, she endured the ongoing pain with little help or clear explanations from doctors and managed her deteriorating mental health via medication and one-on-one monthly counseling sessions. The mastectomy on top of an ongoing depression shook her confidence and quality of life, but as she narrates below, her health situation only worsened after the passing of the storms and the long delay of reliable and caring medical attention. "M" refers to Marisol while "I" refers to interviewer.[2]

Excerpt 1
This was chaos

66	M:	est- >esto fue un caos< (.)
		thi- this was chaos
67		sa ↑bes >antes yo estaba< <u>antes</u> estaba mal,
		you know before that I was down in the dumps
68		>pero estaba con mi tratamiento<
		but I was receiving my treatment
69		y ↑sí me ayudaba un montón↓
		and yes it helped me a lot
70		>ahí todo se ↑viró<
		then everything went upside down
71		>que se ↑complicó< pues ↑<u>María</u>
		what complicated things well Maria
72		y estaba recién opera' de de prácticamente de °lo del seno°
		and I was recently operated of of the- practically- of the- of that breast thing

---

[2] Transcription conventions can be found in the appendix.

73	>°que todavía no lo había superado°<
	which I had still not gotten over
74	Que: °eso fue lo que pasó°
	that was what happened
75	desde ahí pa' acá °como que- >como que he ido pa' ↑atrás°<
	from there on like- like my health has gotten worse
	[. . .]
423	y ese mes pues traté de <u>llamar y llamar</u> y no
	and that month well I tried to call and call and no
424	nadie cogía el teléfono
	no one picked up the phone
	[. . .]
452	>pero después de ahí< (1.0)
	but after that
453	no pude com- no he podido comunicarme con ellos
	I couldn't com- I haven't been able to communicate with them
454	y no no están- no están ahí
	and no- they're not there- they're not there
455	sae' que no sé (.) si fue que ellos cambiaron el teléfono
	you know I don't know if they changed their telephone number
456	n- a raíz de lo de la tormenta >o no sé<
	because of the storm or I don't know
457	>la cosa es< me quedé
	the thing is that I'm not with-
458	no estoy yendo al psiquiatra
	I'm not going to the psychiatrist
459 I:	°wuao°
	Wow
460	no- °no estoy yendo al psiquiatra° no-
	no- I am not going to the psychiatrist no
461	>no estoy tomando nada< (1.0)
	I am not taking anything (1.0)
462	°y yo estuve mucho tiempo⁰°
	and I was getting treatment for a long time-
463	°estuve como cuatro años con mi (.) tratamiento°
	I had it for about four years

In assessing the situation and the chaos that hurricane María unleashed, Marisol has a few primary goals; in the interview context, her immediate interactional goal revolves around the joint action of talking with us about her helpseeking practices after the hurricane (i.e., turn-taking, sequence organization). She acts on this by sharing the story about her unsuccessful medical helpseeking with us. In fact, we can observe how she interactionally manages her health issues by talking around the stigmatizing label of depression ("*antes estaba mal*" or "before I was down in the dumps", line 67, instead of "I was depressed") and vaguely refers to her mastectomy as "*lo del seno*" ("the breast thing", line 72). She also interactionally manages her accountability dealing with her illness by narrating her trajectory, the actions she took, the results and outcome of the actions taken. For instance, she stresses the action taken in greater emphasis when she says and repeats the word "call" in line 421 ("I tried to call and call"); she rationalizes the results of the action when she tells us "they" (presumably the psychiatrist and/ or counselors) are not there in line 454; she further rationalizes this by presenting the possibility that they may have changed their number as a result of the storm (line 455); and finally she provides an outcome to her health situation – I'm not going to the psychiatrist, I'm not taking anything (lines 458, 460–461).

Her story, however, is not only about the inability to secure treatment to continue receiving anti-depressants and monthly counseling sessions to have a better quality of life, but also about making sense of her lived experience; in essence, it is about what she does with the words she uses to talk about her health situation and her health perceptions and ideologies. Through her first-person account of past events as well as through the informal register and lexical choices made (e.g., "things went upside down", "things got complicated", lines 70–71), she requests for help in the then-and-there moment (i.e., "I tried to call and call", line 423), as securing help would allow her to meet her own goal of feeling better (lines 68–69). When help is not returned, she frames the multiple constraints of agency and of accessing treatment and medication for depression to an external actor (lines 66, 71–72, 454: it was chaos, it was María, it was being recently operated, it was them not being there). Even the use of whispering while discussing the topic of depression, her mastectomy (lines 72–74), and her termination of treatment (lines 460–463) suggests there is a sense of fragmentation and agentive angst in her story – revealing the sensitive and unresolved nature of her health. While she provides a rationale and a justification for her helpseeking story (she called for help, but no one answered), it is indicative of the multiple constraints to the distribution of agency in the narrative world. That is, while there could have been multiple stakeholders that could have acted in unison with Marisol to provide her the help she needed in the narrative world (and at the same time share with her the elements of agency), there are none. Her lack of flexibility to control others' actions is the crux of the matter.

At another level, the reflexive quality of her language also exposes macro dynamics about her accountability and flexibility regarding her health, helpseeking, and healthcare that were key to her experience before and after hurricane María. As Enfield (2017) explains, distributed agency is anchored in time, and the components of accountability and flexibility can take micro-seconds (as in the turn-taking in talk) or a much longer time scale to materialize. In terms of Marisol's story, the agency attributed to the hurricane as responsible for her situation seems to be amiss for other agentic persons and artifacts in the story world that do not materialize. For instance, an already weakened and underprepared social health structure prior to María may have been the trigger and catalyst leading to her negative outcome and the eventual termination of her much-needed treatment. Had a more reliable social safety net been available, or had governmental health agencies, medical groups or other health organizations established a protocol for those most vulnerable, perhaps Marisol's story would have been different. One could also suggest that a weakened or frayed preventative care system may be held accountable for not providing expert advice or expert knowledge regarding treatment after the storm. Perhaps the construction and ideologies of health care practices as one wherein the patient is responsible and accountable for their own health (i.e., discourses of health as a personal choice or ideology of health as patient driven) may have led to faulty expectations on behalf of the network of mental health care providers. In the end, vulnerabilities in the social and medical health care system equally account for Marisol's diminished or perhaps limited ability to make healthcare and helpseeking choices after the storm. The series of cascading events that led to a seeming dead end in terms of treatment demonstrates her thwarted flexibility. These actions laid the ground for her vulnerability and disempowerment well before the hurricanes. In this sense, we can say that agency is distributed along a chain of events and circumstances within the economic and sociohistorical context prior to and after the storm's path. The effects of the different social factors and social personae and their course of action led to the disaster-related effects of termination of treatment, worsening health outcomes, and deteriorating quality of life. This example demonstrates mobilization of helpseeking on behalf of Marisol, but massive failure on behalf of the health care system.

3.2 El Viejo and Lilian: The physical barriers to care

Excerpt 2 presents the case of an older married couple, El Viejo (73, a retired construction and agriculture seasonal worker) and Lilian (76, the principal family caregiver), living in one of the rural barrios outside of the center of their town which suffered many landslides during the heavy rainfalls brought by hurricane María and remained without running water or electricity upwards of five months. A year post-hurricane María, the road to their home – a narrow, winding one-laner typical of rural roads of the mountainous interior – still contained traces of the storm's path: bare hillsides with dead Norfolk pines, uprooted trees, and broken wooden electricity posts. New foliage and growth covered the mountainside. We learned that the road leading up to Lilian and El Viejo's home was divided into sectors named after the different families that lived in the area. In the past, all the sectors shared common kinship ties but at the time of our interview, many of these kinship ties had weakened or disappeared. And although younger generations remained and distant cousins moved in, not all sectors have exercised kinship collaboration and camaraderie.

We also observed the varying states of the many two- to three-story cement homes and a few wooden structures. Some had been remodeled and repainted, while others still bore the impact of the hurricanes in the facade. Most houses in this area (as in most mountainous areas of Puerto Rico) do not rest on a foundation but on concrete columns anchored into the slopes; incomplete constructions abound with exposed cinderblock walls that have yet to be plastered. Lilian and El Viejo's home, a two-story dilapidated cement structure built piecemeal on a lush mountainside facing the town, accommodated them as well as an older daughter with developmental disabilities. The lower level accommodated another adult daughter (working as a domestic in the capital city of San Juan) and her children. A different structure at the far end of the house accommodated a granddaughter (working as a nurse tech in the southeastern coastal town of Guayama) and her husband. A short distance away and on the same shared cement road that led one outside of the property to the main road, lived an older, estranged niece of the older woman in an equally dilapidated two-story cement home with what seemed to be an abandoned car and a handful of dogs tied to chains. This extended family lived in what was formerly land belonging to Lilian's parents – with her being the main inheritor, the connection to the other kin living in this area, and the matriarch of the family.

Lilian and El Viejo both had Plan Vital (the government-run health insurance plan) and reported multiple chronic health conditions for which they were prescribed multiple medicines. When asked about their general health outcome and asked to compare it with others their same age, they remained optimistic even though they both rated their health as poor; their source of optimism was that they had better health when compared with others their same age – even though they report discontinuation of medical help from specialists after the storm. Their medical helpseeking story is one of multiple physical, infrastructural challenges to obtain medicines or see their doctors after the event.

In the following excerpt, they explain the problem with excess mud that accumulated in the road that led to their home and the uprooted trees that blocked the path to anyone. They explain that it took them one week to clean the road from their home to the main municipal road; to clear a path once on the main road, they paid a private company to help cut down trees with a chain saw and clear the road of debris and mud because they couldn't be sure when their municipality was going to send the emergency cleaning brigades. The municipality did not show up until a month later further demonstrating structural holes in its civil response team (Cruz Rodríguez and López de Victoria 2019). The work of cleaning the main road took an additional week. Meanwhile, they had to wait so that they could travel to the downtown area to get medicines. Once they had access to the main road, new obstacles arose. El Viejo told the following story (note that *P2* refers to El Viejo while *I* refers to interviewer):

Excerpt 2
We were in a bit of a rough spot

41	P2:	*nos las vimos un poquito ↑fea*
		we found ourselves in a bit of an ugly situation
42		*eh (.) nos quedamos sin paso*
		uh uh we had no access to the road
43		*(.) hubo que que hace- ↑hacer fuerzas por ahí >sin poder<*
		There was a need to- to gai- gain strength without having it
44	I:	*mjum*
		Uh huh
45	P2:	*e:h valga que lo entre los vecinos unos de acá y unos de allá*
		Uh goodness between the neighbors some from here and others from there
46		*pues hicimos brecha y >después que abrimos camino<*
		well we made an opening and then we opened the path
47		*pues se normalizó ↑un poco*
		well everything became a bit more normal
48		*porque ↑no teníamos agua*
		because we didn't have water
49		*entonces y yo >con ese jeepito que tengo ahí<*
		and I- with that little jeep I have here
50		*>cargaba agua todos los días pa' la casa< y ↑las pasamos (.)*
		I carried water to the house every day and we survived
51		*.hh pero ↑gracias a Dios de ahí en fuera hh. (.) diría que la pasamos bastante bien*
		But thank God from there on I would say that we got through it okay
52		*>porque no nos faltó comida< pa este*
		because we did not need food
53		*pues no .hh este este se sufrió como ↓loco*
		because no- uh- uh- there was lots of suffering
54		*↓pero nada °hasta ahora h. Papito Dios siempre ha estado ahí h. ↓y nos ha cuidao'°*
		But nothing up to now the heavenly Father has always been there and taken care of us

---

In this excerpt, El Viejo tells his story, predominantly from a first-person plural perspective in an informal register, while using mostly past tense verbs with the occasional "se" impersonal/ passive voice construction. At first, he responds to the interviewer's question, "who needed medical help after the storm?", using first-person plural pronoun "we" in the conjugated reflexive, past tense verb "*nos las vimos*" ("we found ourselves", line 40). El Viejo's response seems to suggest that his story was going to revolve around a highly difficult or perhaps extreme experience wherein the family sought medical help, but his turn develops into talk about the other difficult and taxing consequences of the storm (the road being impassable, being without water, working with neighbors, and enduring suffering; lines 42, 48, and 53). The shift in story line evokes the many difficulties experienced by many in this region living without safe access to water because the water system operated by the Puerto Rico Aqueducts and Sewers Authority require electricity to distribute. As El Viejo explains, not having water (for five months) meant traveling to a water oasis on a regular basis to provide his home with access to drinking water, something that must have been incredibly difficult for El Viejo, a 73-year-old living with debilitating arthritis. Arguably, the change of topic is justified given the metaphorical and literal "ugliness" (line 40) palpable in their neighborhood. These obstacles were more pressing than health and medical concerns.

The interactional goals in the story world, the lexical choices made, and the intonational features of his talk invite a more profound analysis of this excerpt. Interactionally, his goal is to talk about the emergency that demanded his community act to survive. The discursive features that underpin these acts of solidarity in clearing a path – mostly demonstrated by first-person plural "we", past tense, and impersonal, passive voice "se" constructions – by far do the work of highlighting how the emergency turned into an act of altruism and social cooperation between neighbors "from here and there" (line 45) in the face of suffering and adversity while engaging the listener in the act. Unlike Marisol's assessment of chaos after the storm, here El Viejo seems to present the same event differently, highlighting the distributed sense of agency and flexibility among the neighbors while softening the effects and taking on a more proactive yet at times impersonal (and at times optimistic) stance. Although he describes the situation as being a "a bit" ugly for them (line 41), he downplays or softens the significance of the event repeatedly through interactional resources such as diminutives (e.g., "poquito", "jeepito", "papito") and extreme case formulations (Pomerantz 1986), such as "*siempre*" (always), indexing a relaxed, yet tenacious persona in the story world. Then when he then uses the deictic marker "there" preceded by preposition "around", the details of his story – embedded in the agentless, impersonal constructed structure "there was a need to gain strength" to clear the road (line 43) – again mitigate and distance the "extremeness" of this life-threatening event. These strategies seem to do the job of managing his accountability and flexibility in the face of a life-threatening disaster, but they also serve to manage his narrative persona who is now observing these past events from a here-and-now lens with us. Finally, in the coda-like assessment in line 53 "*se sufrió como loco*" ("there was lots of suffering"), a construction which reduces the prominence of the speaker (Martínez-Linares 2009), he reinforces this experience and its telling followed by an appeal and an affirmation to larger cultural and social logics: "*papito Dios siempre ha estado ahí y nos ha cuidado*" ("God is always there and takes care of us", line 53). Their suffering then draws on larger social orders and cultural logics of faith, which affirm his religious views and belief system and his positive outlook that is reflected in his narrative when he says "*la pasamos bastante bien*" ("we got through it okay", line 51). Although immediate access to the medical help they needed was not possible because of the many physical obstacles, his solidarity with others in the community and his faith in God maintained him grounded and optimistic, searching for the necessary energy to carry on in the face of adversity.

3.3 Lilian's waiting game

In the next excerpt, Lilian, El Viejo's wife, focuses on telling her medical help-seeking experience after the storm. Note that "L" refers to Lilian while "P2" refers to El Viejo.

Excerpt 3
We had to wait

67	L:	>*primero era que estaba obstruida*<
		first it was that the road was obstructed
68		>*después era que había mucho lodo* <
		then it was that there was too much mud
69		*y no se podía ir en carro al pueblo*
		and you could not go to town in a car
70		>↑*y después de esto pues fui*< .hh *a la farmacia*
		and then after that I went to the pharmacy
71		*no tenía* ↑*luz. Se dañó la*=
		and they didn't have electricity. The electric generator=
72	P2:	=*Ah sí*=
		Ah yes
73	L:	=↑*se dañó la planta y tuvimos que esperar*
		The electric generator got damaged and we had to wait
74		*porque yo tengo mis recetas allá en esa (.) farmacia*
		because I have my prescriptions there in that pharmacy
75		*pues no podía ir a comprar al menos que comprara este sin receta (.)*
		so I couldn't buy them unless I paid for them out of pocket
76		*y y así para ir al médico pues también a esperar (.) un* ↓*poco.*
		and and like that as well to go to the doctor we had to wait a bit too

---

While the interactional goals of El Viejo's story were circumscribed to the community efforts to dissipate the effects of the storm on everyday activities and their livelihood, Lilian's story not only repeats the assessments previously made by her husband (in a more distant and generalized manner), but she also focuses on exposing what helpseeking was like two to three weeks post-María – equivalent to the time it took her husband and the neighbors to clear the roads and travel by car to the town's center. Using lists to interactionally manage the telling as well as make more generalizable her story (Jefferson 1990; Potter 1996), she reveals the difficulty helpseeking represented for her in the story world given the economic limitations she previously reported in the interview. Interestingly, this is not the only list in this rather brief, matter-of-fact narrative. At first, she lists the physical obstacles to getting to the pharmacy (the obstructions on the road, too much mud; lines 67–68). Then she lists a new series of obstacles in the pharmacy (no power and a broken generator; lines 71–73) that hinder her ability to receive her medication; in order to do so, she would have had to go to a different pharmacy and pay for these out-of-pocket, something that would be extremely onerous given her limited income. These events – while confirming the difficulties in getting medication – also suggest what Potter (1996) characterizes as commonplace or normal constructions of events or actions in talk. Arguably, Lilian interactively managed and displayed a sense of generalizability of the events because anyone who lived through María very likely lived through very similar or at least relatable events. Perhaps the sense of normalcy in this waiting game (as everyone else had to wait too) helps to lend more credibility to their experience as to a certain degree, it could be said these events not only relate to her individually but to the wider community, so it is important to list these so as to establish accountability in the narrative and here-and-now story world as well as to establish accord by any possible naysayer. While she manages the discursive space to justify her actions that resulted in a waiting game, her actions and agency seem thwarted by her limited flexibility. Ultimately, not having her medication could have had some very detrimental effects on her health, not to mention further complications on other chronic illnesses.

3.4 Having no choice

In the next excerpt, we present the helpseeking story shared by Elsie, a 71-year-old retired teacher, who along with her husband, Ramón, a 72-year-old retired industrial mechanic, required acquiring medication weeks after the storm's passing. Both are middle class older adults living in a rural neighborhood not too distant from the urban center, which historically was created from a special municipal housing program stimulating homeownership from local citizens (c.f. Picó 2006). In the 1970s, this municipal program sold parcels of land to underemployed or low-income families, like Elsie and Ramón, so that they could construct their homes. Unlike the houses in Marisol's subdivision (most of which were owned by those with the ability to pay for living in a middle-class neighborhood), the barrio where Elsie lived had a very diverse composition, with some middle class and others living below the poverty level. In the case of Elsie and Ramón, their two-story cement home was in the hilly area of the neighborhood, above the hustle and bustle of the streets with access to the main road. This choice, as they commented, was both a blessing and a curse given the difficulties they had accessing the road after the storm. Their home, unlike Lilian and El Viejo's, was built on a foundation and could better withstand the impact of the storms and the 2020 earthquakes.

Elsie and Ramón both had private health insurance and reported multiple chronic health conditions, with Elsie taking upwards of five different medicines daily and Ramón requiring asthma treatment. When asked about their health, Elsie reported a poor general health outlook while Ramón reported a very good health outcome, despite having had a very serious asthma attack during the passing of the storm. Although she reported being and feeling prepared for the storms and not having had a major health event afterwards, one of her controlled medicines ran out weeks post-María. She also had to wait weeks to be able to travel to the pharmacies in town, only to wait in the hours-long queues to talk to a pharmacist. In the excerpt that follows, she explains what she experienced in the process of trying to acquire said medication in a chain pharmacy to ultimately travel to a different pharmacy to acquire it. "E" refers to Elsie.

Excerpt 4
I had to pay

54 E: *Este em- (tsk) y entonce:s este un medicamento no lo tenían disponible*
        Uh mhm (tsk) and then one of the medicines was not available
55   *Me tuve que ir a la farmacia de la comunidad*
        I had to go to the community pharmacy
56 I: *Okey*
        Okay
57 E: *.hh y la farmacia de la comunidad no tenía sistema ni nada ↑*
        And the community pharmacy didn't have the billing system or anything
58   ↑*y me cobraron el medicamento*
        and they billed me the medicine
59 I: *O:key*
        Okay

60	E:	*(tsk) En Walgreens me cogieron el seguro*
		(tsk) In Walgreens they accepted my insurance
61		↓*pero (.) farmacia de la comunidad* ↓*lo tuve que pagar*
		but (.) in the community pharmacy I had to pay out of pocket
62	I:	*Okey*
		Okay
63	E:	*La farmacia del pueblo pues lo tuve que pagar*
		at the community pharmacy I had to pay ok
64		*porque no-* ↓*que no tenía y que sistema*
		because supposedly they did not have the billing system
65		*y lo tuve que pagar <u>porque la necesidad</u>*
		and I had to pay because of the need

To understand Elsie's story, it is important to point out the broader social contexts at play during this time. While the storm's winds destroyed many homes, it also rendered the retail industry, including pharmacies, inoperable for an extended period. In the case of chain pharmacies which were operating after the storm, such as the one mentioned in this excerpt, these had better access to much-needed resources (i.e., diesel, power generators, security), yet confronted serious problems in delivering prescription medicines. That is, a supply chain disruption given the impassable road conditions and the limited port capacity in the metropolitan port authority translated to lack of a reliable medicine supply chain to many pharmacies (Hernández and Mufson 2017; Kim and Bui 2019). Faced with an increasing public health crisis, the local government deregulated many of the everyday health protocols via executive and administrative orders; the federal government lifted the Merchant Marine Act of 1920 (also known as the Jones Act) for ten days. While the federal response to the hurricane intended to bolster much-needed relief headed to the island, this may not have been as effective for persons like Elsie. Notwithstanding the major mismanagement at the local level, the local response – in particular the passing of Administrative order 2017-10-00 – helped relax the requirement to present current prescription when refilling medications at any pharmacy (2017). At a time of crisis, the actions taken by the local government were supposed to afford patients, like Elsie, the flexibility to purchase medicines elsewhere if they possessed evidence of their prescription (e.g., an empty medicine bottle with a recent prescription date); given the constraints with communications and technology, these processes were not without major barriers, as can be observed in Elsie's story.

It is also important to point out the pivotal role community pharmacies played locally immediately after the disaster (Melin and Conte 2018; Melin et al. 2018; Zorrilla 2017). Once the local government passed Administrative Order

2017-10-00, community pharmacies became de facto "first responders" as they were quick to provide services to anyone in need, agreeing to dispense medication without an advance verification of the patients' insurance coverage or assurance of receiving payment from patients. Their services were quickly advertised in local radio programming and newspapers as an alternative to the larger chain pharmacies (Soto 2017), and news of their solidarity with everyday citizens traveled widely and swiftly through word-of-mouth as people waited in hours-long queues in chain pharmacies and supermarkets, gas stations, and banks. Chain pharmacies, on the other hand, were reported as shuttering their doors while they awaited insurance policies to take effect. Not surprisingly, purchasing one's medicines and products through a community pharmacy became an issue of pride for many and quickly began evoking discourses of nationality, solidarity, sustainability, and empowerment in the face of adversity, which provoked a newfound relevance in local community and in movements of *auto-gestión* (autonomous organization) in agriculture (Garriga-López 2019), community kitchens (Roberto 2019), and cooperative-based electric microgrids (Massol-Deyá 2019). In the case of pharmacies, they were accepting risks, which in some cases could amount to not receiving payment from the third-party payer because of inaccurate reporting of coverage. Nevertheless, refilling a medication at a different pharmacy from one's own during this time sometimes meant making hefty out-of-pocket cash payments as most pharmacies were unable to process deductibles through the web-based billing system due to the massive power outages and lack of internet. And with most Puerto Rican banks imposing limits on cash withdrawal to $200 per day, many were further constrained to purchasing a limited number of medication or go without.

With these points in mind, we turn to Elsie's narrative. Demonstrating the canonical Labovian narrative structure (Labov and Waletzky 1967), Elsie transports her audience to a there-and-then narrative world using her voice as narrator to tell her version of the events, the action-steps that followed, her perceived obligations, and the decisions she made to obtain her medication. Her interactional goals – responding to our questions by telling her helpseeking story after the storm – also include airing out grievances in the process of obtaining her medication in addition to allocating blame to the community pharmacy.

In the case of the linguistic devices used in her story, most notable is the repetition of deontic modality through the use of *tener que* (had to); not only is it strategically used to convey the sense of obligation from the opening and closing of this particular story, but it is used as a way to account for Elsie's critical stance (and perhaps surprise) towards the event as well as a way to justify her criticisms. This is coupled with the repetition of the action *"lo tuve que pagar"* ("I had to pay for it", lines 61 and 63), the rise and occasional drops in intonation in her speech in lines 57–58, 61, and 64, as well as the greater emphasis in talk in lines 58 and 65 when she complains about being billed the medication to later make the assessment, "*porque la necesidad*" ("because of the need"). The rise of intonation in line 58 is also formulated so as to display affect acoustically in the form of surprise and frustration towards unjustly being charged for medication that should have been covered by her medical insurance.

Of most interest in this excerpt, however, is Elsie's rhetorical strategies to build a case for agency, accountability, responsibility, and blame in the process of helpseeking post-disaster, with blame being particularly crafted through the use of a passive-like speaker formulation, extreme case formulation, repetition, and voicing. Starting in line 55, Elsie constructs and manages her there-and-then persona in the excerpt by casting herself as one having little (or no) choice in the matter of picking the community pharmacy referred to in the excerpt. In line 57, she places blame on the community pharmacy through the combined use of the negative particle "no" in "*no tenía sistema*" ("they didn't have the billing system"), and the extreme case formulation "*ni nada*" (literally meaning "nor nothing", but translated to "or anything"), which together work to strengthen her complaint narrative and to legitimize her point of view of being unfairly charged. Later in lines 60–61, she juxtaposes the actions of her primary pharmacy (described as a passive, unaccountable actor which accepts the insurance but lacks the medicine) to the actions of the community pharmacy to further manage and construct her powerlessness in the transaction and her right to complain. Later, in line 64 Elsie uses a non-quotative reported speech formula in the form of hearsay in "*que no tenía y que sistema*" ("that supposedly they did not have the billing system") implying skepticism in the response and questioning the reasons behind the billing of the medicine. All in all, Elsie's complaint, as accomplished through these rhetorical strategies and the thrice repeated phrase marked by the deontic modal *tener que* in "*lo tuve que pagar*" ("I had to pay for it", lines 61, 63, and 65), establishes to her here-and-now audience that she has a right to complain because ultimately her own actions were an obligation: she had no choice but to pay for the medication as it was a priority for her health and quality of life. In the end, she accounts for her actions, her powerlessness, and victimhood, but also holds accountable and responsible the community pharmacy as the public's expectations of these pharmacies post-disaster is to be more flexible in times of crisis, especially considering the many reports of patients not being charged for their medicine.

While the linguistic devices and rhetorical strategies featured in Elsie's telling make us empathize with her and her levels of frustration, powerlessness, and anger in obtaining prescription medication, it is also worth noting the unnamed actors in this story or those that fail to be accounted for in this trying account of helpseeking. First, her own pharmacy is not held accountable for not having provided her the medicine in the first place or for not having had the flexibility to verify at another pharmacy branch. Had they preemptively held stock of their inventory prior to the storm, contacted other branches, or taken account of the pre-existing failures in local infrastructure and prepared, perhaps they would have been able to remedy the situation swiftly. A second unaccounted actor in this narrative is the local government. Their lack of preparedness prior to the storm and their poor mitigation response post disaster threatened the very livelihood of many post-disaster. Their inaction exposed many to unhealthy and inhumane living conditions. And although these inactions could have been the consequence of willfully ignorant leaders (or worse, terribly callous and indifferent ones), clear mechanisms should be in place to remedy these situations of chaos and crisis. In essence, the lack of altruism and solidarity and the acts of willful ignorance crafted through attribution of blame to negligible actors are a reflection of wider systemic problems and inadequacies in preparedness and mitigation strategies post-disaster, ultimately indexing the local government's very palpable acts of negligence and systemic social harm. Said unaccounted actors reveal that at a localized level, the lack of preparation and response plan on behalf of prescribers, third-party payers, and pharmacies with those most vulnerable in times of crisis must be addressed and accounted for. In the context of post-disaster recuperation, Elsie's story then not only serves to reiterate the disarticulated and irresponsible response on behalf of local government, but also calls into question the role that all prescribers, third-party payers, and pharmacies have in the context of crisis and disaster. In other words, not only do community pharmacies have the responsibility to vouch for the dire needs of those with health care needs, but so do all service providers, health insurance companies, and governmental public health agencies. All in all, Elsie's tone of irritation and frustration in asking older adults to pay full amount for their much-needed medicines in a pharmacy echoed a general sentiment in the population: pharmaceutical treatment should never come at the expense of the patient who is already pressed and stretched economically. Not only did the lack of response on behalf of these unmentioned actors exacerbate acute and chronic health conditions in public health in general, but also were acts of structural violence further unleashing greater waves of crisis, disaster, and violence in an already disenfranchised community.

4 Discussing the barriers, the obstacles, and the inaction after the hurricanes

Using a discourse analytic lens to examine and tease apart the issues related to helpseeking immediately after the hurricanes of 2017, we demonstrated the complex interactions and accounts experienced by Marisol, El Viejo, Lilian, and

Elsie. The barriers and obstacles to medical helpseeking in the aftermath of a near category five hurricane demonstrate the multiple constraints and differential levels of agency distributed unevenly across persons' networks of care and kinship ties.

In the case of Marisol, she was constrained not only by the multiple health situations which restricted her ability to act on her own behalf, but by her limited flexibility to petition others to act on her behalf, particularly her kinship ties and physicians. These chains of actors could have afforded her the flexibility necessary to control actions and decisions on timely medical treatment. Not having a reliable network of kinship ties on top of the lack of reliable and timely medical team and safety net that would afford her a better quality of life led to a negative health outcome, the termination of treatment, and a deteriorating quality of life.

In the case of El Viejo, Lilian, and Elsie, they all seem to be able to wield their flexibility through new connections with neighbors, alternative means to accomplish their goals, and distributed agency through their ties with others and their networks of care. Ultimately, their action steps and strategies in medical helpseeking in health and illness through the descriptions of their own and others' behaviors as manifested in the linguistic resources used and the choices made encode differential degrees of accountability, flexibility, and agency. They (including El Viejo) had to problem-solve in difficult circumstances, without access to the local mechanisms normally resorted to in times of need. In the case of Elsie, her problem-solving resulted in a temporary 'work-around' to access health care, new collaborations with local pharmacies, and possible manipulations of the system. In the case of El Viejo and Lilian, their problem-solving resulted in new collaborations with neighbors. In this sense, agency is best understood as distributed unevenly across networks of persons, organizations, and places.

For the older adults presented in this chapter experiencing changed patterns of adaptation, social equilibria, or 'new normals' in routine health care, these changes were not welcome at first. As time passed, these shifts sometimes led to stabilizing yet temporary pathways to helpseeking (as seen in Elsie's experience); however, for some, these led to destabilizing, long-term ailments/disability experiences that have worsened health outcomes (as in the case of Marisol). Yet others' health helpseeking pathways may have settled into relatively reliable patterns that only partially meet their needs (as with El Viejo and Lilian).

A common thread among all three women's narrative however was the urgency to access prescription medicine to continue managing their health and offset any other future health-related complications. The drastic shift in everyday ordinary actions, such as visiting one's doctor, making a call to a pharmacy, purchasing a refill via health insurance, makes more tangible the conditions of imbalance, characterized by social and economic inequalities. While Marisol's narrative seeking prescription medicines and medical help from her team of psychologists and psychiatrist lays bare the frayed yet multilayered dynamics of medical helpseeking in times of disaster and crisis for those most vulnerable, Lydia and Elsie's narratives display negotiation and resistance as they navigated through a frayed landscape peppered in layers of responsibility, accountability, flexibility, and blame.

At a more profound level, those actors in the chain of events that wield more knowledge and power yet remain unnamed due to inaction or maladaptation are telling about (1) the sense of loss of accountability and (2) the multi-layered inadequacies and failures in preparedness response, disaster recovery, and recuperation at a local level that is normalized after disaster (Oliver-Smith and Hoffman 2019). In these narratives, those who were responsible or should have been accounted for remained mostly in the shadow, and, to a certain degree, protected from being held accountable for the lack of preparedness, recovery, and recuperation efforts after the storms. In this sense, the voicing of disaster and the language to talk about disaster presented here lay bare the concealed inefficiencies, assumptions, and inequalities of long-standing social organization, which are further heightened by neo-liberal practices of governments, themselves characterized by systems of blame that "are reorganized in ways that now distribute responsibility to all 'active' citizens" (Arribas-Ayllon et al. 2013: 6).

5 Our understanding and recommendations of health care practices in times of crisis

In this chapter, we have had occasion to mention that our understanding of agency and health helpseeking in times of crisis emerged out of real, tangible sociohistorical contexts and conditions which have been documented and explained through the cases herein presented. The stories that Marisol, El Viejo, Lilian, and Elsie told demonstrate helpseeking pathways that were exacerbated by the physical destruction of the hurricane, but more so by an uncoordinated and (arguably) underfunded response by the local and United States government. Although the stories discussed in this chapter present the varying levels of difficulty in accessing beneficial medical helpseeking pathways immediately after or even a few weeks after the storms, these issues are still very much present four years post-disaster. This has given us the opportunity to reflect on recommendations and critical components necessary in health care actions and practices prior to a disaster and in times of crisis.

Based on our interviews, we have come to understand that health care providers and prescribers are important first actors in the chain of events that lead to successful and stabilizing pathways to healthcare for older adults. We recommend health care providers and prescribers establish proactive emergency protocols to be in place prior to the emergency event, disaster, or crisis. This should include establishing mandated routine visits for those with chronic health conditions prior to and early in the storm season, keeping a paper-based prescription copy in the patient's records for emergency cases, and establishing a more extensive next of kin list on the patient's record in case of inability to contact the patient. Second, our data also reveals that pharmacies are key sites where successful helpseeking mechanisms and strategies must be practiced. As such, we echo others' recommendations (Melin et al. 2018) of establishing mechanisms and assurances for the reimbursement of prescription medication. Given the many difficulties experienced by our collaborators in accessing medication refills from pharmacies, these protocols are instrumental to the management of health conditions and must therefore be available and in place before an emergency. More specifically, third-party payers should establish an emergency protocol which should be activated by all pharmacies prior to the event and afterwards, but especially in case of systemic communication failures. We underscore the importance of these mechanisms and recommendations in light of the data herein presented, but, more importantly, stress these be mandated by local governmental agencies as this would alleviate issues such as inaccessible or lost patient dosage information, damaged, lost or perishable medications (insulin), problems with health insurance, out-of-pocket payment for prescription medication, among others.

6 Concluding remarks

In this chapter, we have presented the results of an ongoing project where older adults talk about their experiences seeking medical or social help at different times after the passing of hurricanes Irma and María to explore the role of language as a medium for social action and as a response to the lack of government aid at a time of crisis. As we noted at the beginning of this chapter, we aimed to show that applied linguistics research and the microanalytic lens shed on collaborative acts of helpseeking displayed through performativity, indexicality, and talk-in-interaction has much to contribute to the study of aging, illness, and health in the context of disaster and crises. Examining how older adults talk about helpseeking strategies after compounded crises, we discussed how distributed agency within each case may at times lead to flexibility, accountability, and blame. We also discussed ways in which blame is constructed and managed: through the rhetorical and linguistic strategies used in the unsaid and the unaccounted for in the context of medical helpseeking. From a first glance, what these strategies reveal is a mix of ad hoc and sometimes stabilizing pathways to health care for older adults after hurricane Maria, but many a times a barrier to health and quality of life. Impaired access to care in situations such as the ones presented in this chapter lead to exacerbations of chronic conditions. At a more profound level, the experiences revealed by our collaborators are embedded, transmitted, and constituted in discourse and linguistic practices. Language, thus, is the site where framing, naming, rationalizing, legitimizing, acting (or not acting), silencing, and voicing the ailing body is made possible. From it, health and illness in bodies are made palpable, tangible, corporeal.

Moreover, our own experiences in navigating the social and health context after the hurricanes through language have taught us that it is important to critically interrogate and address the social, political, and linguistic nuances of health care policies in times of crisis and disaster. As evinced in these life experiences narrated in this chapter, we conceptualize pathways to health care in older adults in the context of crises and depleted resources as more than just a series of steps and strategies: it is an everyday struggle, with increasing levels of exclusion and disenfranchisement from the systems that purportedly provide health and quality of life to older adults. Investments in networks of care, in social safety nets, in systems that strengthen public education, public health, infrastructure, supply chain distribution, and the centralization and concentration of help and resources in the aftermath are equally important for Puerto Rico's landscape. Most importantly, older adults should not be asked to come to terms with multiple and varied contingencies as was the case after hurricane María and Irma.

Last but not least, our research has focused on real-world, authentic interactions with older adults living in a non-English context to shed light on the importance of applied linguistic research outside of the mainstream cultural settings. Understanding the underlying challenges and actual practices in health care contexts outside of the United States or Europe allow for intercultural opportunities to widen the field of applied linguistic research – an important site to better understand and promote continuity of care in health care contexts.

Appendix: Transcription conventions

Adapted from Hutchby & Woofit 1998; Jefferson 2004.

(0.5)	silent gap in tenths of a second
(.)	silent gap less than one tenth of a second
.h	in-breath; additional hhh indicate elongating the in-breath
h.	out-breath; additional hhh indicate elongating the out-breath
° °	spoken more quietly than the surrounding talk
> <	spoken more quickly than the surrounding talk
:	preceding sound or letter has been stretched; more colons indicate greater stretching
↑↓	<u>falling or rising</u> intonational shift in what follows
=	spoken sounds follow immediately on one another
<u>underline</u>	greater emphasis than surrounding talk

References

Agha, Asif. 2007. *Language and social relations*. Cambridge University Press.
Ahearn, Laura M. 2010. Agency and language. *Society and language use* 7. 28–48.
Arribas-Ayllon, Michael, Srikant Sarangi & Angus Clarke. 2013. *Genetic testing: accounts of autonomy, responsibility and blame*. Routledge.
Austin, John L. 1962. *How to do things with words*. Oxford University Press.
Bonilla, Yarimar. 2020. The coloniality of disaster: Race, empire, and the temporal logics of emergency in Puerto Rico, USA. *Political geography* 78. 102181.
Bonilla, Yarimar & Marisol LeBrón. 2019. *Aftershocks of disaster: Puerto Rico before and after the storm*. Haymarket Books.
Candlin, Christopher N. & Sally Candlin. 2003. 8. Health care communication: A problematic site for Applied Linguistics research. *Annual Review of Applied Linguistics* 23. 134–154.
Chafe, Wallace. 1994. *Discourse, consciousness, and time: The flow and displacement of conscious experience in speaking and writing*. Chicago & London: The University of Chicago Press.
Cruz Rodríguez, Gabriel & Patria López de Victoria. 2019. Bridging resources after a catastrophe: A case study on paramedics and their roles after hurricane María. Paper presented at the American Anthropological Association (AAA) and the Canadian Anthropology Society (CAS) Annual Meeting, Vancouver, Canada.
De Fina, Anna & Alexandra Georgakopoulou. 2011. *Analyzing narrative: Discourse and sociolinguistic perspectives*. Cambridge University Press.
Duranti, Alessandro. 2004. Agency in language. *A companion to linguistic anthropology*. John Wiley & Sons.
Enfield, Nicholas J. & Paul Kockelman. 2017. *Distributed agency*. Oxford University Press.
Enfield, Nicholas J. & Jack Sidnell. 2017. *The concept of action*. Cambridge University Press.

Enfield, Nick J. 2000. The theory of cultural logic: How individuals combine social intelligence with semiotics to create and maintain cultural meaning. *Cultural Dynamics* 12(1). 35–64.

Enfield, Nick J. 2017. Elements of agency. *Distributed agency*, 3–8.

Fcc-gov. 2017. *Hurricane Maria Communications Status Report for Sept. 21.* https://docs.fcc.gov/public/attachments/DOC-346840A1.pdf.

Garriga-López, Adriana. 2019. Puerto Rico: The future in question. *Shima* 13(2). 174–192.

Groleau, Danielle, Allan Young & Laurence J. Kirmayer. 2006. The McGill Illness Narrative Interview (MINI): an interview schedule to elicit meanings and modes of reasoning related to illness experience. *Transcultural Psychiatry* 43(4). 671–691.

Hernández, Arelis R. & Steven Mufson. 2017. Getting relief supplies to Puerto Rico ports is only half the problem. *The Washington Post*.

Hutchby, Ian & Robin Wooffitt. 1998. *Conversation analysis: Principles, practices, and applications*. Cambridge: Polity.

Jefferson, Gail. 1990. *List construction as a task and resource*. Lanham, MD: University Press of America.

Jefferson, Gail. 2004. Glossary of transcript symbols with an introduction. In Gene Lerner (ed.), *Conversation analysis: Studies from the first generation*, 13–34. Philadelphia: John Benjamins.

Kim, Karl & Lily Bui. 2019. Learning from Hurricane Maria: Island ports and supply chain resilience. *International Journal of Disaster Risk Reduction* 39. 101244.

Kishore, Nishant, Domingo Marqués, Ayesha Mahmud, Mathew V Kiang, Irmary Rodriguez, Arlan Fuller, Peggy Ebner, Cecilia Sorensen, Fabio Racy & Jay Lemery. 2018. Mortality in Puerto Rico after Hurricane Maria. *New England Journal of Medicine* 379(2). 162–170.

Kockelman, Paul. 2007. Agency: The relation between meaning, power, and knowledge. *Current Anthropology* 48(3). 375–401.

Labov, William & Joshua Waletzky. 1967. Narrative analysis: Oral versions of personal experience. *The Journal of Narrative and Life History* 7(3). 3–38.

Martínez-Linares, María Antonia 2009. From hiding the speaker to persuasion: "se"-passive and "se"-impersonal constructions. In Victoria Guillén-Nieto, Carmen Marimón-Llorca & Chelo Vargas-Sierra (eds.), *Intercultural business communication and simulation and gaming methodology*, 223–260. Bern, Switzerland: Peter Lang.

Massol-Deyá, Arturo. 2019. The energy uprising: A community-driven search for sustainability and sovereignty in Puerto Rico. In Yarimar Bonilla & Marisol LeBrón (eds.), *Aftershocks of disaster: Puerto Rico before and after the storm*, 298–308. Chicago, Il.: Haymarket Books.

Melin, Kyle & Nelly Conte. 2018. Community pharmacists as first responders in Puerto Rico after Hurricane Maria. *Journal of the American Pharmacists Association* 58(2). 149.

Melin, Kyle, Wanda T. Maldonado & Angel López-Candales. 2018. Lessons learned from Hurricane Maria: Pharmacists' perspective. *Annals of Pharmacotherapy* 52(5). 493–494.

Mora, Marie T., Alberto Dávila & Havidán Rodríguez. 2017. *Population, migration, and socioeconomic outcomes among island and mainland Puerto Ricans: La Crisis Boricua*. Lexington Books.

Ochs, Elinor & Lisa Capps. 2009. *Living narrative: Creating lives in everyday storytelling*. Harvard University Press.

Oficina del Comisionado de Seguros (ed.), CN-2017-221-D. 2017. *Huracan María – pago de primas, manejo de despacho de medicamentos, servicios fuera de puerto rico, proveedores fuera de la red, preautorizaciones, referidos y reclamaciones de proveedores, asegurados y suscriptores*. Puerto Rico: Gobierno de Puerto Rico

Oliver-Smith, Anthony & Susanna M. Hoffman (eds.). 2019. *The angry earth: Disaster in anthropological perspective*. Routledge.

Perreira, Krista, Rebecca Peters, Nicole Lallemand & Stephen Zuckerman. 2017. Puerto Rico health care infrastructure assessment. *Health Policy Center*.

Picó, Fernando. 2006. *Historia general de Puerto Rico*. Ediciones Huracán.

Pomerantz, Anita. 1986. Extreme case formulations: A way of legitimizing claims. *Human Studies* 9. 219–229.

Potter, Jonathan. 1996. *Representing reality: Discourse, rhetoric, and social construction*. London: SAGE.

Potter, Jonathan & Margaret Wetherell. 1987. *Discourse and social psychology: Beyond attitudes and behaviour*. Sage.

Ramanathan, Vaidehi. 2014. Contesting chemotherapy, amputation, and prosthesis. *The Routledge handbook of language and health communication*. 123.

Riessman, Catherine Kohler. 2008. *Narrative methods for the human sciences*. Sage.

Roberto, Giovanni. 2019. Community kitchens: An emerging movement? In Yarimar Bonilla & Marisol LeBrón (eds.), *Aftershocks of disaster: Puerto Rico before and after the storm*, 309–318. Chicago, Il: Haymarket Books.

Sacks, Harvey, Emanuel Schegloff & Gail Jefferson. 1974. A simplest systematics for the organization of turn-taking for conversation. *Language* 50(4). 696–735.

Santos-Lozada, Alexis R. & Jeffrey T. Howard. 2018. Use of death counts from vital statistics to calculate excess deaths in puerto rico following Hurricane Maria. *JAMA* 320(14). 1491–1493.

Sarangi, Srikant. 2012. Practising discourse analysis in healthcare settings. *The SAGE handbook of qualitative methods in health research*. 397–416.

Schegloff, Emanuel A. 2007. *Sequence organization in interaction: A primer in conversation analysis I*. Cambridge University Press.

Schrauf, Robert W. 2016. *Mixed methods: Interviews, surveys, and cross-cultural comparisons*. Cambridge University Press.

Schrauf, Robert W., Patria López de Victoria & Brett Diaz. 2020. Linguistic stance: An integrative paradigm for mixed methods social science. *Language in Society* 49(2). 257–281.

Searle, John R. 1975. Indirect speech acts. In P. Cole & J. Morgan (eds.), *Syntax and Semantics, 3: Speech acts*, 59–82. New York: Academic Press.

Searle, John R. 1976. A classification of illocutionary acts. *Language in Society* 5(1). 1–23.

Searle, John R., PG Searle, S Willis & John Rogers Searle. 1969. *Speech acts: An essay in the philosophy of language*. Cambridge university press.

Silverstein, Michael. 1976. Shifters, linguistic categories, and cultural description. *Meaning in anthropology*. 11–55.

Silverstein, Michael. 2003. Indexical order and the dialectics of sociolinguistic life. *Language & Communication* 23(3–4). 193–229.

Soto, Miladys. 2017. Más de 400 farmacias de la comunidad ya ofrecen servicio. *Metro*. Puerto Rico.

Strauss, Susan & Parastou Feiz. 2013. *Discourse analysis: Putting our worlds into words*. Routledge.

Strauss, Susan, Parastou Feiz & Xuehua Xiang. 2018. *Grammar, meaning, and concepts: A discourse-based approach to English grammar*. Routledge.

Tashakkori, Abbas, R. Burke Johnson & Charles Teddlie. 2020. *Foundations of mixed methods research: Integrating quantitative and qualitative approaches in the social and behavioral sciences*. SAGE Publications, Incorporated.

Teddlie, Charles & Fen Yu. 2007. Mixed methods sampling: A typology with examples. *Journal of Mixed Methods Research* 1(1). 77–100.

Tracy, Karen & Jessica S. Robles. 2013. *Everyday talk: Building and reflecting identities*. Guilford Press.

Zorrilla, Carmen D. 2017. The view from Puerto Rico – Hurricane Maria and its aftermath. *New England journal of Medicine* 377(19). 1801–1803.

Section 4: **Applied linguistics and health interventions**

Emily M. Feuerherm, Bonnie McIntosh
Chapter 8
Beyond "Limited English Proficient" in health care policy, practice, and programs

1 Introduction

Despite policies that are intended to increase multilingual access to health care, health research has shown that monolingual practices continue to negatively impact patients' health in the US (Wilson et al. 2005; DuBard and Gizlice 2008). Applied linguists are uniquely positioned to advocate for health equity through interdisciplinary and collaborative work with healthcare providers, researchers, and community organizers (Showstack et al. 2019; Feuerherm et al. 2021). We will address health policies, practices, and programs in this chapter by focusing on a community-based health literacy intervention in Flint, Michigan.

We begin by setting the stage and introducing the story of the public health emergency commonly known as the Flint water crisis (FWC). We then provide background information related to social determinants of health and health literacy, while connecting this to the Flint community with demographic information. Following this, we compare the language policies to the practices of distributing reliable and valid health information successfully during such a local crisis. We provide anecdotes from our research participants about their experiences during the FWC to show instances of policy failures in ensuring accessibility of information. These stories come from the experiences of three immigrant women from Mexico who came to a community-based health literacy intervention called Health and ESL Literacy Program (HELP). In order to protect the identities of the immigrant women we did not digitally record the classes or the women's voices, and we use pseudonyms when presenting their experiences. The details come from the researchers' notes, including written field notes and reflections

---

Acknowledgments: We are grateful to our research assistants (Olusola Atoyebi, Bianca Ramirez, Reese Gunn, and Danielle Hankerd), community partners, and participants of this research study. This research would not have been possible without the support of our funders, the Michigan Institute of Clinical Health Research (funded by the National Institute of Health, UL1TR002240) and the Flint Truth and Action Partnership Project (funded by the Kellogg Foundation).

Emily M. Feuerherm, University of Michigan-Flint
Bonnie McIntosh, ACE Community Health

https://doi.org/10.1515/9783110744804-009

from each of the three ESL teachers and two community partners who provided public service translation and interpreting. The participants' stories tell us about systemic linguistic oppression during a public health crisis, the divergence in cultural practices that worsened their experiences, and the ongoing trauma that continues to interfere with their daily lives. Their stories are a local example of the failings of our national and state-wide public policies to achieve civil rights and health equity for minoritized language speakers.

Our chapter then traces the steps that a multi-disciplinary community-based research team took in building interventions focused on the dual public health crises of the FWC and the COVID 19 pandemic. Partnerships between applied linguistics and health are gaining momentum and we will discuss our process for developing a language and literacy education program for adults that addresses the concerns of the community. We outline not only the successes of the program, but also the obstacles that we faced and sometimes overcame. Community-based research is founded upon long-standing relationships and the common goals of a community. Therefore, this chapter reflects only a portion of the larger and ongoing projects.

2 Setting the stage

Even before the city of Flint exposed its citizens to lead through their drinking water, commonly referred to as the Flint water crisis (FWC), the city was "synonymous with faded American industrial and automotive power" (Young 2013: 2). The birthplace of General Motors, Flint reached its peak in the 1960s, and was followed by years of decreases in industrialization, investment, and population. However, this is only one part of Flint's history that set the stage for the water crisis. As the Michigan Civil Rights Commission (MCRC 2017) says of the Flint Water Crisis, "one cannot understand Flint's current distress without understanding the central role of race. There were and still are racialized policies, practices, cultural norms and institutional arrangements that help create and maintain racially disparate outcomes" (p. 10). Antidiscrimination rights in US policies include protections for race, color, and national origin (e.g. The Civil Rights Act of 1964), and yet MCRC found that history of institutional and structural racism were the underlying causes of this public health emergency. Flint is what is known as a "majority minority" city meaning that there are more people of color in the city than there are white people.

Although the MCRC focuses on the role of race, it also states that English fluency and citizenship status were important factors that contributed to increased harm for Flint residents who speak minoritized languages (MCRC 2017: 8). English language fluency was a key determinant in early knowledge of the lead-poisoned water and access to health information and services. This demographic and economic background is important because it sets the stage for health disparities experienced by citizens of Flint.

2.1 Social determinants of health (SDOH)

The social determinants of health (SDOH) are complex and interconnected. SDOH "are nonmedical factors that influence health outcomes" (World Health Organization n.d.). They "are conditions [in the environments] in which people are born, grow, work, live, and age," in addition to broader structural factors and systems that influence the circumstances of day-to-day lives (World Health Organization n.d.). Factors and systems include economic and political systems, development, as well as social norms and policies (World Health Organization n.d.). SDOH are cut from present day and historical allocations of money, power, as well as community, national, and global resources (Schillinger, 2020). That is, social structures and economic systems are multifarious yet interconnected and they influence health inequities because they comprise the physical and social environments, health services, and political environment (Schillinger 2020).

SDOH can contribute to health disparities and inequities among racial and ethnic groups. Additionally, immigrants, refugees, indigenous peoples, and other ethnic minoritized groups have experienced health disparities that can be traced to a history of social and linguistic segregation (Chang 2019; Showstack et al. 2019). In US policies and medical practice and research, the term "limited English proficient"[1] is often used to identify people who speak a language other than English at home, though linguists would choose other terms such as minoritized language speakers, multilingual speakers, emergent English speakers, or in some cases English (language) learners.

Speaking a minoritized language in the U.S. has been identified by public health research as a barrier to quality of care for patients (Wilson et al. 2005) and language and literacy are important issues related to SDOH (Feuerherm et al. 2021; Rowlands et al. 2015). Minoritized language speakers have been associated with decreased cancer screening adherence, less self-management of asthma,

---

[1] The phrase "Limited English Proficient" will be used in this chapter with quotation marks to indicate its use in policies, though the authors will otherwise choose terminology that does not have the deficit implications of this phrase.

and poorer glycemic control among diabetics (Wagner 2019). Further, research on U.S. Hispanic[2] people who elected to answer questions on a survey in Spanish reported poorer health status, an absence of health insurance, lack of a family doctor, and not seeking a doctor because of healthcare costs compared to Hispanic people who chose to respond in English (DuBard and Gizlice 2008). Additionally, an estimated 50% of Hispanic patients have problems accessing and using reliable health information, and it is estimated to cost the United States between $106 and $236 billion annually in preventable health costs (Wagner 2019). These examples of research shows how language is part of the SDOH.

2.2 Health literacy and SDOH

Health literacy relates to an individual's ability to obtain, process, and understand health information and services that they need to make appropriate health decisions (Sørensen et al. 2012). The role of health literacy in SDOH continues to evolve. Recent research has increasingly shown the important connections between SDOH and health literacy. Rowlands et al. (2015) model how social determinants of health connect with health literacy, specifically highlighting the importance of the environment within which people collect health information. Their model is patient-centered and participants in the study described how work and income influence the way you live your life, but knowledge and skills (including health literacy) can be used to counteract adverse social determinants. Another model connecting SDOH to health literacy synthesizes research from multiple disciplines and shows SDOH as a starting point for which health literacy becomes a barrier or pathway to better health (Schillinger 2021). These models show that health literacy is a target for intervention efforts to reduce health disparities.

For multilingual speakers, English fluency and literacy[3] may serve as obstacles to health literacy, since so much of our health literacy in the US is English-centric. Research shows that people with emergent health literacy may have adverse experiences with their health and wellness, lengthier hospital stays, challenges with the self-management of chronic conditions, increased use of emergency medical care, and greater all-cause mortality rates (Wagner 2019). Researchers have indicated that when compared to adults with a high level of health liter-

---

2 Here we have chosen to use "Hispanic" because that is the language used in the US Census.
3 Fundamentally, fluency is the overall command of the language while literacy is the ability to engage with written forms of the language.

acy, adults with a low health literacy level had a hazard ratio of 1.26 for all-cause mortality (Bostock and Steptoe 2012); that is because adverse health outcomes are associated with difficulties reading and following medical instructions and health messages (Wagner 2019).

2.3 Language and policy

Speakers of minoritized languages are supposed to be protected by national antidiscrimination policies particularly when it comes to health and education, but the policies are too easily overlooked and lack teeth for regular enforcement. When looking more specifically into the underlying ideologies that undergird US antidiscrimination law, language sits in a complicated position. It is not explicitly identified as a protected identity, though it is subsumed under the protections against national origin discrimination, making it "illegal to discriminate because of a person's birthplace, ancestry, culture or language" (US Department of Justice 2015). Antidiscrimination laws in the US are set within ideologies of immutability, meaning those aspects of a person's identity which cannot be changed or altered (Kibbee 2016). So, the US Civil Rights Act (1964) protects from discrimination on the basis of race, color, sex, religion, (dis)ability, and national origin. This ideology of mutability means that the home language is not protected on its own grounds because it is seen as something that can be changed or altered by learning. In this case mutability is conflated with voluntary or involuntary action: immigrants in the US whose native language is not English are expected to learn English because they have chosen to immigrate. This perspective ignores the many factors which may prevent learning the local language such as the time and circumstances of immigration, accessibility of resources, and wish to maintain the heritage language.

The practices on the ground during the FWC erased the linguistic diversity of the community and assumed a monolingual community of English speakers. For our research participants, the pressures of working multiple jobs, family obligations and caring for children and grandchildren, and the lack of local educational resources for learning English were obstacles to meeting this ideological expectation of learning English. This does not mean that immigrant families in Flint (or elsewhere in the US) are unwilling to learn English, but it does mean that there are on-the-ground barriers to learning which the national US policies and ideologies of mutability cannot account for. Additionally, one of the women, Juana, was pre-literate in her first language. Artieda's (2017) data on first language (L1) literacy suggests that "L1 literacy acts as a threshold for academically disadvantaged learners, who may not be able to profit from education in a second language until they have reached a minimum level of literacy in their L1" (174), meaning that people like Juana would benefit from becoming literate in their L1 before or alongside learning English. With such obstacles to learning, accessibility of health information becomes that much more important, as does the use of translations and interpreters.

The US Civil Rights Act of 1964 requires recipients of federal financial assistance to provide "reasonable steps" for meaningful access for people with "limited English proficiency." The vagueness of this policy means that it has been variously interpreted at the state, local, and institutional level leading to vast differences between the services which count as "reasonable" and "accessible." The Affordable Care Act also incentivizes the use of "language services, community outreach, and cultural competency trainings" at the national level in order to reduce health disparities (Affordable Care Act 2010: 78). This act also sets guidelines on dissemination of health care documents, and data collection and evaluation that considers the primary language of the individual in order to address underserved populations that are the result of language barriers. Additionally, the National Standards for Culturally and Linguistically Appropriate Services (CLAS) outlines expectations for agencies receiving federal funds to provide understandable information for minoritized language speakers and further proposes that health information and care should be responsive "to diverse cultural health beliefs and practices, preferred languages, health literacy, and other communication needs" (US Department of Health and Human Services, CLAS Standards n.d.). This includes providing free language assistance (e.g. interpreting and translation) from qualified individuals for those who are identified as having "limited English proficiency." Nevertheless, there continues to be a wide range of support levels for minoritized language speakers and in the case of a public health emergency such as the FWC, there is increased risk that a community's multilingualism is overlooked. Applied linguists involved in critical and engaged language policy have advanced our understanding of how even well-intentioned policies can maintain inequitable power distributions or leave gaps in the protections against discrimination (Davis 2014; Davis and Phyak 2017; Ramanathan 2013). Importantly, they also show us how local activists and researchers address these policies on local and national scales.

2.4 Community partner: La Placita

La Placita is a 501c3 non-profit that was formally established in 2014 from a group of volunteers who had been loosely working together in Flint since the 1980s to serve the Latinx community in Flint. The FWC was an important reason for establishing a formal status and structure as it was immediately clear that the Spanish-speaking community of Flint was in need of more advocacy and resources to address the public health crisis and raise awareness of multilingualism in Flint. Grassroots responses, like those of La Placita, included translations and interpreting to make information accessible. These responders organized local outreach in culturally and linguistically sensitive ways, empowering members of the community to participate in their own information sharing and healing. Bilingual volunteers went to homes of Latinx residents to share information and resources such as water filters, bottled water, and other health information about the dangers of lead poisoning. These initial home visits were a result of the extended social networks of La Placita and word-of-mouth reports that families lacked knowledge about and resources for the FWC.

Meanwhile, policy makers and governmental agencies struggled to catch up, turning to these grassroots organizations for translations, interpreting, and outreach to the community. This is a common problem in communities where linguistic diversity is overlooked and communities are made to advocate for themselves (see also Tipton 2017). In 2017 the MCRC noted that these grassroots efforts had "resulted in tangible changes including providing information in multiple languages and clarifying that proof of citizenship was not required to receive bottled water" (8) and that "also less tangible changes in the way uniformed personnel were deployed so as to not frighten people who need assistance in a way that prevents them from getting it" (9). For example, La Placita recruited bilingual youth to go door-to-door in neighborhoods with a greater number of Latinx residents in order to inform and distribute information to all families with the hope of identifying more Latinx residents previously unidentified by La Placita. As described by MCRC, the city had sent out uniformed officers and other personnel to go door to door, which caused fear in the communities and prevented families from receiving the help that was being offered. La Placita's use of bilingual youth rather than people in uniforms was a more culturally and linguistically sensitive means of information distribution, and is how one of our research participants, Leticia, learned about the water. Unfortunately, this didn't happen until almost a year after the first announcements and warnings of the FWC had been made in English. La Placita has continued to serve the Flint community offering support and programming in relation to the FWC, translation and interpreting services, grant-funded support for Flint residents to pay their bills, a weekly food pantry, and advocacy for the Latinx community at local, state, and national scales. It is a well-known organization in the city of Flint which people usually discover through word-of-mouth and the vast connections it has with other local organizations. Unfortunately, in the past few years the organization has struggled to find enough grant funding to continue to offer all of its programming and has had to cut back on the number of staff it employs. Nevertheless, the organization continues to serve and advocate for Flint's Latinx residents to the best of its ability and through its network with researchers and other organizations.

2.5 Experiences of the flint water crisis

The FWC is a striking example of how social determinants of health (including the social, political, economic, and linguistic issues) exacerbated the public health crisis and caused increased harm to certain populations within the city. According to the US census (July 1, 2019), nearly 40% of Flint's population lives at or below the poverty line. Much of the residual wealth from the automobile industry can still be found in Genesee County, but not within the city limits. At the same time, the residual costs of brownfields, urban blight, and crumbling infrastructure continue to be borne by those who live within the city limits. A century of racially-based policies and practices such as redlining, white flight, and razing and re-developing Black neighborhoods led to this city-wide health emergency (MCRC 2017). Neighborhoods most impacted by the water crisis were those with more abandoned houses, more people of color, and more people living below the national poverty line (Sadler et al. 2017). These environmental and economic factors are not only issues that led to the FWC, but also added to disparities in health equity for those living in the city, making it more difficult to overcome the man-made public health crisis of the FWC.

As a typical US city in the Midwest, Flint has some linguistic diversity, but the majority of the population is English-speaking. Immigrant languages (especially Spanish and Arabic) and American Sign Language make up the majority of languages other than English found in this area. According to the US census population estimates from July 1, 2019, Flint had a population of 95,538 with 4.5% identifying as Hispanic or Latino, 0.5% Asian, and 0.0% Native Hawaiian and other Pacific Islander, making Hispanic and Latino the largest population of people other than White and Black/African American. The census also estimates that 2% are foreign born and 3.8% speak a language other English at home (U.S. Census Bureau 2019). These population statistics, alongside experiential observation, indicate that Spanish is the most common foreign language found in Flint. Our research subjects are all Spanish-speaking immigrants living within the city of Flint. Feuerherm and Oshio (2020) discuss a community-based needs analysis which showed that there was a lack of language education resources during the FWC, alongside growing concerns around health among Flint's immigrant population, particularly for Latinx immigrants.

In the midst of the FWC, immigrants and linguistic minorities were erased from the conversation of harm and health effects, as information was distributed in English, without translations or interpretations for several months. Our informants told us that they first heard about the problems with the water through La Placita, a grassroots organization and the authors' long-term research partner. One woman, Rosa, had heard that there was a problem with the tap water and had been boiling her water, as this is what she did in Mexico when water was dangerous. However, boiling does not get rid of lead and can actually increase the likelihood of being poisoned by even higher amounts of lead as the boiling water evaporates and concentrates the lead. Another woman, Leticia, had been totally unaware of any problem with the water until volunteers from La Placita showed up on her doorstep to test her water and give her bottled water and filters. She later discovered that her house had high levels of lead in the water and reported that she continues to experience many of the symptoms of lead poisoning such as high blood pressure, headaches, and joint and muscle pain. There is no cure for lead poisoning, so Leticia will need to manage these symptoms for the rest of her life. All of the women agreed that they had experienced hair loss, increased stress and depression, memory loss, rashes and other skin irritations, and a lack of sleep since the beginning of the FWC. Rosa stated that she has no appetite, and only eats when forced to by her children. None had taken a blood-lead test to identify their level of exposure, though all had likely been exposed to lead through their water. Critical to their experience was the fact that information about the lead in the water was inaccessible to them for much longer than other Flint residents because of the language barrier and lack of multilingual health information, which increased their risk of acute and chronic lead poisoning. These anecdotes make clear that the intersection between SDOH, language spoken, literacy and especially health literacy in English are all factors which worsened the effect of the FWC on these women. Without grassroots organizations like La Placita intervening and advocating for this community the adverse impact could have been even worse.

3 Community-based participatory action research

Community-Based Participatory Action Research (CBPAR) in public health focuses on using an equitable process of a community-driven partnership to design and implement a research project, as well as to report findings back to a community. This partnership includes community members, organizational representatives, and researchers. This process includes: (1) acknowledging the community as a unit and individuals; (2) building upon existing community strengths and resources; (3) enabling shared partnerships on all phases of the research project life cycle; (4) combining knowledge and action for shared advantages; (5) encouraging a mutual learning and empowering course that tackles social inequities; (6) is a recurring and iterative process; (7) speaking to health from an ecological and positive viewpoint; and (8) distributing results and knowledge to all partners (Israel 2012).

Improving health literacy demands a systems approach (Sørensen et al. 2012). It requires a community-driven and participatory approach that combines multiple components. The National Action Plan to Improve Health Literacy (U.S. Department of Health and Human Services 2010) highlights that community-based English-language classes can help people in cultivating health literacy through education (Soto Mas et al. 2014; 2015). English as a second language (ESL) lessons that emphasize health topics can have a progressive impact on participants' health literacy (Soto Mas et al. 2015) health knowledge (Elder et al. 2000), and health behaviors (Santos, et al., 2014). Experimental and quasi-experimental evidence indicates that programs integrating Health Literacy and ESL can considerably increase health literacy levels and English language proficiency amongst Spanish-speaking adult program members (Soto Mas et al. 2018).

This has implications for SDOH because educational programming can address both language and health literacy barriers, as discussed earlier. Further, evidence indicates that ESL classes are seen by Latinx immigrants as a way to add economic and social opportunities to their lives, which again have implications for SDOH: if economic status and social opportunities are increased, then adverse effects of SDOH may possibly be decreased. This connection has been demonstrated for other programs, such as adult basic skills (ABS) research which shows that regular and extended participation in educational programs yielded higher future earnings (Reder 2014). Additionally, research found that implementing an ESL health literacy curriculum in community settings (e.g. colleges, faith-based sites, and worksites) can simplify program recruitment and retention, thereby reaching and retaining more people (Soto Mas et al. 2018). Despite this promising evidence related to health literacy and ESL programs, a barrier in continuing these types of programs is related to funding issues, mainly in U.S. states with no political health literacy legislation or a systems approach to health literacy effort (Wagner 2019). Considering the evidence for how educational programs can intervene and advance people's economic and health status, it would make sense for more funding to be allocated in support of policies such as the National Action Plan to Improve Health Literacy and adult basic skills programs that include ESL classes.

3.1 Language policy arbiters for advocacy and action

Our Health and ESL Literacy Program (HELP) was designed to take action on the outcomes from the FWC in a localized way by operationalizing the CBPAR process. The top-down nature of policies, such as antidiscrimination laws or language policies, are meant to organize and control the systems and practices on the ground. However, Johnson and Johnson (2014) show that language policy *arbiters*–the people who have power over how a policy is created, interpreted, or appropriated– impact the practices at multiple scales. A national policy will be interpreted at the state level, then passed down to the local policy arbiters. At each scale, the language policy arbiters are interpreting and implementing policies. When policies are insufficient or ineffective in reducing harm to (linguistic) minorities, such as what happened during the FWC, grassroots advocates are pivotal for challenging these policies.

Our community-based research combines grassroots advocacy, local policy action, and linguistics research in addressing the effects of the FWC on local Latinx immigrants. The core research team consists of:

- Feuerherm: an applied linguist and university professor and her research assistants. She organizes the language curriculum and is the Principal Investigator on the project.
- McIntosh: a public health advocate, community partner, and Principal at ACE Community Health and her research assistants. She advises on public health policy, health resources, health communication, and dissemination.
- Olivares: an immigrant and long-time resident of Flint who established La Placita and her staff. She coordinates between the research team and the Latinx community in Flint, provides translation and interpreting, and monitors the research and advocacy efforts for linguistic and cultural appropriacy.

This team has used community-based participatory action research (CBPAR) to develop health and local policy interventions to address the harm caused by the FWC. Our team is an example of how CBPAR combines the capacities and expertise of community members in constructing a research and action plan. The expertise of Feuerherm in applied linguistics and McIntosh in public health, and as a community partner, are additive in their potential to impact individuals, communities, and health outcomes. Olivares and her staff are an invaluable resource for local knowledge and importantly provide support and guidance for working with the Latinx community in general and undocumented immigrants in particular. In addition to the core team, we also have a community advisory board that consists of other stakeholders in the research project and the lives and experiences of the Latinx community of Flint. The advisory board includes representatives from multiple sectors including health, education, non-profit community organizations, and transportation. It is summarized in Table 1 below:

Table 1: Community Advisory Board.

Sector	Organization	Details
Education	Flint and Genesee Literacy Network	Supports and coordinates providers of literacy-based programming
	Richfield Public School Academy	Flint school grades K-8 with the most English learners
Health	Health Alliance Plan	Low-cost insurance plans and community health programming
	Healthy Flint Research Coordinating Center	Community resources for health and research including a community ethics review board and open data repository
	Genesee Health Plan	Los-cost insurance plans and community health programming
	United Healthcare	Health insurance
Community organizations and businesses	Flint Fresh	Local distributor of fresh, local, low-cost produce to Flint residents through boxed deliveries and mobile food carts serving food deserts
	Latinos in Michigan TV	Spanish-language news outlet focused on state-level news
	Latinx Technology and Community Center	Educational programs for all ages, translation and interpreting, computer lab, a food pantry and community garden
	Michigan Transportation Authority	Public transit including busses and smaller vehicles
	Red Cross	Disaster relief and prevention

The community advisory board functions as support for the core research partners and the project as a whole. They provide information on local resources, review and make suggestions on the research process and development, and help with recruitment and dissemination of findings. Our community advisory board does not participate directly in the research, but are important partners in identifying and sharing resources, recruiting participants, and pushing for local policy changes based on our research. In their review of community advisory boards, Newman et al. (2011) list the benefits of working with an advisory board as well as the processes for establishing and sustaining one. We have seen small indicators of improvement in the recognition of the linguistic, cultural, and educational diversity of our community because of the advisory board. Health care providers and Flint Fresh have recognized that language and literacy can change people's access to their services, and have asked us to create Spanish language videos to help new clients access their services and information. Flint Fresh has also asked for recommendations for culturally appropriate fruits and vegetables to increase the variety of their produce. These small, local changes in practice by local policy arbiters are examples of the rippling effect CBPAR can have on communities.

3.2 CBPAR challenges

CBPAR also presents many challenges related to time and funding, two related issues with which we experienced particular difficulties. Although we began planning this project in 2017 after conducting the community needs analysis discussed in Feuerherm and Oshio (2020), it was not until 2020 that we were able to begin implementing our plans. Those three years of preparation included lengthy funding applications with slow turn-around times, as well as institutional review board and bureaucratic processes not designed with community partners in mind. The university required increased oversight on this project because of NIH funding, working with multiple community partners to ensure no conflicts of interest, and working with a particularly vulnerable population (undocumented immigrants with low literacy). Because of these delays, one of the partners, Olivares, was almost unable to participate and the HELP program has struggled to recruit participants as the urgency has waned.

These setbacks mirror Carrera et al.'s (2019) findings that Flint community members were distrustful and resentful of government agencies and universities because they felt that these organizations were slow in addressing the problems from the FWC. Meanwhile, local nonprofits and faith-based institutions consistently received high levels of trust. The fact that La Placita had high levels of interest in the program early on, but had to keep postponing the start of the program meant that their relationship with Feuerherm and CBPAR hurt rather than helped the organization's reputation in the community. This is something that researchers and institutions should be aware of before engaging in any CBPAR research and ensure that any plans for research projects are able to quickly move through institutional procedures for research with community partners and human subjects. Further, Feuerherm had no experience conducting a clinical health trial and had to rely extensively on McIntosh to navigate the requirements such as registering with clinicaltrials.gov. While this was a significant learning experience that built trust between the partners, it also meant that the PI (Feuerherm) was not initially aware of the additional work conducting a clinical health trial entailed. Any applied linguist interested in clinical health research, even when the intervention is purely educational, should seek out information and training on how to conduct a clinical trial before they begin.

4 Health and ESL literacy program

HELP is a health literacy program focused on preventing lead exposure that uses a translingual approach to teaching ESL. The National Action Plan to Improve Health Literacy (2010) includes seven broad goals to engage organizations and individuals in a multi-sector effort to improve health literacy in the US. This policy includes expanding local efforts to provide adult ESL education and culturally and linguistically appropriate health information and services. HELP aligns with The National Action Plan to Improve Health Literacy and uses a community-based participatory research approach for the design, implementation, and evaluation that integrates health systems thinking. In particular, with this policy as a framework, HELP was designed to combine literacy, health literacy, and linguistically and culturally appropriate health information about lead poisoning to Latinx immigrants in Flint. It was supposed to begin on March 20, 2020, but this coincided with the beginning of the Coronavirus pandemic in the US and statewide stay-at-home orders, as well as a pause on in-person human-subject research. Thus the program was postponed indefinitely. When La Placita's clients were asked if they would be interested in learning online rather than in-person, their reaction was profoundly negative. This was until December of 2020, after they had seen and experienced online education for their children and grandchildren attending K-12 schools.

The first pilot program for HELP ran for 6 weeks from May to July 2021 in an online format. The course consisted of weekly health topics broken down in Table 2:

Table 2: HELP Curriculum Topics for Health.

1: Is my water safe?	1. Describe experiences during the water crisis 2. Identify current health needs 3. Develop personal goals for the program
2: Testing water	1. Describe how to get and use free water tests 2. Describe how to get and use free water filters 3. Practice using and discussing water tests and filters

Table 2 (continued)

3: Blood-lead test	1.	Discuss when, where, and how to get tested for lead
	2.	Manage health after lead-exposure: identify community resources
	3.	Practice making appointments and talking with health professionals
4: Nutrition	1.	Identify healthy and unhealthy foods at home
	2.	Reading and interpreting food labels
	3.	Develop a plan for healthy eating
5: Nutrition	1.	Discuss recommended diets for general health, diabetes, or heart disease
	2.	Evaluate barriers to good nutrition
	3.	Develop ideas and resources to overcome barriers
6: Review	1.	Evaluate your goals and learning
	2.	Give examples of how to find and evaluate health information
	3.	Practice sharing health information reliability

These health topics would be discussed together using a mix of English and Spanish. Any local resources that were shared, such as phone numbers or locations for water testing, filters, and bottled water were first tested by the research staff to identify which services were available in English and Spanish. While not all resources had bilingual staff, the receptionist at Flint's city hall in charge of distributing water testing kits and filters was bilingual and an excellent resource for related services available in Spanish in other regions of the city. This was a big change from before the FWC, where information in Spanish was scarce and reliant upon non-profit organizations for translation and interpreting. Nutrition topics were given two weeks because although there is no cure for lead poisoning, ensuring good nutrition with plenty of iron, calcium, and vitamin C can reduce lead absorption (U.S. Environmental Protection Agency October 2019). Additionally, Olivares informed the research team that diabetes, high cholesterol, and high blood pressure were common concerns for the Latinx population, so we wanted to address healthy diets specific to those diseases (e.g. the Diabetes Plate Method). Importantly, much of Flint is considered a food desert, so we worked with our community advisory board member – Flint Fresh – to create a culturally appropriate box of fresh fruits and vegetables to be delivered to the participants.

HELP also included language and literacy education. The program separated learners into 3 levels according to literacy and English fluency. These levels were established using the Fostering Literacy for Good Health Today (FLIGHT)/Vive Desarollando Amplia Salud (VIDAS) test (Ownby 2015). This health literacy test can be administered in either English or Spanish and we additionally sought students' own reflections on their placement into the levels to ensure that they agreed that they were placed at a level that was not too difficult or easy. The program levels participants were placed into were: (1) Basic literacy focused on building literacy in the first language (Spanish) with some spoken English; (2) Beginning ESL included English literacy and A1-2 level of English instruction; (3) Intermediate ESL continued to advance English literacy and fluency. The health topics were still included in these lessons, such as making doctor appointments or following instructions for medication, but were not exclusively focused on lead exposure prevention. We used a translingual approach to teaching English where we scaffolded learning by using Spanish and encouraging code mixing/switching when a word or concept was not known in English. All of the teachers spoke at least an intermediate level of Spanish and staff from La Placita were on hand to support by interpreting as needed.

4.1 The pilot program

The first session of the pilot program had three participants, one in each level, so we do not have robust data yet to quantitatively measure the impact of the program on health knowledge or behaviors. Another limitation to the program was the online modality. There were many sessions where the first 15–30 minutes were spent troubleshooting issues with zoom as participants connected through their phones. Using a phone for online education is not ideal since the screen is so much smaller; any screen sharing of slides or the whiteboard feature must be large in order to be visible on a phone screen. Additionally, had the program been in-person it would have meant that participants would not be so easily distracted from the course by their surroundings. For example, Juana had a full house of children and grandchildren during most of the classes and was often required to excuse herself to help her family. Rosa called in to the class from work one day, and participated in the lesson while simultaneously cleaning a building. Although we believe an in-person course would have improved the interactions, it may have simultaneously limited participants' ability to attend.

The courses were structured so that the beginning of the course was focused on health topics such as lead exposure prevention. The first part of the lesson was bilingual in English and Spanish and used visual support through slides that included both English and Spanish information. A certified medical interpreter from La Placita was present to ensure that information was being accurately imparted in both languages. Following the health lesson, the three teachers and students would divide into their levels (using Zoom breakout rooms) to discuss topics relevant to health literacy at the appropriate levels. Again, slides would be used as visual support and English and Spanish were used as appropriate or needed. The basic level focused on literacy in Spanish, the beginning level instructed beginning English literacy on health-related topics with some Spanish language support, and the intermediate level focused on evaluation of health information and more advanced English literacy on health topics. Health topics and resources included in the curriculum were first evaluated for their accuracy, relevancy, reliability of the source, and appropriateness of the language (using plain English/Spanish) by our public health professional and advisor at ACE Community Health.

An important aspect of health literacy is finding and evaluating health information. This topic was most extensively explored at the intermediate level, but we included aspects of it in the health lessons at the beginning as well. From our field notes, our participants knew how to find and evaluate health information theoretically, but through discussion it was clear that this was complicated by the lived experiences of the three women. For example, Juana's experiences with health professionals had been complicated by mistrust and perceived discrimination, an all-too common experience for people of color (Jaiswal 2019; López-Cevallos et al. 2014). Because of this, she said she did not trust her doctors and would seek second opinions when anything was very concerning to her. Rosa was similarly mistrustful of government agencies and health recommendations, joking that until the US government gave her "papers" she was not going to trust what they said. Joking aside, it is common among Flint residents to be skeptical of the state and local governments when it comes to public health, since the FWC was a man-made crisis denied at first by the local government. And lastly, although participants recognized Facebook as an unreliable source for health information, they used it as a source of information anyway. For example, Rosa said that she had not gotten the COVID-19 vaccine because of the negative reports she had read on Facebook. In response, Olivares and Feuerherm shared their reasons for getting vaccinated and provided information about how to get a vaccine even when you don't have health insurance or a social security number. It is evident from just these small experiences that evaluating health information is complicated by several factors and may take more than a 6-week health literacy course to fully address.

5 Conclusion

The top-down nature of policies, such as antidiscrimination laws or language and literacy policies, are meant to organize and control the systems and practices on the ground. When policies are insufficient, ineffective, or overlooked, such as what happened during the FWC, grassroots advocates are pivotal for challenging these policies and practices. Grassroots advocacy and linguistics research go hand-in-hand in addressing language accessibility when using a CBPAR approach to program development. Social determinants of health, health literacy and limited English language fluency are connected and influenced by allocations of money, power, and resources (e.g., community, national, and global). A systems approach is needed to overcome health inequities in social determinants of health that are associated with limited English proficiency, health literacy, and literacy. This is a role for interdisciplinary research teams that combine expertise from linguistics, communication, anthropology, and/or education with health professionals in order to research and address the role of language and literacy in health outcomes. Linguists in particular can advocate for a move away from monolingual ideologies in our policies and practices, as represented by the "limited English proficient" label, to more inclusive language that highlights the linguistic diversity of our communities and prioritizes diverse access points for multilingual community members.

US antidiscrimination policies (Civil Rights Act, CLAS Standards, Affordable Care Act, and National Action Plan to Improve Health Literacy) offer a bird's-eye view of how to increase equity and accessibility for health. However, language policy arbiters make on-the-ground decisions which impact patient's experiences of health and health care. More research is needed to understand the intersections between language, literacy, and health, and the best practices for building increased equity, stronger programs, and better advocacy for speakers of minoritized languages. More programs like HELP are needed so that when a public health emergency occurs, such as the COVID-19 pandemic, communities are prepared to respond quickly and efficiently in many languages.

We conclude by offering recommendations for other researchers interested in building an interdisciplinary team and contributing to research and action at the intersection of language, literacy, and health.

- For researchers new to CBPAR and clinical trials, familiarize yourself with the process and expectations this research approach entails. Overestimate the amount of time the research will take, and plan ahead for delays.
- When building a research project, include experts from interdisciplinary fields and community stakeholders (such as a community advisory board) and take time to build trust and identify skills and expertise relevant to the goals of the research agenda. This allows for greater impact and wider dissemination.
- Ensure that information is accessible to all community stakeholders and that voices from diverse community stakeholders are heard. This is an imperative practice to use in health care policy development for community programs.

References

Artieda, Gemma. 2017. The role of L1 literacy and reading habits on the L2 achievement of adult learners of English as a foreign language. *System*, 66. 168–176. DOI https://doi.org/10.1016/j.system.2017.03.020.

Bostock, Sophie & Andrew Steptoe. 2012. Association between low functional health literacy and mortality in older adults: Longitudinal cohort study. *British Medical Journal*, 344, e1602. 10.1136/bmj.e1602

Carerra, Jennifer, Kent Key, Yvonne Lewis, Woolford, S., Bailey, S., Hamm, J., . . . Calhoun, K. 2019. Community Science as a Pathway for Resiliency in Response to a Public Health Crisis in Flint, MI. Social Sciences. Special Issue – Engaged Scholarship for Resilient Communities. Retrieved from https://michr.umich.edu/resources/2020/2/18/community-voice-on-the-flint-water-crisis-a-trust-study.

Chang, Cindy D. 2019. Social determinants of health and health disparities among immigrants and their children. *Current Problems in Pediatric and Adolescent Health Care* 49(1). 23–30. doi:10.1016/j.cppeds.2018.11.009.

Davis, Kathryn A. 2014. Engaged language policy and practices [Thematic issue]. *Language Policy* 13(2). 83–100. doi:10.1007/s10993-013-9296-5.

Davis, Kathryn A. & Prem Phyak. 2017. *Engaged Language Policy and Practices*. New York, NY: Routledge.

DuBard, C. Annette & Ziya Gizlice. 2008. Language spoken and differences in health status, access to care, and receipt of Preventive Services among us Hispanics. *American Journal of Public Health* 98(11). 2021–2028. doi:10.2105/ajph.2007.119008.

US Department of Justice. (August 6, 2015). Federal protections against national origin discrimination. https://www.justice.gov/crt/federal-protections-against-national-origin-discrimination-1#:~:text=Federal%20laws%20prohibit%20discrimination%20based,%2C%20ancestry%2C%20culture%20or%20language.

Elder, John P., Jeanette I. Candelaria, Susan I. Woodruff, Michael H. Criqui, Gregory A. Talavera & Joan W. Rupp. 2000. Results of language for Health: Cardiovascular Disease Nutrition Education for latino English-as-a-second-language students. *Health Education & Behavior* 27(1). 50–63. doi:10.1177/109019810002700106.

Feuerherm, Emily & Toko Oshio. 2020. Conducting a community-based ESOL programme needs analysis. *English Language Teaching Journal* 74(3). 327–337. https://doi.org/10.1093/elt/ccaa011

Feuerherm, Emily M., Rachel E. Showstack, Maricel G. Santos, Glen A. Martinez & Holly E. Jacobson. 2021. Language as a social determinant of health: Partnerships for health equity. In Doris S. Warriner & Elizabeth R. Miller (eds.), *Extending Applied Linguistics for Social Impact: Cross-Disciplinary Collaborations in Diverse Spaces of Public Inquiry*, 125–148. New York, NY: Bloomsbury.

Israel, Barbara A., Eugenia Eng, Amy J. Schulz & Edith A. Parker (eds.). 2012. *Methods in community-based participatory research for health*. San Francisco: Jossey-Bass.

Jaiswal, Jessica. 2019. Whose responsibility is it to dismantle medical mistrust? Future directions for researchers and health care providers. *Behavioral Medicine* 45(2). 188–196. doi:10.1080/08964289.2019.1630357.

Johnson, David Cassels & Eric J. Johnson. 2014. Power and agency in language policy appropriation. *Language Policy* 14(3). 221–243. doi:10.1007/s10993-014-9333-z.

Kibbee, Douglas A. 2016. *Language and the Law: Linguistic inequality in America*. Cambridge, UK: Cambridge University Press.

López-Cevallos, Daniel F., S. Marie Harvey & Jocelyn T. Warren. 2014. Medical mistrust, perceived discrimination, and satisfaction with health care among young-adult rural Latinos. *The Journal of Rural Health* 30(4). 344–351. doi:10.1111/jrh.12063.

Michigan Civil Rights Commission. Feb. 17, 2017. The Flint water crisis: Systemic racism through the lens of Flint. Retrieved from https://www.michigan.gov/documents/mdcr/VFlintCrisisRep-F-Edited3-13-17_554317_7.pdf

Newman Susan D., Jeannette O. Andrews, Gayenell S. Magwood, Carolyn Jenkins, Melissa J. Cox & Deborah C. Williamson. 2011. Community advisory boards in community-based participatory research: A synthesis of best processes. *Prev Chronic Dis*, 8 (3):A70.PMID: 21477510; PMCID: PMC3103575.

Ownby, Raymond L. 2015. *FLIGHT/VIDAS user manual*. Fort Lauderdale, FL: Enalan Communications, Inc.

Ramanathan, Vaidehi (ed.). 2013. *Language policies and (dis)citizenship: Rights, access, pedagogies*. Bristol: Multilingual Matters.

Reder, Stephen. 2014. *The impact of ABS program participation on long-term economic outcomes*. US Department of Education, Office of Career, Technical, and Adult Education. Retrieved from https://lincs.ed.gov/publications/pdf/ABS_EconomicOutcomes.pdf

Rodriguez, Elias. (June 11, 2021). EPA, Newark to discuss lead in drinking water. *US Environmental Protection Agency*. https://www.epa.gov/newsreleases/epa-newark-discuss-lead-drinking-water

Rowlands, Gillian, Adrienne Shaw, Sabrena Jaswal, Sian Smith & Trudy Harpham. 2015. Health literacy and the social determinants of health: A qualitative model from adult learners. *Health Promotion International*. doi:10.1093/heapro/dav093.

Sadler, Richard Casey, Jenny LaChance & Mona Hanna-Attisha. 2017. Social and built environmental correlates of predicted blood lead levels in the Flint Water Crisis. *American Journal of Public Health* 107(5). 763–769. doi:10.2105/ajph.2017.303692.

Santos, Maricel G., Margaret A. Handley, Karin Omark & Dean Schillinger. 2014. ESL participation as a mechanism for advancing health literacy in immigrant communities. *Journal of Health Communication* 19(sup2). 89–105. doi:10.1080/10810730.2014.934935.

Schillinger, Dean. 2020. The Intersections Between Social Determinants of Health, Health Literacy, and Health Disparities. *Studies in Health Technology and Informatics, 269*, 22–41. 10.3233/SHTI200020

Schillinger, D. 2021. Social determinants, health literacy, and disparities: Intersections and controversies. *Health Literacy Research and Practice*, 5(3), 234–243. doi: 10.3928/24748307-20210712-01.

Showstack, Rachel, Maricel G. Santos, Emily Feuerherm, Holly Jacobson & Glenn Martinez. (Dec. 9, 2019). Language as a social determinant of health: An applied linguistics perspective on health equity. American Association of Applied Linguistics, PAEC Briefs. Retrieved from https://www.aaal.org/news/language-as-a-social-determinant-of-health-an-applied-linguistics-perspective-on-health-equity

Soto Mas, Francisco, C. Cordova, A. Murrietta, H. E. Jacobson, F. Ronquillo & D. Helitzer. 2014. A multisite community-based health literacy intervention for Spanish speakers. *Journal of Community Health* 40(3). 431–438. doi:10.1007/s10900-014-9953-4.

Soto Mas, Francisco, Cheryl L. Schmitt, Holly E. Jacobson & Orrin B. Myers. 2018. A cardiovascular health intervention for Spanish speakers: The Health Literacy and ESL curriculum. *Journal of Community Health* 43(4). 717–724. doi:10.1007/s10900-018-0475-3.

Soto Mas, Francisco, Ming Ji, Brenda O. Fuentes & Josefina Tinajero. 2015. The Health Literacy and ESL study: A community-based intervention for Spanish-speaking adults. *Journal of Health Communication* 20(4). 369–376. doi:10.1080/10810730.2014.965368.

Sørensen, Kristine, Stephan Van den Broucke, James Fullam, Gerardine Doyle, Jürgen Pelikan, Zofia Slonska & Helmut Brand. 2012. Health Literacy and Public Health: A systematic review and integration of definitions and models. *BMC Public Health* 12(1). doi:10.1186/1471-2458-12-80.

Tipton, Rebecca. 2017. Interpreting-as-conflict: PSIT in third sector organisations and the impact of third way politics. In Carmen Valero-Garcés & Rebecca Tipton (eds.), *Ideology, Ethics and Policy Development in Public Service Interpreting and Translation*, 38–62. Bristol, UK: Multilingual Matters.

U.S. Affordable Care Act of 2010, 42 USC 18001. Retrieved from https://www.govinfo.gov/content/pkg/PLAW-111publ148/pdf/PLAW-111publ148.pdf

U.S. Census Bureau. July 1, 2019. *QuickFacts, Flint city, Michigan*. Retrieved from https://thinkculturalhealth.hhs.gov/clas/standards

U.S. Department of Health and Human Services. n.d. *National culturally and linguistically appropriate services standards*. Retrieved from https://thinkculturalhealth.hhs.gov/clas/standards

U.S. Department of Health and Human Services, Office of Disease Prevention and Health Promotion. *Healthy People 2030*. Retrieved from https://health.gov/healthypeople/objectives-and-data/social-determinants-health

U.S. Department of Health and Human Services, Office of Disease Prevention and Health Promotion. n.d. *Language and Literacy*. Retrieved from https://health.gov/healthypeople/objectives-and-data/social-determinants-health/literature-summaries/language-and-literacy#top

U.S. Civil Rights Act of 1964, Pub.L.88-352, 78 Stat. 241.

U.S. Department of Health and Human Services, Office of Disease Prevention and Health Promotion. 2010. *National Action Plan to Improve Health Literacy*. Retrieved from https://health.gov/our-work/health-literacy/national-action-plan-improve-health-literacy

U.S. Department of Justice. 2000. *Federal protections against national origin discrimination*. Retrieved from https://www.justice.gov/crt/federal-protections-against-national-origin-discrimination-1

U.S. Environmental Protection Agency. October 2019. *Fight lead poisoning with a healthy diet: Lead poisoning prevention tips for families*. Retrieved from https://www.epa.gov/sites/default/files/2020-01/documents/fight_lead_poisoning_with_a_healthy_diet_2019.pdf

Wagner, Teresa. 2019. Incorporating health literacy into English as a second language classes. *HLRP: Health Literacy Research and Practice* 3(3). doi:10.3928/24748307-20190405-02.

Wilson, Elisabeth, Alice Hm Chen, Kevin Grumbach, Frances Wang & Alicia Fernandez. 2005. Effects of limited English proficiency and physician language on health care comprehension. *Journal of General Internal Medicine* 20(9). 800–806. doi:10.1111/j.1525-1497.2005.0174.x.

World Health Organization. (n.d.). *Social Determinants of Health*. Retrieved from: https://www.who.int/health-topics/social-determinants-of-health#tab=tab_1

Young, Gordon. 2013. *Teardown: Memoir of a vanishing city*. Berkeley: University of California Press.

Lisa Mikesell
Chapter 9
Designing health interventions on transdisciplinary research teams: Contributions of LSI scholarship

1 Introduction

In this chapter, I make a case for how communication scholars of language and social interaction (LSI) are particularly well positioned to contribute to the engaged work of transdisciplinary teams designing and developing health interventions. For many communication scholars who work in health contexts, designing interventions is often a major undertaking of our teams. However, before interventions can be conceptualized, let alone developed, implemented, and evaluated, there is much work to be done. First, the utility, feasibility and effectiveness of interventions is significantly benefitted when we first invest the time to deeply understand the local context and culture, work practices, and perspectives and experiences of diverse stakeholders (Wight et al. 2016; see Fadem 2021), areas of study that are the cornerstones of much communication-centered and LSI research. Additionally, the processes by which health interventions come to be realized (e.g., how diverse stakeholders are engaged in the research and design processes, how design decisions are actually made in real time) are ripe areas of investigation that contribute to both LSI scholarship and applied goals. Lastly, once a health intervention is fully conceptualized and designed, its impact is likely to shape the communicative, interactional, and relational processes between patients, families, and providers (see Mikesell et al. 2018). These processes significantly contribute to the illness experiences of families and the work experiences of clinicians, and thus should not be overlooked as important outcomes in their own right.

Transdisciplinarity calls for the close collaboration of experts from different disciplines and methodological backgrounds with the goal of moving beyond or 'transcending' individual disciplinary perspectives. According to Park and Choi (2006: 359), *multidisciplinarity* is additive and "draws on knowledge from different disciplines but stays within the boundaries of those fields" (e.g., when a patient is treated by multiple experts), while *interdisciplinarity* is integrative and

---

Lisa Mikesell, Department of Communication, Rutgers University

https://doi.org/10.1515/9783110744804-010

"analyzes, synthesizes and harmonizes links between disciplines into a coordinated and coherent whole" (e.g., when different medical experts work together to develop a single treatment plan). *Transdisciplinary* teams, on the other hand, do more than apply different disciplinary perspectives to a problem or object of study. They "[integrate] the natural, social and health sciences in a humanities context, and in doing so [transcend] each of their traditional boundaries" (e.g., when clinical team members acquire expertise of other specialists and share roles). Transdisciplinary work offers "holistic schemes that subordinate disciplines, looking at dynamics of whole systems" (Park and Choi 2006: 255) and are thus particularly apt for the development and design of health interventions, which must consider the lived histories of diverse stakeholders, their experiences addressing health concerns and navigating health care systems, the sociophysical particulars of health care environments, and best scientific approaches for establishing and implementing evidence-based practice. Such work requires a deeper shared understanding of the epistemological and methodological traditions from the natural, social and health sciences, while attending to the humanistic elements of health care delivery.

As an LSI scholar who worked for several years in health services research and continues to work on research teams with clinicians and practitioners of various kinds, I'd like to emphasize that, although transdisciplinary collaborations are certainly not without their challenges, they are tremendously rewarding when the research is "owned by co-creators who believe in its purpose and product," a characteristic that communication scholars Simpson and Seibold (2008: 268) argue defines the best engaged scholarship. Transdisciplinary work developing interventions often calls for an engaged approach to scholarship which entails "being immersed in the lives of real-world groups and organizations and involved in close work and learning with stakeholders" (Barge, Simpson and Shockley-Zalabak 2008: 243). This immersion has been growing in popularity in health services and public health research in the form of community engagement (Mikesell, Bromley and Khodyakov 2013) and has always been present to some degree within the discipline of communication. Simpson and Seibold (2008: 266), for instance, begin their essay on the co-creation of engaged scholarship by explicating the primary concern of the field. As they describe it, "[t]he field of communication has been concerned – at least since the writing of Plato's *Republic* – with the dilemmas people face as they coordinate action in their lives and work." In transdisciplinary work, the efforts of engagement take place between those who may most closely identify as "researchers" and those who identify as "community partners" but also between academic researchers from different disciplines.

In this chapter, I explicate how LSI scholars are particularly well positioned to contribute to the engaged work of transdisciplinary teams when designing health interventions. Given LSI scholars' careful attention to what interactants themselves orient to as meaningful and their close consideration of how interactants come together to manage the moment-by-moment collaborative achievements of everyday actions and institutional tasks, their approaches can reveal how co-members on transdisciplinary teams accomplish research tasks and manage role sharing and how clinical staff and patients manage institutional goals, while also accounting for what is interactionally at stake for these participants as they coordinate and negotiate tasks and challenges. Although my scholarship has drawn significantly on Conversation Analysis (CA) and I will make reference to its practices, I try to present a broader perspective that is applicable to the multiple traditions within LSI (e.g., ethnography of communication, discourse analysis), what Sanders (2005) refers to as a "multidisciplinary confederation" of LSI, whose work shares a broad but common interest in revealing the situated practices of human interaction through which participants achieve social order and thus accomplish aspects of their interpersonal and institutional lives.

Each tradition within LSI constitutes both a theoretical orientation and a methodological approach. As Raclaw (2015: 1) describes for CA, the theoretical focus "is on the local production of social order, and in particular on the ways in which participants organize their contributions to an episode of talk as vehicles for the production of social action." Methodologically, CA "provides the analysts with a set of tools for describing the structural characteristics of talk in interaction" – the conversational machinery – and "allows the analyst to examine the participants' own displayed understandings of these processes within the course of the unfolding interaction" (Raclaw 2015: 1). It is through these social actions managed within talk-in-interaction that participants reach mutual understanding, conduct social and institutional activities, and achieve both interactional and institutional order (Mondada 2012). Accordingly, I argue that bringing LSI expertise to transdisciplinary health intervention research is beneficial throughout the process of designing a health intervention, from defining the problem in need of intervention to investigating its impact. In doing so, I reflect on the ways that health contexts can provide rich sites of inquiry for communication/LSI scholarship as well as how our backgrounds in LSI contribute to the applied problems that are also of interest to our clinic and patient partners.

In what follows, I explore the importance of LSI scholarship throughout the entire process of the development of an intervention – from the early conceptualization of a potential intervention through to implementing the intervention in a clinic context. In the three sections that form the core of this chapter, I discuss how LSI scholarship has the capacity to contribute to health care intervention research before, during, and after development. More specifically, I explicate how LSI scholarship has the capacity to contribute to health care intervention research

(1) by sensitively attending to stakeholder perspectives, the local context, culture and work practices that are crucial to understand *before* an intervention is conceptualized, (2) by accounting for the interactional practices by which interventions come to be realized through the collaboration of diverse stakeholders *during* the conceptualization and design of an intervention, processes which tend to be backgrounded and often remain behind-the-scenes in the reporting of most health intervention research (Chandler et al. 2013), and (3) after development by closely investigating how interventions that target a particular outcome (often clinically defined) simultaneously shape clinic communication and interactions and thus impact participants' everyday experiences within healthcare organizations. I believe that understanding these contributions may be especially helpful for students and new scholars to better articulate the value that they bring to engaged, transdisciplinary teams developing health interventions and enable them to more readily reflect on how their work simultaneously contributes to the aims of their research partners and the aims of their home discipline.

2 Our work *before* an intervention is conceptualized

Although public health and health services researchers have made the case that the process of designing health interventions is as important as the process of evaluating them, they also recognize that there is little guidance regarding the former (Armstrong et al. 2008; Wight et al. 2016). Chandler et al. (2013: 374), for instance, note that in comparison to the amount of investment made in evaluating complex health interventions, "less attention has been paid to how such interventions are designed and to reflecting on how this design process works in practice." My experience similarly reflects this tendency. I have often been asked to join teams only after the intervention has been conceptualized and designed, when the team determines (or a grant reviewer has recommended) that they should investigate the intervention's impact on patient-provider communication or patient experience to help evaluate its effectiveness. This means by the time I am consulted, the problem from the perspective of the research team has already been defined and the components of the intervention targeting the problem have already been established.

However, LSI scholars can and should contribute, not only to the efforts evaluating the outcomes of an intervention, but also to explicate the communication landscape, institutional practices, clinic culture, and stakeholder perspectives well *before* an intervention is fully conceptualized. When "the processes undertaken and people, agendas and disciplines that have influenced the design of complex health care improvement interventions" are not made explicit, we impede "the ability to interpret how findings of intervention effects could be inferred from one setting to another..." (Chandler et al. 2013: 374). Such efforts can also help avoid using unnecessary resources to evaluate and implement a poorly designed intervention (Wight et al., 2016) or an intervention designed to meet a problem that was not well-defined from the perspectives or lived experiences of the stakeholders. LSI scholars are trained to closely examine the communicative and interactional practices by which participants – which may be the co-members of the transdisciplinary research team, the practitioners of the health care clinic, and/or the patients and family – come together to achieve demonstrable goals. As such, they not only identify the on-the-ground processes that directly influence the development of health interventions, but they also reveal the varying (and often disciplinary) assumptions that participants bring to interactions that are easily overlooked when such differences do not cause explicit disagreements or conflict. In such cases, it may initially appear that the design tasks are achieved without complication, only to have these differing assumptions later surface, revealing how an intervention is flawed or not adequately meeting stakeholder needs.

For example, drawing on LSI approaches to examine the institutional interactions that constitute a work culture before an intervention is conceptualized can help identify challenges, gaps, and perspectives of participants as they are engaged in their work practices *in situ* (as opposed to their rationalized retrospective reflections, which often neglect important and practical aspects of work). Such efforts not only bring a real-world lens to defining challenges in need of intervention but also to identifying barriers and facilitators that may impact the success of an intervention later designed to address those challenges. Such work also contributes to LSI scholarship, which itself has an established and growing tradition of drawing on its approaches to change institutional practices (see Antaki 2011). Perhaps most apparently, this work contributes to the relevance and impact of epistemic asymmetries – for example, the variable knowledge domains of clinicians as compared to patients or research partners – that are often commonplace to institutional interactions (Sidnell 2012; see also Park 2012; Weiste, Voutilainen, and Peräkylä 2016).

In several LSI traditions, including CA, this careful, close attention to the practices that accomplish institutional work requires video-recordings and as little interference as possible by the researchers. In the illustrative case below, however, I illuminate how our LSI training to attend to participants' meanings as they are demonstrated *in situ* and in relationship to their interactional goals can contribute to a more grounded definition of the problem in need of resolution, even before any recordings of workplace interactions are conducted. This more ethnographic approach to examining complex institutions has been contentious in CA because, as Mondada (2013: 4) notes, "it is seen as running the risk of imposing exogenous categorical and typological characterizations on the setting, the participants, or the activity before examining the details of talk and conduct." However, Mondada (2013: 4) also reminds us that ethnographic observations have benefited CA studies by "provid[ing] information about the research site and serv[ing] as a form of proto-analysis helping to identify the relevant activities in situ . . ." In the following case study, I hope to show how LSI sensibilities, even before formal data collection, can be helpful for defining the problem in need of resolution, a necessary step in the development of a successful intervention.

2.1 Illustrative case

One project I recently worked on in collaboration with user-centered designers and clinicians treating patients with acute leukemia illustrates the value of LSI perspectives during our early collaboration on this team that aspired to transdisciplinary goals. This value was especially evident when we first began exploring the boundaries of the problem to be addressed (see Fadem 2021). Our clinic partners had reasonably developed clear understandings of the problem they perceived to be most in need of resolution. Clinicians described to us the delicate and challenging conversations they had with patients about whether to continue with chemotherapy or receive a bone marrow transplant. They described transplant as a particularly difficult decision because it is often the only chance for curative treatment; however, the outcomes are uncertain and come with high risks, including death, that are hard to predict. While oncologists may be able to tell patients if they are 'good' candidates for transplant based on their health status and history, even ideal candidates may experience adverse outcomes. Additionally, predicting which adverse outcomes a patient is likely to experience and when is next to impossible.

From clinicians' perspective, as reported to us, the problem seemed clear: Despite a mandatory educational course on the risks and outcomes of transplant for all patients and caregivers, numerous conversations with their care team, and signing a consent form that detailed the possible risks of transplant, patients were coming to clinicians after receiving transplant claiming that they were unaware of the various complications that they were now facing. Clinicians were understandably concerned about patients experiencing decisional regret. They perceived the problem needing resolution to be one of poor decision making and so described wanting to design a "decision support tool" to help provide patients with more precise and accurate risk information along with video recorded testimonials of patients' experiences of common adverse outcomes. They believed that systematically communicating this information would translate to families being able to make more informed decisions and be more prepared for what might happen post-transplant.

At this early stage of the project, we were simply learning about our partners, our mutual perceived needs and how we might most effectively share roles and work together. While this early period may be perceived as preliminary and occurring before official data collection (i.e., for many LSI traditions this means audio/video recording institutional practices), as LSI scholars, these interactions were nevertheless ripe for our analytical expertise. For instance, I wrote the following in fieldnotes after our initial meetings with the clinic team describing my early observations in the clinic:

Example 1
Patients do not seem to use the same terminology or terms as clinicians to make reference to the adverse events they experience post-transplant. When providers explain potential adverse outcomes to patients, they use non-descript terminology presumably common to the medical community (e.g., dry eyes) and mitigate the possibility of outcomes given that they are hard to predict. For example, one provider described a possible outcome as "you might, for example, get dry eyes. That could be a possible event that indicates graft-versus-host-disease (GVHD).[1]" However, when patients talk about the experience of such outcomes, they often express surprise, not at getting dry eyes per se but about how it feels and how much impact it has on their ability to live and function. Effectively, this experience is not "dry eyes" as one might understand it void of context, because dry eyes is an experience most people could likely imagine or connect some prior experience to in order to make sense of it. But post-transplant, dry eyes is debilitating. Often one can't read, can't work. This is not a minor inconvenience but significantly life altering.

The clinic team presented the problem as one of *decision making* and the solution as *information-based*: If families receive more personalized risk and experiential information about adverse outcomes, they believed the decision itself would be easier and patients would experience less negativity post-transplant. My early understanding reflected in my fieldnotes in some ways corroborates clinicians' perspective – it did seem patients could be better prepared for what they might experience post-transplant, something clinicians were concerned about. However, this reflection also subtly questions whether the challenge is one of decision making per se by beginning to pinpoint the nature of the challenge from the patient per-

---

[1] GVHD and how to recognize it following transplant are crucial for patients to understand and is often emphasized during patient-provider interactions both leading up to and following transplant.

spective, not so much as an *information gap* preventing informed treatment decisions but as an *intersubjectivity gap*, that is, a gap in mutual understanding that often arises because it is difficult for patients and families to apply clinical glosses of possible outcomes to the particulars of one's life and lived experiences. Such a gap prevents a functional understanding of adverse events when they are eventually experienced. Remaining sensitive to these subtle distinctions in how participants variably defined the problem for which we were aiming to design a solution suggested that a solution delivering more pre-transplant information alone may not be sufficient.

Indeed, patients already received a considerable amount of information before making a decision, so much so that some described the quantity as overwhelming. Similarly, the cancer center had already designed and implemented an information-based solution in the clinic that aligned with their understanding of the problem as a matter of decision-making: a mandatory 3 hour-long education course about transplant. Our early observations of the education course demonstrated that it was primarily didactic and seemed systematically designed to fill these perceived information gaps. However, this information-based solution was not adequate (Bontempo et al. 2020). When talking with patients and observing them talk with other families during and after the education course, they often expressed feeling plagued by so much information and had difficulty emotionally processing the negativity of the class, which one patient described as "a thousand ways to die." The challenge for patients thus seemed to be one not of information quantity, but of translating the information in a way that they could effectively make sense of in the context of their lives without losing hope (see Fadem 2021; Fadem and Mikesell 2022). Thus, while providers wanted to communicate medical realism to support better decision-making (i.e., pre-transplant), patients needed to experientially understand their post-transplant experiences without being drained of optimism (see Kim et al. 2020).

During this early phase of the project, we talked with and observed clinicians, patients and families but did little recording of institutional interactions for transcription and analysis. While the heart of CA's analytical work begins with the detailed, close transcription of recorded interactions, a process that facilitates unanticipated discoveries of communicative practice, my CA training nevertheless contributed to this early attention to important distinctions in participants' perspectives of the problem at hand. When learning about a new context and its workings, it can be easy to take the first expert perspective you learn – in our case that of clinicians – as a more-or-less definitive representation of the problem. Had we had done this, we may have easily concluded that patients' complaints of feeling unprepared for adverse outcomes corroborated providers' understanding of the problem. However, LSI's orientation to "unmotivated looking" (Sacks 1984) and analytic prioritization of what is demonstrably meaningful for participants in these institutional interactions helped prevent us from non-reflectively using clinicians' reports as a ready-made framework for interpreting patients' and families' experiences and how they attribute meaning to them. Our analytic focus was attuned to how participants agree and disagree, solve problems, and respond to questions to achieve their in-the-moment goals, a sensitivity that allowed close attention to participants' perspectives, not only as they rationally and retrospectively reflected on them in response to traditional needs assessment interview questions (see below), but as they managed them *in situ*.

In health intervention research, problem definition is typically the starting point for developing an intervention. For example, needs assessment surveys and interviews are often the recommended first phase in which we ask stakeholders about how they perceive the major challenges they are facing and then use these understandings to consider our initial designs (Wight et al. 2016; see Cavanaugh and Chadwick 2005). This process typically entails interviewing different stakeholders to provide a thematic synthesis of their rationalized perspectives. However, thematic analyses of such interviews, as we know from Potter and Hepburn's (2005) work on interviews as an interactional phenomenon, can easily miss the interactional context in which those perspectives are produced. In this case, even before we systematically brought our LSI analytical tools to recordings of interactions in the clinic, our professional sensitivity to the subtleties of language when interacting with patients and families drew our attention to what was meaningful to participants and how problems were being oriented to differently by different participants. As noted, identifying such differences in intersubjectivities can be hard to capture using traditional methodological approaches that do not (arguably, cannot) elicit participants' sociocultural and sense-making practices that are organically and implicitly drawn on to navigate their worlds. Yet, they are crucial to explore since they reveal moments of misalignment between stakeholders (of which they may not be conscious) that fundamentally shape how a problem gets defined as well as subsequent intervention planning. As LSI scholars, we must bring the rigor and insights of our disciplinary approaches, not only to the investigation of the intervention's impact on outcomes, but also to the examination of the social, institutional and sensemaking practices that define a context well before an intervention is conceptualized and its design discussed. In doing so, we can also advance the scholarship within our field that explicates the practices by which epistemic asymmetries are negotiated and intersubjectivity is reached while simultaneously contributing to better translation and possible up-scale of interventions (see below).

3 Our work *during* the process of designing an intervention

Close attention to the details of interaction is not only helpful for defining a problem in ways that are most meaningful for participants. It is also helpful for investigating the interactional practices by which our transdisciplinary teams and partners work together and by which we invite stakeholders to participate in research efforts. Given LSI scholars' backgrounds in social science and the humanities, we often work on teams that address complex interventions entailing multiple intersecting components that may be difficult to tease a part and thus evaluate for their unique contributions to outcomes (Campbell et al. 2000). Examples include: psychotherapeutic interventions to address the needs of a particular disorder and developmental age (e.g., Chung, Mikesell, and Miklowitz 2014), patient support tools such as the one described above (e.g., Kim et al. 2020), or mobile health applications to improve patient/family reporting of clinically relevant information (e.g. Mikesell et al. 2018; see below).

When complex health interventions are described in publications, the components of the intervention and the underlying intentions/rationale for their development are often reduced to a few sentences in the methods section, but the processes that underlie the development are rarely described and are even less commonly treated as part of systematic data collection and analysis. However, because complex interventions are multifaceted with many components, it is especially critical that we attend to the interactions that result in actual design decisions. These interactions constitute the processes by which various stakeholders are engaged and invited to share perspectives and by which research partners manage design tasks. They also constitute the moments when mutual agreement is reached amongst collaborators. Thus, rather than exclusively relying on theoretical models and clinical priors to explicate how discrete design components are likely to achieve the aims of the intervention, we can also detail the fine-grained interactional practices that support or hinder transdisciplinary teamwork that (dis)align with theoretical explanations and ultimately influence design choices.

3.1 Illustrative case

This case draws on the same bone marrow transplant project introduced above. Early in the process the research partners attended a patient advisory meeting that the clinic director had organized with former patients who had received transplant. This meeting included the clinic team (the director, two oncologists, a resident, a nurse, two transplant coordinators), five former patients who had undergone transplant, and three social science researchers that included a user-centered designer and two communication scholars trained in LSI. The clinic director organized the meeting to present his intentions to design the decision support tool to assist patients making this high-risk medical decision as well as some preliminary ideas about what such a tool might look like. The aim of the meeting was to elicit patients' early feedback and guidance.

Patient, family, and community advisory boards are an increasingly common component in health research, particularly in patient-centered outcomes research utilizing engaged approaches (e.g., community-based participatory research; Mikesell, Bromley, and Khodyahov 2013; Newman et al. 2011; Oldfield et al. 2019). Although there is very little systematic research explicating the mechanisms by which patient and community engagement may be effective (Oldfield et al., 2019), many scholars have written on the challenges of bringing together stakeholders with differing perspectives and expertise for the purposes of research and have offered recommendations and guidelines for how stakeholder engagement processes can be improved. For example, recommendations include clarifying purpose, function and roles; establishing operating principles and procedures; and evaluating partnership processes (Newman et al. 2011). However, far fewer studies consider stakeholder engagement as a set of situated communication practices deployed to accomplish institutional and interpersonal agendas. Below we examine a 3-minute segment of this patient advisory meeting to explore the insights that LSI approaches might offer for understanding stakeholder engagement as situated practices and thus from a grounded, rather than abstracted, perspective.

The extract below took place between minute 7 and 10 of the meeting. Before this point, the clinic director, from the podium at the front of the conference room, had described the purpose and functionality of the envisioned decision support tool and presented some possible information it could contain. Following laughter in response to a playful joke the director had just made (not shown), he shifts course of action in line 1 to elicit feedback about the ideas he has just presented. He first indicates the interactional organization for this new phase of the meeting: he will present his questions and then 'open it up for discussion' (lines 1–2). Remaining at the podium, he presents a series of questions in a fairly lengthy spate of talk (lines 2–20) and then moves to transition to an open dialogue but without much success (lines 20–22).

Example 2
Patient Advisory Meeting, 7:13-10:01
(DIR=director, RS=researcher, TC=transplant coordinator)

```
01  DIR:  So the questions that I have an- and then we can just open it
02        up for discussion, i:s .hh would a tool like this be beneficial.
03        Or would it have been beneficial or helpful as you were making a
04        decision. .hh Uh: how can we determine how beneficial it i:s, .hh
05        uh:: what do you wish (0.1) you and your cohort uh knew before
06        transplant. And what prepared you the best, if anything for the
07        uncertainties that go alo:ng with transplant. And everyone in
08        this roo:m has had- everybody who goes through transplant has had
09        uncertainties. .hh Uh: everybody has had uh: y'know their paths
10        uh .hhh obstructed with one thing and had ta-uh move arou:nd onto
11        a different path. .hh Uh what information do you wish you would
12        have been provided and wasn't.=Is this too much information for
13        many people, .hh and what type of questions should we ask
14        patients and caregivers as part of this initiative.=.hhh We plan
15        on .hh asking them s:o uh they can talk specifically about
16        chronic graft versus host dis>ease<,=acute graft versus host
17        >disease<,=conditioning problems,=relapse,=irreversible
18        toxicity,=even families and friends of people .hhh who didn't
19        survi:ve. But the question is what types of general questions,
20        what types of other questions should we be asking. And uh I'd
21        just like to open it up to: discussion and (to) see if anyone has
22        anything to say.
23        (.)
24  DIR:  Uh or advice.=An' I don't know if anyone- if- if you want to
25        chime in no:w. [addressed to social scientists]
26        (0.3)
27  RS1:  .tsk u[:m
28  RS2:        [(*Fir-) is it okay if I take notes?
29        (.)
30  RS2:  .hh(h)(h)
31  DIR:  Yea.
32  TC1:  Robert, I think it- I think it would be good to go back to the
33        [questions. ( )
34  TC2:  [to the [questions.
35  RS1:          [Y(h)e(h)a(h) huh.
36  TC1:  Because that was a lot.
37  TC1:  And just address it question by question ( ).
38  DIR:  I will say that one thing so fa:r uh:: any- any funding we have
39        for this is coming from our yearly bicycle ra:ce [name of race].
40        (4.2)
41  DIR:  And that's why it's part of the uh (0.5) (welcome).
42        (4.1)
```

```
43  RS1: So maybe [we could just-
44  DIR:         [So do you think a tool like this could be
45       he_lpful?
46       (2.1)
47  PAT: I have a que_stion. (.) If- if you were fo_llowing that too:l,
48       (0.2) a::nd (.) for the pa_tient or the pe_rson that's going o_n
49       the:re, and circumstances cha_:nge for some re_ason, you could-
50       what do you do, just flip through to another- to one other kind
51       of scena_rio?
52  DIR: No, e- are you saying if somebody deve_lops chronic gra_ft versus
53       ho_st disease?
54  PAT: Yea, because we're coming o_n to this, right, to get informa_tion,
55       right? *Uh*
56  DIR: Yea. This is usually at the sta_:rt of the proce:ss.
57       [An e_ducational tool.
58  PAT: [At the start of the process.
```

Close attention to the details of this exchange reveals the interactional machinery of patient advisory meetings that can help maximize their impact. Patient advisory meetings aim to solicit patient perspectives and experiences to inform and guide research and, in this case, the development and design of an intervention. However, during the meeting when the director moves to solicit patient perspectives, he delivers a series of questions one right after the other that he would like addressed. He then works to transition from this lengthy prologue/presentation to a dialogue. How to transition from one course of action to another is challenged. Given the number of participants present, rather than select a next speaker, which would facilitate turn transition but call out a specific participant to comment first and possibly cause discomfort for that individual, he describes the new course of action he would like everyone to attend to ('open it up to discussion'). This marks a shift from the prologue to a dialogue and opens the floor to 'anyone' (line 21), leaving the fourteen participants to work out who should respond first.

The interactional puzzle is how to facilitate a collaborative discussion amongst so many participants who are meeting for the first time for this very particular purpose. In light of Aakhus' (2007: 112) work, this seems a candidate for communication design when we might intervene "into some ongoing activity through the invention of techniques, devices, and procedures that aim to redesign interactivity and thus shape the possibilities for communication." In everyday interactions as well, participants (re)design communication in how they collaborate, solve problems, and deploy and manipulate language to achieve their ends (Aakhus and

Jackson 2005). Thus, in this extract above, we can see how the director attempts to "design" communication for the purposes of shifting the course of action to an open discussion as compared to, for instance, the transplant coordinator who proposes a different approach to this problem.

After the director has indicated a shift to open discussion, at the first hearable point of completion (line 22), there is no immediate uptake from the audience (whether verbally or nonverbally by hand raising) and the director continues his turn with an increment ('uh or advice.'). He then latches a hedged alternative course of action, offering to turn the floor to the researchers on the team, which he does by gazing toward the researchers and identifying them collectively as "you" (lines 24–25). This, too, appears rather unsuccessful. Researcher 1 delays her turn (line 27), which is overlapped by researcher 2, who asks a procedural question about his role as a researcher in this meeting (line 28). This move interrupts the progressivity of the course of action the director is working to get underway (i.e., opening up a dialogue) and incidentally may also work to get the researcher off the hook for having to respond. A transplant coordinator then addresses the director with an address term (line 32; a pseudonym) and offers a suggestion for how to organize the transition to this new course of action that might more effectively facilitate an open dialogue – 'to go back to the questions' and present them 'question by question.'

Here, the transplant coordinator engages in meta-talk that indicates how she understands the nature of interaction that is more likely to achieve the aims of an open discussion and that would serve the broader goals of a patient advisory meeting. This is notably in contrast to the implicit understanding of communication that the director orients to in his prologue when he presents several questions in list form before moving to open it up for comments from the participants. He essentially treats interaction as a form of information exchange (see Ruben 2016) whereby questions are posed to seek information which then can be readily answered in the act of information provision. However, information exchange and conversational exchange are quite different forms of engagement, an understanding that the transplant coordinator demonstrably recognizes. The director's move to explicitly invite participants' responses could reasonably be understood as fulfilling the recommendations for advisory boards (see Mikesell et al. 2013: e5) such as "address[ing] partner concerns and challenges," "seek[ing] community advice or approval on research decisions," and "help[ing] researchers ascertain the needs and wishes of partners." However, from an LSI approach, we can observe how this is an interactionally achieved matter. We can see that the precise situated actions employed to achieve these abstracted communicative tasks of addressing partner concerns, seeking advice, and ascertaining partner needs are critical to the outcomes of stakeholder engagement during advisory meetings.

Practically speaking, advisory board meetings require careful consideration regarding how they themselves are designed, and LSI brings insights about best practices for inviting participants' perspectives in these settings. For LSI scholarship, these endeavors can contribute to the body of work exploring how activity transitions are managed in institutional contexts (e.g., Mori 2021; Robinson and Stivers 2001). Additionally, as can be observed in the transcript, we see that when a patient asks her question (lines 47–51), she presents a hypothetical dilemma in which a patient might find themselves, which displays her understanding of the potential uses of such a tool. Specifically, she appears to consider a patient post-transplant who might run into unexpected challenges (that the clinical director understands to be GVHD) as the intended target for the intervention. In doing so, we see how she and the clinic director are differently oriented to what is at stake. While the director is focused on the design of the tool, the patient reflects on what patients experience and how they make sense of it. She also makes available that she understands a likely use of the tool to be helping patients to process unexpected hurdles and challenges *post*-transplant. As such, we see how her displayed understanding differs from that of the clinical director's understanding that the tool would be for making treatment decisions that occur at the "the start of the process" (line 56).

The role of LSI researchers during intervention development is multifaceted. LSI scholars may identify practices that hinder or facilitate engaged scholarship and thus contribute to designing more effective interactions involving diverse stakeholders and team members. However, in doing so, they can also reveal what different stakeholders are oriented to, thereby revealing participants' priorities and what matters for them. This last endeavor is ongoing throughout the development of an intervention, just as we saw earlier that remaining sensitive to participants' orientations was important for defining the problem from multiple perspectives. In this interaction, after the patient presented her question, the clinic director directed the conversation back to his understanding of what is at stake – the tool for decision making – thereby limiting the interactional space for the patient to develop and explicate what is meaningful for her. LSI scholars can more strategically attend to these moments and follow up on them to draw out such perspectives that are meaningful to intervention planning and development.

4 Our work *after* the design of an intervention

Unsurprisingly, healthcare interventions aim to positively impact health outcomes in some way. Health communication scholars often aim to understand the pathways from communication to outcomes and are thus most often interested in how communication processes impact proximal and intermediate outcomes that in turn impact health outcomes (Street 2013). However, we might work with teams who are less interested in redesigning communication per se and more interested in intervening on the proximal (e.g., trust and rapport) or intermediate (e.g., self-care skills) outcomes that impact health. Regardless of the assumptions about this causal pathway that team members may bring to transdisciplinary teams, with complex interventions, "the interpretation of findings is frequently dependent on a range of contextual factors, irrespective of study design" (Armstrong et al. 2008: 104) that LSI scholars are well-suited to consider.

When we intervene in healthcare, whether we intervene directly on communication, proximal outcomes, or intermediate outcomes, we often create feedback loops that also require our attention. That is, regardless of where on the pathway we intervene – from clinic communication to health outcomes – our interventions often simultaneously reshape the interactional environment in which patients, providers and caregivers interact. In the illustrative case below, I describe an intervention designed to improve ADHD medication adherence that alters in-clinic conversations with providers in unanticipated ways. Because interventions have impacts beyond the outcomes that we target when we develop design components, it is paramount that we also pay careful attention to how interventions shape clinic interactions and patient-provider relationships that so critically define healthcare experiences. Those interactions constitute the processes by which healthcare is delivered and information is exchanged, but they also constitute the milieu that defines the work experiences for providers and illness experiences for patients and families. And as several have argued, considering these interactions and the relationships they sustain is as important as considering the mechanisms hypothesized to directly underlie a desired health outcome (Brody 1999; Holt-Lunstad, Smith, and Layton 2010; see also Mikesell 2013).

4.1 Illustrative case

Because the bone marrow transplant support tool has yet to be fully designed, I will introduce a different intervention for this illustrative case. The intervention was developed to help parents of children recently diagnosed with ADHD retrospectively report on their children's experiences when taking stimulant medication for the first time. Medication titration is a complex process: The goal is to identify an appropriate stimulant and dose for a particular child that reduces ADHD symptoms without causing unmanageable side effects. Thus, these pediatric psychiatry consults aim to document changes in ADHD symptoms and medication effects as the child experiences small incremental increases in doses of stimulant medication over time. However, because clinic visits are sometimes weeks apart, parents and children are frequently asked to report on their experiences well after they have occurred. Clinicians recognized this challenge, and the clinic team developed an mHealth web-based application for parents to report daily observations and experiences in real-time at home on their mobile phones. This information was then aggregated and presented in longitudinal graphs for clinicians to access on an iPad, to which they were able to make reference during their clinic visits with families as they determined appropriate (see Mikesell et al. 2018).

After its development, the mHealth tool was piloted in two community health clinics in South Los Angeles/North Compton. While our team agreed on various quality improvement outcomes that were important to document (e.g., medication adherence rates), we were also interested in how the intervention shaped clinic communication and we video recorded a series of clinic visits to observe how clinicians were drawing on the tool in real-time with families. One of our main findings was that psychiatrists most frequently referenced the tool in clinic visits to verify or confirm the accuracy of the parent reported data, particularly parents' reports of medication adherence.

A typical case is shown in the following extract. Here, the clinician begins a new sequence inquiring about medication adherence. She starts the sequence with an open-ended interview question (*How is-*), which gets reformulated as a yes-no interrogative (YNI) (line 1; *Is he remembering to take it everyday.*). Before mom can respond, however, the clinician latches (i.e., quickly articulates) the start of a follow-up question, another YNI (lines 1–2; *Are there-*), which she abandons in order to reference the data that is visible to her in the tool. In doing so, she produces an evidential assertion (*'looks like'*; Heritage and Stivers 1999) to present her observation of the mom's reported adherence (line 2; *looks like there's a couple days you forgot. Maybe.*) Upon no uptake from mom (line 3), she continues reporting the dates that medication appears to have been missed (*like (1.2) the fourteenth or the thirteenth*). Mom disconfirms this and corrects that "we took it everyday" (line 6).

Example 3

```
ADHD Stimulant Medication Titration Visit
01 DOC: How is- >is he< remembering to take it everyday::y.=Are
02      there- looks like there's a couple days you forgot. Maybe.
03      (0.6)
04 DOC: Like (1.2) ((looking at tool)) the fourtee:nth or the
05      thirtee:[nth
06 MOM:         [We took it everyday.
07 DOC: Oh you [did.
08 MOM:        [It's just that- (0.5) I forgot to
09 DOC: Oh to put it in,
10 MOM: To put it in.
11 DOC: I can put it in.
12 MOM: Yea because we've taken it- he's taken it everyd[ay.<Sometime
13 DOC:                                                 [mm hm
14 MOM: I'm like I'm gonna do it.<I'm gonna do it. .hh and then I get
15      caught up in doing this [that and the other.
16 DOC:                         [Oh I kno:w.
17 MOM: And then when the day go by it's like oh(h): go(h):d I can't
18      go back and say oh we missed it yesterday.
19 DOC: Yea.
```

From an LSI perspective, we can begin to wrestle with the interactional consequences for how the tool is organically being utilized. On the one hand, the tool enables the clinician to verify the reported data and thus achieves an important clinical aim (i.e., ensuring accurate clinically relevant information). On the other hand, the clinician demonstrates trouble formulating the question about adherence. Her incremental repairs move from an open-ended question to formulating a YNI to presenting an observation of the tool's data for mom's (dis)confirmation. These many reformulations increasingly constrain the mother's responses (Boyd and Heritage 2006; Stivers and Hayashi 2010). Presenting information that is presumably already known to the parent and provider (i.e., the information reported in the tool) for (dis)confirmation, rather than asking an open-ended question that presents the information as unknown to the provider, is perhaps not a surprising tendency that we observed across the data. As Goodwin (1979) and others have shown, participants in naturally occurring interaction generally do not tell others what they already know or ask questions for which they already know the answers. Since the providers already have the information in the mHealth app, asking for it in an open-ended question may seem inappropriate and not well designed for the recipient (see Heritage 2011).

However, drawing on the tool to seek confirmation rather than asking open-ended questions may have interactional consequences that require careful consideration. Reorganizing question-answer sequences more typical of a clinical interview into a series of observations drawn from the tool for parents to confirm or disconfirm runs the risk of reducing, and possibly eliminating, opportunities for families to narrativize their experiences. In primary care contexts, patients have been found to value opening questions that allow them to narratively define, on their terms, their illness experiences. When providers ask opening questions that allow patients to engage in these illness narratives without constraint, they report higher satisfaction with their visits (Robinson and Heritage 2006). Additionally, presenting 'evidence' of possible missed doses as documented in the tool makes conditionally relevant (Schegloff 1968) an account from mom: If the doses were, in fact, missed, an account for why the doses were missed is due. If the doses were not missed, an account for why they were not inputted into the mHealth tool becomes relevant. Indeed, after mom corrects the inaccuracy of the reported data, she moves to provide a rather extensive account explaining why she was unable to input medication adherence on those days (lines 8–18). Thus, presenting observations from the tool may not only reduce opportunities for families to narrativize their medication experiences (narratives that may also provide clinically relevant information for clinicians that goes otherwise unarticulated), it may also result in families being publicly called out for poor documentation of medication adherence which they may feel the need to justify, in turn possibly straining the patient-provider relationship.

As LSI scholars, we have a unique vantage point from which to consider the processes by which we intervene in healthcare contexts with a special sensitivity to how interventions restructure the interactions and communication landscape in both anticipated and unanticipated ways. That unique vantage point requires that we attend to the real-world discourse practices that are deployed by participants that may bolster or diminish patient autonomy, facilitate or impede shared decision making, engage or disengage cultural appropriateness, and attend or disattend to recipients' epistemic stances. It also provides a lens as to how stakeholders in these interactions discursively show – demonstrably reveal to others through their discourse and interactional practices – what is meaningful for them in these moments. Our approaches provide a powerful and finely-focused lens with which to understand patients' and families' health-related experiences, decisions, and how clinic conversations support or interfere with their goals. Thus, when it comes to designing health interventions, transdisciplinary collaborations between LSI scholars, healthcare practitioners and clinical researchers provide opportunities to consider more carefully how intervening not only has the potential to impact health outcomes as we typically define them (e.g., remission, pain control, survival, functional ability, medication adherence), but also identify opportunities to improve the experiences of patients and families as they interact with healthcare providers and systems.

5 Reflections on intervention design

The illustrative cases presented above aimed to demonstrate how collaborations that include LSI scholars can contribute to the applied aims of designing health interventions. More specifically, I made the case that LSI scholarship can provide valuable insights that help illuminate the varied and overlapping perspectives of stakeholders, particularly regarding how they understand and define the problem in need of intervention and display that understanding *in situ*. As such, even before formal data collection begins, LSI scholars' sensitivities to how participants navigate institutional tasks and activities help reveal rich understandings of stakeholder challenges and thus contribute to ecologically grounded conceptualizations of design components to address them. These are valuable first steps in the process of conceptualizing an intervention that will address stakeholder needs as they are experienced on the ground. Indeed, in the case of the bone marrow transplant project, these early contributions significantly shifted the conceptualization of the tool from one strictly of "decision support" aimed at filling in information gaps pre-transplant to one of "sensemaking support" aimed at helping patients and families to process and interpret new information and challenges in the context of their lives throughout the transplant journey (Fadem 2021; Fadem and Mikesell 2022).

I also showed how LSI approaches are beneficial for explicating the processes by which stakeholders are engaged, particularly in the form of patient and community advisory boards, which have become a well-recognized component for many types of health research. While various recommendations have been made to improve the process of how to incorporate and convene advisory boards in health research, these recommendations have been conceptual rather than offering concrete practices for research partners. While such recommendations are needed, LSI approaches, in contrast, can ground these abstract recommendations in situated practices that help provide clear guidance for designing interactions that can effectively realize the aims of advisory boards. This work suggests that advisory boards would benefit when the transdisciplinary team engages in deliberative design tasks for soliciting information from stakeholders and in post-advisory board debriefings to consider how the designed interactions may have constrained stakeholder perspectives in unintended ways. In our case, engaging in such a design task may have encouraged us to 1) elicit authentic patient experiences of what they need and not only their reflections about what a pre-determined tool might provide them and 2) deliberately allow for more interactional space with which to articulate these experiences before returning to a pre-determined meeting agenda. Engaging in these design tasks are also likely to contribute to transdisciplinary team building because they provide time for co-researchers to understand and share roles. As shown in the illustrative case of the advisory board, the social science researchers did not take on leadership roles during this meeting and one researcher demonstrated how he was figuring out in the moment what constituted his role when his participation was sought.

Lastly, I showed how LSI approaches can illuminate how an intervention may alter the situated communication practices that take place once it is implemented. This work can show how an intervention may have unintended consequences that may fundamentally shape clinic and healthcare experiences and also suggests ways to potentially alter or improve practitioner training with an intervention. In the case of ADHD medication titration, a CA-based solution might be a simple recommendation for practitioners to begin visits without first relying on or presenting the data in the tool. This solution can thus address the potential problem of eliminating families' medication narratives, while also providing clear training protocols for practitioners who demonstrably struggled with how to formulate opening questions most appropriately.

Although not the focus of this chapter, I also suggested that engaged collaborations that aim to be transdisciplinary are likely to reap the most benefit as they facilitate productivity on teams that include members of different disciplines with varying epistemological and methodological backgrounds. Most, if not all, LSI scholars working in health contexts have experienced the challenge of translating their approaches to their colleagues. Similarly, LSI scholars may lack understanding of the practical challenges and institutional constraints practitioners are facing. Transdisciplinarity encourages co-researchers to move beyond their disciplinary traditions by working to internalize the perspectives of their colleagues. Securing a commitment to transdisciplinarity early in the collaboration can help address tensions that naturally arise when bringing together members from seemingly disparate traditions. Although this requires more time investment up front, successful efforts are likely to lead to the conceptualization and development of interventions that are both humanistic and evidence-based.

6 Reflections on the disciplinary aims of LSI

While transdisciplinarity asks researchers to share the perspectives and roles of their team members, it does not require the abandonment of one's own disciplinary training and values. And it is worth reflecting on how these transdisciplinary collaborations can also contribute to the disciplinary aims of LSI scholars (see Ford 2012). Thus far, I have only touched upon this value such as the work on epistemic asymmetries and how distinct territories of knowledge of clinicians and patients are negotiated in medical interactions, how activity transitions are interactionally managed in institutional contexts, and how health interventions shape institutional talk between patients and providers, which is a growing and rich area of CA research (Maynard and Heritage 2005; see also Robinson 2011 explicating the relationship between CA and health communication; Robinson and Heritage 2014 on 'conversation analytic intervention'). Perhaps the area of CA research that is most clearly informed by these efforts is the work of *applied CA*.

Antaki (2011) identifies at least six meanings of applied CA: social-problem (a perspective on macro-societal issues), communicational (a complementary or alternative analysis of 'disordered' talk), diagnostic (correlating sequential features of talk with clinical disorders), institutional (an illumination of routine institutional work), foundational (respecifying an intellectual field of study), and interventionist (solving pre-existing problems collaboratively). While designing health interventions on transdisciplinary teams may reasonably be identified as an example of *interventionist applied CA*, the work of CA scholars as discussed above shows how other forms of applied CA – namely, *institutional* and *foundational* applied CA – may equally contribute to the interventionist agenda.

As Antaki (2011: 8) describes, interventionist work applies CA "to an interactional problem which pre-existed the analyst's arrival; it has the strong implication that a solution will be identified via the analysis of the sequential organization of talk; and it is undertaken collaboratively, achieved with people in the local scene." While I hoped to make the case that LSI expertise is indeed crucial for developing solutions to many problems in healthcare, I also hoped to show how LSI scholars can contribute to defining the problem in the first place. While many examples of interventionist CA have taken the problem presented by practitioners as given (perhaps more likely on interdisciplinary teams), many (though not all) health contexts could benefit from transdisciplinary collaborations that form much earlier in the process of developing interventions and whose members are open to reimagining the problem at the outset.

This work of LSI *before* the conceptualization of health interventions might be best described as what Antaki (2011: 1) refers to as *institutional* applied CA "where [CA] illuminates the workings of society's institutions." When we consider how participants in institutional contexts design their turns and sequentially organize their talk to achieve institutional business, we are provided a window into how participants socially construct and negotiate coherent sets of institutional norms through their moment-to-moment actions. As shown in the first illustrative example above, uncovering the daily work of providers as they communicated risk with patients and how patients responded provided traction on the problem from both clinicians' and patients' perspectives. Institutional applied CA does not aim to solve institutional problems but rather aims "to see how the institution manages to carry off its work..." (Antaki 2011: 1). In doing so, the values and presumptions that participants bring to these contexts can be revealed. Uncovering how the daily work of an institution is achieved can thus identify where gaps in participant orientations exist and can in turn inform how problems are practically defined. Such an enterprise, while itself is not oriented to intervening per se, nevertheless, can ultimately contribute to the process and planning of interventions.

LSI scholarship *during* the conceptualization and design of health interventions might be best described as *foundational,* where we "'apply' CA to other disciplines and respecify their fields of study, chalk off old problems as meaningless, and identify new and more interesting ones, with a CA solution" (Antaki 2011: 3). For example, in the second illustrative case, I discussed a commonly recognized problem of how to utilize and conduct advisory boards to best incorporate the expertise of non-researchers. In public health, various challenges regarding how to best center patients and other non-researchers in the research process have been frequently discussed (Mikesell et al. 2013). In the case above, I reconstituted this problem typically addressed in the field of public health as a communicative one for which CA is able to illuminate mechanisms that enable or stall participation. Reconceptualizing these known challenges of community engagement (Mikesell et al. 2013) through the lens of CA in turn helps consider solutions that may have thus far been overlooked, such as how to design communicative tasks for stakeholders that are more likely to elicit genuine understandings. Like the institutional work taking place *before* the conceptualization of the intervention, this foundational work itself may not directly achieve interventionist aims but nevertheless can contribute to broader interventionist goals.

The work discussed above that comes *after* the conceptualization and development of an intervention may indeed be most aptly understood within the *interventionist* applied CA agenda. Although interventionist applied CA typically arises when practitioners are facing a recognized difficulty in the delivery of their services that the tools of CA might help address (Antaki 2011), I showed how CA may also help to identify how an intervention, developed to resolve one sort of difficulty, can unintentionally lead to other difficulties (or successes) that may or may not be recognized by practitioners or the institution. In this way, interventionist applied CA has the potential to help develop solutions to known problems *and* help identify unexpected problems that may also be resolved by CA-based solutions once interventions are put into practice.

There is benefit to understanding the boundaries of foundational, institutional and interventionist applied CA as distinct domains of CA scholarship. However, when we consider how CA might contribute to transdisciplinary health intervention research, from the early conceptualization through to the development and implementation of health interventions, we can observe how these differing domains of applied CA can each inform the broader aims of interventionist work in distinct ways. Overall, this chapter emphasizes that transdisciplinary health intervention research is complex and its boundaries considerably more expansive than many might typically presume, extending from well before the conceptualization of an intervention to well after its development. Given LSI scholarship's orientations to situated practices that constitute the flow of institutional work – whether that work involves practitioners collaborating in clinic, academic and clinic co-researchers negotiating the aims of an intervention, or patients and providers communicating during clinic interviews – LSI can contribute in fundamental ways to the various sequential phases comprising transdisciplinary health intervention research.

References

Aakhus, Mark. 2007. Communication as design. *Communication Monographs* 74 (1). 112–117.
Antaki, Charles. (ed.). 2011. *Applied conversation analysis: Intervention and change in institutional talk*. Palgrave Macmillan.
Armstrong, Rebecca, Elizabeth Water, Laurence Moore, Elisha Riggs, Luis G. Cuervo, Pisake Lumbiganon & Penelope Hawe. 2008. Improving the reporting of public health intervention research: Advancing TREND and CONSORT. *Journal of Public Health* 30 (1). 103–109.
Barge, James K., Jennifer L. Simpson & Pamela Shockley-Zalabak. 2008. Introduction: Toward purposeful and practical models of engaged scholarship. *Journal of Applied Communication Research* 36 (3). 243–244.
Boyd, Elizabeth & John Heritage. 2006. Taking the history: Questioning during comprehensive history taking. In John Heritage & Douglad W. Maynard (eds.), *Communication in medical care*, 151–184. New York: Cambridge University Press.
Brody, H. 1999. The doctor as therapeutic agent: A placebo effect research agenda. In Anne Harrington (ed.), *The placebo effect: An interdisciplinary exploration*, 77–92. Cambridge, MA: Harvard University Press.
Campbell, Michelle, Ray Fitzpatrick, Andrew Haines, Ann Louise Kinmonth, Peter Sandercock, David Spiegelhalter & Peter Tyrer. 2000. Framework for design and evaluation of complex interventions to improve health. *BMJ* 321 (7262). 694–696.

Cavanaugh, Sue & Keith Chadwick. 2005. *Health needs assessment: A practical guide*. London, NICE. https://ihub.scot/media/1841/health_needs_assessment_a_practical_guide.pdf (accessed 9 May 2021).

Chandler, Clare, I. R., Helen Burchett, Louise Boyle, Olivia Achonduh, Anthony Mbonye, Deborah DiLiberto, Hugh Reyburn, Obinna Onwujekwe, Ane Haaland, Arantxa Roca-Feltrer, Frank Baiden, Wilfred F. Mbacham, Richard Ndyomugyenyi, Forence Nankya, Lindsay Mangham-Jefferies, Sian Clarke, Hilda Mbakilwa, Joanna Reynolds, Sham Lal, Toby Leslie, Catherine Maiteki-Sebuguzi, Jayne Webster, Pascal Magnussen, Evelyn Ansah, Kristian S. Hansen, Eleanor Hutchinson, Bonnie Cundill, Shunmay Yeung, David Schellenberg, Sarah G. Staedke, Virginia Wiseman, David G. Lalloo & Christopher J. M. Whitty. 2013. Examining intervention design: Lessons from the development of eight related Malaria health care intervention studies. *Health Systems & Reform* 2 (4). 373–388.

Choi, Bernard. C. K. & Anita W.P. Pak. 2006. Multidisciplinarity, interdisciplinarity and transdisciplinarity in health research, services, education and policy: 1. Definitions, objectives and evidence of effectiveness. *Clinical and Investigative Medicine* 29 (6). 351–364.

Chung, Bowen, Lisa Mikesell & David Miklowitz. 2014. Flexibility and structure may enhance implementation of family-focused therapy in community mental health settings. *Community Mental Health Journal* 50 (7). 787–791.

Egbert, Maria. 2011. Conversation analysis applied to user-centered design: A study of the who 'the user' is. In Charles Antaki (ed.), *Applied conversation analysis: Interventions and change in institutional talk*, 207–221. Palgrave Macmillan.

Fadem, Sarah. 2021. *Design for sensemaking in complex and ambiguous medical situations*. New Brunswick, NJ: Rutgers University dissertation.

Fadem, Sarah & Lisa Mikesell. 2022. Patient and provider perspectives on the impacts of unpredictability for patient sensemaking: Implications for intervention design. *Journal of Patient Experience* 9. 1–7.

Ford, Ceclia E. 2012. Clarity in applied and interdisciplinary conversation analysis. *Discourse Studies* 14 (4). 507–513.

Goodwin, Charles. 1979. The interactive construction of a sentence in natural conversation. In Geroge Psathas (ed.), *Everyday language: Studies in ethnomethodology*, 97–121. New York: Irvington Publishers.

Hannawa, Annegret F., Leonarda Garcia-Jimenez, Carey Candrian, Constanze Rossmann & Peter J. Schulz. 2015. Identifying the field of health communication. *Journal of Health Communication* 20. 521–530.

Heritage, John. 2011. The interaction order and clinical practice: Some observations on dysfunctions and action steps. *Patient Education and Counseling*, 84. 338–343.

Heritage, John & Tanya Stivers. 1999. Online commentary in acute medical visits: A method of shaping patient expectations. *Social Science & Medicine* 49. 1501–1517.

Holt-Lunstad, Julianne, Timothy B. Smith & J. Bradley Layton. 2010. Social relationships and mortality risk: A meta-analysis review. *PLoS Medicine* 7 (7). e1000316.

Kim, Sunyoung, Beatrice Trinidad, Lisa Mikesell & Mark Aakhus. 2020. Improving prognosis communication for leukemia patients facing complex medical treatment: A user-centered approach. *International Journal of Medical Informatics* 141. 104147.

Maynard, Douglas W. & John Heritage. 2005. Conversation analysis, doctor-patient interaction and medical communication. *Medical Education* 39 (4). 428–435.

Mikesell, Lisa. 2013. Medicinal relationships: Caring conversation. *Medical Education* 47. 443–452.

Mikesell, Lisa, Elizabeth Bromley & Dmitry Khodyakov. 2013. Ethical community-engaged research: A literature review. *American Journal of Public Health* 103 (12). e7–e14.

Mikesell, Lisa, Alethea F. Marti, Jennifer R. Guzmán, Michael M. McCreary & Bonnie Zima. 2018. Affordances of mHealth technology and the structuring of clinic communication. *Journal of Applied Communication Research* 46 (3). 323–347.

Mondada, Lorenza. 2013. Conversation analysis and institutional interaction. In C. Chapelle (ed.), *The encyclopedia of applied linguistics*, pages. Oxford: Wiley.

Mori, Junko. 2021. Between researchers and practitioners: Possibilities and challenges for applied conversation analysis. In Silvia Kunitz, Numa Markee & Olcay Sert (eds.), *Classroom-based conversation analytic research: Theoretical and applied research*, 407–415. Springer Nature.

Newman, Susan D., Jeannette O. Andrews, Gayenell S. Magwood, Carolyn Jenkins, Melissa J. Cox & Deborah Williamson. 2011. Community advisory boards in community-based participatory research: A synthesis of best processes. *Preventing Chronic Disease* 8 (3). A70.

Oldfield, Benjamin J., Marcus A. Harrison, Inginia Genao, Ann T. Greene, Ellen Pappas, Janis G. Glover & Marjorie S. Rosenthal. 2019. Patient, family, and community advisory councils in health care and research: A systematic review. *Journal of General Internal Medicine* 34. 1292–1303.

Potter, Jonathan & Alexa Hepburn. 2005. Qualitative interviews in psychology: Problems and possibilities. *Qualitative Research in Psychology* 2. 281–307.

Raclaw, Joshua. 2015. Conversation analysis, overview. In Karen Tracy, Cornelia Ilie & Todd Sandel (eds.), *The international encyclopedia of language and social interaction*, 219–229). John Wiley.

Robinson, Jeffrey D. 2011. Conversation analysis and health communication. In Teresa Thompson, Alicia Dorsey, Katherine Miller & Roxanne Parrott (eds.), *Handbook of health communication* 2nd edn., 501–518. Mahwah, NJ: Lawrence Erlbaum.

Robinson, Jeffrey D. & John Heritage. 2006. Physicians' opening questions and patients' satisfaction. *Patient Education and Counseling* 60. 279–285.

Robinson, Jeffrey D. & John Heritage. 2014. Intervening with conversation analysis: The case of medicine. *Research on Language and Social Interaction* 47 (3). 201–218.

Robinson, Jeffrey D. & Tanya Stivers. 2001. Achieving activity transitions in physician-patient encounters: From history taking to physical examination. *Health Communication Research* 27 (2). 253–298.

Ruben, Brent. D. 2016. Communication theory and health communication practice: The more things change, the more they stay the same. *Health Communication* 31 (1). 1–11.

Sanders, Robert E. 2005. Introduction: LSI as a subject matter and as a multidisciplinary confederation. In Kristine L. Fitch & Robert E. Sanders (eds.), *Handbook of Language and Social Interaction*, 1–14. Mahwah, NJ: Lawrence Erlbaum.

Schegloff, Emmanuel A. 1968. Sequencing in conversational openings. *American Anthropologist* 70. 1075–1095.

Schegloff, Emmanuel A. 2007. *Sequence organization in interaction*. Cambridge University Press.

Simpson, Jennifer L. & David R. Seibold. 2008. Practical engagements and co-created research. *Journal of Applied Communication Research* 36 (3). 266–280.

Stivers, Tanya & Makoto Hayashi. 2010. Transformative answers: One way to resist a question's constraints. *Language in Society* 39. 1–25.

Street, Richard L. 2013. How clinician-patient communication contributes to health improvement: Modeling pathways from talk to outcome. *Patient Education and Counseling* 92. 286–291.

Weiste, Elina, Liisa Voutilainen & Anssi Peräkylä. 2016. Epistemic asymmetries in psychotherapy interaction: Therapists' practices for displaying access to clients' inner experiences. *Sociology of Health & Illness* 38 (4). 645–661.

Wight, Daniel, Erica Wimbush, Ruth Jepson & Lawrence Doi. 2016. Six steps in quality intervention development (6SQuID). *Journal of Epidemiology and Community Health* 70. 520–525.

Brett A. Diaz
Conclusion

1 Introduction

The preceding chapters of this volume have demonstrated that health research, education, and policy is an area of attention that is diverse, professionally and intellectually rich, and full of reasons for optimism. The importance of language to health can be felt in the unlooked-for ways of speaking and seeing in varied avenues of health research: its role in guiding the development of health professionals, understanding the subtleties needed in crafting life-or-death public health policy mandates, relief efforts in emergency zones, and affordances made to vulnerable populations through community interventions.

The contributors, researchers, and people behind the chapters of this volume are as important to our goals as the data, the analyses, and the scholarly products contained herein. We began this volume with the strongly held position that their voices, histories, and personal insights ought to be valued, up front, and transparently. We also wanted to open a space in which actual dialogue could happen – beyond the intertextual, scholarly conversation in the interstices of these collected chapters. Thus, toward the end of the journey of composing, compiling, and combining the chapters of this volume, we invited our contributors to participate in an informal forum. During this forum, authors were encouraged to share their histories and perspectives in the field. We encouraged them to add personal and unreported details about the paths taken in their research projects. We hoped, ultimately, to glimpse the lives behind the chapters and something of the future of health applied linguistics and communication.

This short concluding chapter, though reflective and less formal than those preceding it, is meant to be a point of inclusion, an invitation for readers to weave their own thread into the tapestry of our profession. We structured it this way in the hope that it can be read and reflected on by people, groups, and communities across health research, education, and policy. This chapter might, for example, serve as an introductory text for students just embarking on their journey in applied linguistics or communication studies. Alternately, the chapter may be of interest to policymakers working in public health organizations, who are interested in learning more about specialists in language and communication, and the questions that they ask. Or, it may serve as a medium of reflection for those

---

Brett A. Diaz, The Wilson Centre, University of Toronto; Centre for Faculty Development, Unity Health Toronto

https://doi.org/10.1515/9783110744804-011

already established in the field, to see themselves and their experiences reflected in the stories of others, and foster feelings of connectedness.

The chapter relates the authors' stories, perspectives, and commitments to health applied linguistics, using their own words. In the first section, the variety of backgrounds and personal paths into the field are discussed. In the second, the contributors discussed challenges and the promise of their current work, and their current situations. In the final section, we focus on potential areas of future interest and work to be done in the field.

In reading this chapter, we invite readers to reflect on their own experience, looking backward and forward to their own practices:
1. How is my current research reflected in these scholars' works?
    a. How might I find a place for my work in health contexts?
2. How has health affected my own life and research?
3. How do I see and understand human communication in relation to health, health professionals, and world events?

Excerpts from the forum have been included here with some light editing for readability. Quotes from our conversation are used with the permission of the contributors.

2 Backgrounds of applied linguists in health research, education, and policy

The backgrounds of people in health contexts are multidisciplinary and broad. As no surprise, there are numerous encounters, intersections, and opportunities in the paths that language and communication scholars take over the course of their professional careers. Thus, some scholars began their careers concentrated in more traditional linguistics areas, such as world languages, language socialization, or neurolinguistics (Excerpt 1). The specific routes vary widely, from entirely new subject areas to natural outgrowths, to staying within the core language science purview. In other cases, they entered the field in what they describe as more direct routes, such as medical anthropology.

(1) *I was working under a neurobiologist, a theorist in neurobiology and evolution of language, but my interests slowly transitioned to thinking more about the kind of applied practical work that I could do with that knowledge. So I started working with neurologists at a neurology clinic and focused my dissertation on frontotemporal dementia. (Lisa Mikesell)*

Still others, formed as language & communication scholars, found themselves immersed in health spaces through community engagement (Excerpt 2).

(2) *[My] dissertation was about a community engaged participatory action research project, that really focused on working with new Iraqi immigrants, refugees and SIV visa holders, as they were kind of getting themselves set up in in the U.S. And we created the refugee, health, and employment attainment program. So, that was the first kind of introduction of health that came. So, we brought in different professionals, doctors, providers, health insurance companies and agents, to kind of help people navigate the process of getting health care taken care of. (Emily Feuerherm)*

A parallel exists between the skills and sensibilities of people like our contributors and those of health professionals when they find themselves concerned with their *own* health issues. In this case, those experiences prompt noticing that leads to questions, and ultimately, seeing health experiences as investigable (Excerpt 3).

(3) *Probably a very typical applied linguistic perspective, that it affects us all. It's a fascinating part of it, the language. The way we talk about our bodies and the way we talk about health shape so much of the kind of treatment we get, and the treatment we give. (Paul McPherron)*

On the side of the applied linguists, scholars may find themselves in unfamiliar, perhaps vulnerable territory. They engage with the health system to receive help, or address a health concern, or to accompany a family member during a difficult time, and so on. Once there, however, they learn, adopt, and exercise the situated practices, activities, and pragmatics of the place (Garfinkel & Sacks 1986; Lynch 2019) – the on-going ways of *being*. Their expertise in communication makes them sensitive to facets of the place, inviting observations, scrutiny, and (ultimately) investigation of how health gets done. They accumulate knowledge and develop insider-insights by becoming research- or education- or policy members of that community through that personal experience.

On the other side, in contrast to applied linguists, health professionals find themselves as patients in their home environments. They usually have power. They usually have knowledge. They have familiarity, built up by the membership practices and norms in which they are enmeshed through formal structure. Yet, when they find themselves in health contexts in a personal capacity, their experience is often markedly different. Health professionals may become aware of the exigencies of context when their power and familiarity is destabilized (Dewar & Frampton 2013; Planetree Foundation 2013). That is, they begin to notice when their professional social orders and their associated practices are *breached* (Garfinkel 1991). In effect, when health professionals experience the *other side* of health seeking for themselves, they become aware of the practices, activities, and realities of engaging in health events in a new way.

The personal experience of health seeking is a powerful catalyst for changing perspectives about what it means to engage in health research, education, and policy. On the one hand, researchers in language, social interaction, and communication, become attentive to the social world underpinning health, and orient to it as a subject of investigation. On the other hand, many in health professions, whether as doctors, nurses, researchers, administrators, or in other roles, begin to recognize the structured nuance and varieties of experience available.

3 Current experiences in health research, education, and policy

Three strong themes emerged during our conversation about what contributors experience in their roles in health research, education, and policy: the communicative medium of health, the stakeholders whom applied linguists serve through their work, and the disciplinary transcriptions that occur. On the one front, there is the necessarily linguistic or discursive character of health interactions that attracts health applied linguists. The analysis of such interactions at fine-grained levels can help their medical colleagues involved in the research to see the value in the work, and enfranchise multidisciplinary cohorts (Excerpt 4). Linguists "hear" medical talk or see medical texts (documents, forms, laptop screens) in different ways, through different lenses, than their medical colleagues, although this does not mean that health professionals are unaware of health-situated language and communication in more or less formal ways. Through their unique positions, health applied linguists invite certain reflexivity, and sensitivities, that can help to bring research teams together around the language and communication of health contexts.

(4) *I found that it's positioning language as both an object of study and the medium of communication, which makes it both fascinating for people in the medical professions, but also somewhat daunting. So largely because we have really credible methodologies, we bring a certain level of insight into language that is really helpful, I think. (Robert W. Schrauf)*

Yet aligning paradigmatically with colleagues can pose its own challenge during the creation of interventions, whether pedagogically or clinically. Getting clinicians, practitioners, and educators to see the value in the work can be a tricky endeavor. In fact, paradigmatic (mis)alignments might occur across several levels of the research, education, and policy spectrum. Two explicit areas of these sorts of negotiations came up during the conversation: health applied linguists' roles in designing interventions, and in shaping education pathways.

Disciplinary boundaries or assumptions, between research team members, has a direct influence on designing health interventions. I use the term "critical" below in two senses – perhaps thought of as big-C, recognizing the effects of power, and little-c, attending to unusual problems and solutions, senses. Because teams are often multidisciplinary, with different rhetorical senses and epistemological legacies, the struggle of the applied linguist to bring their specialized knowledge requires the attentive consideration of norms and assumptions in place. This criticality extends to team members' expectations in designing and carrying out research projects, as presented in Excerpt 5.

(5) *When we design interventions, the clinicians want to design and build things, often with the expectation that "I'm going to communicate less," or communication will somehow easier. And social scientists on the team recognize the outcomes of this are usually that you're sometimes going to be communicating more, but in different, more effective ways. It's very hard to do. It's a very hard negotiation, these frameworks. (Lisa Mikesell)*

The different assumptions of clinicians and health applied communication scholars does not necessarily lead to easy answers or decisions. Rather, expectations about interventions are subtly shifted by dialogue and collaboration during design. These subtle changes set the groundwork for new norms, and continuing development of language and communication sensitivity in health.

Another traditional area in which applied linguists have a major role is training undergraduate, future health professionals who are learning the basic sciences core to future success. For plurilingual students in monolingual education settings, especially technical settings such as STEM, applied linguists can be pivotal (Excerpt 6).

(6) *I'm working on an NSF grant. The idea is to think about students, who come from Spanish speaking families and go into the STEM areas, and who have real difficulties. Trying to convince the biologist [faculty] of these more modern theories when it comes to how to work with people who use the second language, and [not to] go towards that deficit orientation has been a real struggle. (Caroline Vickers)*

Applied linguistics has a rich, if troubled, history with the way that plurilingualism, and plurilingual people, have been positioned in the language sciences (Pennycook 2021; Flores & Rosa 2015; Seidlhofer 2001; Canagarajah 2007; Selinker 1972). Contemporary work in Applied Linguistics has made many contributions to shifting perceptions of language use in education settings. As noted above, modern models of language acquisition, and language and corpus planning (what constitutes the recognized language, and materials produced to support that language), have problematized "deficit models" (Kachru 1991 presented in Seidlhofer 2003: 19–29) that focus on error in language use (Jenkins 2006), and the assumption that multilingual speakers seek to identify with the culture of English language use, including in their goals in academic contexts (Norton 2013).

However, the evolution in thinking about multiple language use is not always reflected in pedagogical models. The critical issue involves the power that language plays in reifying boundaries (otherness) and boundary maintenance. In this case, access to health professions is gatekept by the introduction to and sufficient mastery over basic sciences (STEM). Concomitantly, sufficient mastery over STEM courses in an official, scholastic capacity is contingent on access to language resources and skills to practice and train in higher education. When educators in STEM courses are not well-equipped to work with students from different linguistic backgrounds, the results can lead to exclusion from health professions pathways having little to do with what might be thought of as aptitude, or with intellectual, social, and cultural investment. So, while plurilingualism is without doubt a challenging area for the practice of medicine and health professions generally, language-related complications are faced early in the journey from undergraduate education through postgraduate health professions education.

Beyond education, critical health applied linguists have opportunities to bridge disciplinary boundaries and operate between the institution, the communities, and individuals. As discussed earlier and throughout this volume, work in language and communication opens up avenues for working more closely, and building professional bonds with other researchers. Applied linguists in these areas also build bonds with their participants, community collaborators, and others throughout their studies.

(7) *I've definitely seen that in my own work, making sure that this idea of limited English proficiency gets reframed or rethought about by the people that I'm working with, because I also am working with community partners, who are themselves bilingual, who are having to be advocates and medical interpreters. But at the same time there's some real difficulties.*

> *So these kinds of programs are both full of potential and exciting benefits that you can see, like ripples throughout the community, but at the same time there's a real challenge. (Emily Feuerherm)*

Community health and community action are areas attracting more attention in health research, education, and policy. In Excerpt 6, aspects of language use in education settings and addressing the needs of plurilingual people were considered. In that situation, shifting colleagues' pedagogical models away from deficit-based models was a troubled area. Similar issues are also present in community health settings (Excerpt 7). Communities, whether mono- or multilingual, bear the burden of official language policies (Braley 2010; Ricento 2006; Grin 1998; Spolsky 2004), their underwritten ideologies (Subtirelu 2013; Björkman 2014; Shohamy & Spolsky 2000), and their effects on the material wellbeing of vulnerable people seeking public health services and support (Bowen 2001; Piller 2012).

Language access is one kind of social exclusion that often goes unnoticed yet has consequences for people's access to quality health services. On the one hand, people identify with certain language varieties, as cultural anchors or connections with others. They see their ability to speak and operate within a language as core to who they are. The dark side of these identifiers is that they also create, often covertly, borderlands between the speakers of marginalized languages and the health agents in spaces dominated by an *official* language. As a consequence, limiting language access is at odds with ideas about democratic participation, efficiency, fairness, and other positive aspects of political belonging. Certain ideological camps would argue, and have, that in order for political institutions to function, language must be plain and readily understandable. By implication, citizens must have proper command of that official language, and be able to operate in public spaces using that language. The conundrum is three-fold: one, *a* language is authorized, other languages are not authorized; two, providing language services to minoritized language speakers is not obligatory; three, those that cannot participate in the authorized language are not members, and are subject to erasure from the public discourse.

Critical applied linguists are trained to notice the power differentials created and maintained by language restriction. They have an opportunity to connect with community members, hear their stories and perspectives, and to participate in creating programs to redress linguistic discrimination. Specific interventions and programs can be created, such as creating multilingual health literacy programs and making translation services available, presented by Feuerherm and McIntosh (this volume), and extends to identifying specific aspects of discourse and interaction that best suit the needs of both medical providers and their plurilingual clients, as demonstrated by Vickers and Gobel (this volume). In this way, the languaculture (Agar 1996) of healthcare becomes a medium linking community action programs, community members, and institutional systems and policymakers, and in this context, where critical applied linguists play important roles as culture brokers.

4 Future directions in health applied linguistics and communication

Our conversation ultimately turned to the future and to areas of health that contributors see as potential next steps for health applied linguists and communication specialists. Crises of the last decade have necessitated and invigorated public health conversations, reflecting heterogenous models of public health past and present (Gostin 2001; Hanlon et al. 2011; Fairchild et al. 2010; Rosenberg 2012). In the last two years alone, people have endured crises exacerbated by long-term cultural inequities: disparities linked to racial-class based practices, changes or failures of infrastructure, as in the forced, unplanned shift to remote and virtual services in response to the COVID-19 pandemic, environmental disasters, and the effects of depleted wellbeing, especially mental and social health. In the face of shifting public health norms, health applied linguists have extended their foci beyond traditional spaces for language and communication to imagine how health research, education, and policy can rise to meet emerging needs.

During our conversation, we recognized that a shift to virtual delivery of healthcare and therefore virtual interaction has created opportunities to revise our own practices (Excerpt 8). Utilizing virtual spaces provides an opportunity to share experience and expertise more widely, transporting valuable knowledge to other sectors or communities, thereby building capacity in education and policy.

(8) *Going [virtually] to places that are also struggling with these same issues, and sharing the lessons that we've learned, being able to offer some of the resources and the support that we've been able to build for this program in Flint. [. . .] Before the pandemic, online education teaching was not something that I was really interested in. So, it's definitely been a thing that has a silver lining, and something I'm kind of excited about at the end of the day.* (Emily Feuerherm)

While access to digital resources is by no means universal, digital media has the potential to be more inclusive, with unique educational affordances with fewer restrictions of location, time, and resources. One digital lesson can be distributed to many learning environments; as for example, a virtual conference report can be attended by numerous people, distributed across different communities. Health applied linguists, frequently trained in literacy education, are well-positioned to pivot to this new mode of delivery for health and public health contexts. Moreover, the active shifting of norms of healthcare delivery represents opportunities for research, education, and policy to be mutually informative.

Research in digital health literacy (and again: language access) includes developing online pedagogy and delivery systems, perhaps in the form of curriculum design, based on feedback and dialogue with community leaders. In designing pedagogical interventions, teachers and experts in the field are the key agents, and applied linguists might assist in refining and extending new curricula for the unique linguistic- and social practices of different sites. Similarly, a linguistic-discursive view of health policies draws attention to the distributed nature of communication and participation between communities who may be facing similar conditions (Diaz; Torres; this volume).

Perhaps equally important, being a part of change fuels optimism. As members of teams, health applied linguists not only conduct research in, but also identify with, their participant populations and communities, and thus they help effect change, while being affected themselves. Hence, health applied linguists also attend to issues of equity, diversity, inclusion, and accessibility (EDIA), throughout the health professions pathway, from basic science training through measuring and implementing key initiatives to improve EDIA (Excerpts 12, 13).

(9) *In terms of the diversity equity and inclusion space, the measures are like how many folks of color do we have in that school now? And how many are going into surgery? [Surgery] is a prestigious field. Is that the only outcome we want to look at, or do we want to look at feelings of inclusion and belonging and not being micro-aggressed against constantly? I feel like linguistics has a lot to offer that as well. (Abigail Konopasky)*

(10) *For the time being, I'm really interested in the pipeline: the work in STEM trying to get students from, primarily, bilingual backgrounds interested in the STEM areas. Then, what's the pipeline to get them into the healthcare field? It starts there. It's, if you fail Biology 101, you're going to take a different direction. Mental health is a huge part of that. It's such a huge part of it. That feeling of exclusion, that I don't belong with this cohort of people. Trying to support inclusive efforts, so that people feel like they're part of a community. All of that is just so relevant. (Caroline Vickers)*

To answer the sort of questions raised in excerpt 9, applied linguists bring linguistic and discursive frameworks and tools (both qualitative and quantitative) that deepen our understanding of the demographics, and sometimes exclusionary practices behind admissions to the health professions. While admission statistics cover one aspect, other dimensions of admissions could be addressed by attending to the language of EDIA through case study, institutional ethnography (Smith 2005; Webster et al. 2015), or the language of policy (Torres, this volume). Moreover, language researchers can enrich those text-and-practice based accounts with interviewing. Discipline-specific, discourse analytic methods, such as corpus-assisted discourse analysis or narrative analysis, stitch together policy with insider views and experiences, triangulating official policies with stories of those it affects (Prior, Hughes & Peckham 2012). Chapters in this volume have undertaken some of this work already, providing groundwork for future scholarship, and an open door to the scholarly pathways available.

Our contributors also agreed that language and communication specialists have a unique role to play in addressing mental health in education and communications about mental health more generally (Excerpt 11). We return here to critical issues in mental health and health research, education, and policy. The project of providing empathetic care and education depends on a sophisticated grasp of the mechanisms causing mental strife, the responses evoked, and the ways that those expressions of emotion are evaluated. By paying attention to discursive constructions of mental health, and wellbeing generally, critical applied linguists help disentangle the relations of power that can equally shut down or foster emotions in the trials of health, as professionals, learners, and patients alike.

(11) *We talk about mental health a lot and everybody enjoys and wants to talk about it because we want to help our students but we all feel very stuck in terms of how we talk about it, and what we can actually do for our students. So, I think that's a societal question that will continue to be important, something that linguistic contribute to. (Paul McPherron)*

Mental health discourse must be tended to from a variety of vantage points, and with different sensitivities, both to the positive and negative (Dornan et al. 2015). Health professions education in particular cannot avoid mental health, and expressions of emotion more generally, despite a historical inclination to do so (McNaughton 2013; Helmich et al. 2012; Artino Jr., Holmboe & Durning 2012). Importantly, there are many avenues for addressing mental health and wellbeing, including pedagogical interventions and education sciences, cognitive-psychological and clinical methods, and attending to the impacts on learners that shape the professional identity they eventually embody. Combining this variety and importance means that there are questions and methodological designs that health applied linguists are uniquely ready to meet.

In the closing our conversation, we turned to the increasing prevalence of disasters as dynamic threats to public and personal health, and the associated opportunities for research on language and health (Excerpt 12). Research during disaster recovery and reconstruction can capture dramatic changes in communities and society, interpersonal discourse, and policy response.

(12) *A new context for health applied linguists [is] disaster research. I'm on a grant to look at medical help seeking after hurricanes in Puerto Rico. It's not about doctor patient communication. It's not about medical education. It's a disaster context. Like Covid 19, right? Or lead in the water in Detroit. All those kinds of things open up whole new areas for us in which communication, language description, the way in which people paint realities and interact with one another, all just become really fertile ground for health applied linguists. (Robert W. Schrauf)*

As indicated in Excerpt 12, disaster contexts can have wide-ranging causes, but nonetheless they have important effects on health discourses. On the one hand, communication scholars are equipped to elicit experiences and descriptions of events on the ground, in relatively real time. Proximity to the disaster, with tools ready to describe it, reveals details about disaster experience while the memories are hot. Additionally, the multimodal nature of communication gives us the ability to collect text, speech, video, geo-spatial data, and so on, and align them across levels of discourse. A language and communication focus orients researchers to the interpersonal as well as the institutional and helps understand new ways of being and acting that emerge.

Disaster preparedness, recovery, and mitigation also involve the creation, implementation, and revision of health and governmental policies. At an alternative link in the implementational chain, there is a need to understand the responders and health professionals in disaster areas. Their stories contain essential details about what works, how it works, and where improvements can be made. Health applied linguists can record and organize their stories. Beyond the empathetic, the language of disaster policies can be crafted more carefully by weaving in those exact details, thus better reflecting the everyday ethics (Lambek 2010) of their recipients with attentive modality, content, and evaluative aspects, which are all gleanable through analysis of their language use.

5 Concluding remarks

It is our hope that this volume, through the multiple lenses, places, and concerns presented in its chapters, will serve as a catalyst for future collaboration, investigation, and widened angles of entry to the projects of health research, education, and policy.

Chapters in this volume have covered a variety of topics, locations, and methods, focused through the lens of language use and communicative practices. In the first section, Applied Linguistics and Health Education, our contributors showed the power of functional linguistics in health professions education, and the affordances of discourse analysis to educate health providers on situated practices when providing culturally competent care. In the second section, Applied Linguistics, Translation, and Health, they demonstrated the usefulness of gist translation to provide insights about children's education about dementia in older people, and the processual unfolding of research, identity, and transformation underlying translation in multilingual health projects. In the third section, Applied Linguistics and Public Health, contributors provided inside reflections and analyses of the roles of linguists in unfolding disaster areas, capturing the journeys of people in such fraught situations. Chapters in this section also demonstrated the utility of corpus-assisted discourse analysis in two different contexts, uncovering multiple levels of policy enactment. In our final section, Applied Linguists and Health Interventions, our contributors described improvements to health equity access via community action and remodeling programs of health literacy, and the contribution of language and social interaction scholars to the conceptualization, design, and implementation of health interventions.

Each chapter in this volume represents life and story, relationship and negotiation, of people involved and invisible. Our contributors took up the challenge to make themselves visible in each chapter, in ways that felt authentic to them, reflexively recognizing their craft as writers and authors, while also conveying rigorous, scientific research in health contexts. In this concluding chapter, several authors offered their personal histories, views of the current terrain, and potential future areas for participation and investigation as health scholars. Each point of perspective, past, present, and future, serves as a window into the worlds that health applied linguists and communication workers occupy. If the volume has been successful, readers in applied linguistics will be encouraged to ask new questions, create new projects, and establish new places of work. For readers in adjacent disciplines – clinical medicine, public health, and social science disciplines more generally, we hope that these chapters have provided a glimpse of how linguistic and discursive methods might address the communicative complexities of the spaces in which you work.

Thank you.

References

Agar, Michael. 1996. *Language shock: Understanding the culture of conversation*. New York, NY: William Morrow Paperbacks.

Artino Jr., Anthony R., Eric S. Holmboe & Steven J. Durning. 2012. Can achievement emotions be used to better understand motivation, learning, and performance in medical education? *Medical Teacher*. Taylor & Francis 34(3). 240–244. https://doi.org/10.3109/0142159X.2012.643265.

Björkman, Beyza. 2014. Language ideology or language practice? An analysis of language policy documents at Swedish universities. *Multilingua – Journal of Cross-Cultural and Interlanguage Communication*. De Gruyter Mouton 33(3–4). 335–363. https://doi.org/10.1515/multi-2014-0016.

Bowen, Sarah. 2001. *Language barriers in access to health care*. Transparency – other. Health Canada. https://www.canada.ca/en/health-canada/services/health-care-system/reports-publications/health-care-accessibility/language-barriers.html (27 October, 2021).

Braley, Bruce L. 2010. *H.R.946-111th Congress (2009–2010): Plain Writing Act of 2010*. https://www.congress.gov/bill/111th-congress/house-bill/946 (25 September, 2019).

Canagarajah, Suresh. 2007. Lingua Franca English, Multilingual Communities, and Language Acquisition. *The Modern Language Journal* 91(s1). 923–939. https://doi.org/10.1111/j.1540-4781.2007.00678.x.

Dewar, Belinda & Susan B. Frampton. 2013. Compassion in action. In Susan B. Frampton, Patrick A. Charmel, Sara Guastello & Planetree (eds.), *The Putting Patients First Field Guide*, 69–90. San Francisco: Jossey-Bass.

Dornan, Tim, Emma Pearson, Peter Carson, Esther Helmich & Christine Bundy. 2015. Emotions and identity in the figured world of becoming a doctor. *Medical Education* 49(2). 174–185. https://doi.org/10.1111/medu.12587.

Fairchild, Amy L., David Rosner, James Colgrove, Ronald Bayer & Linda P. Fried. 2010. The EXODUS of public health what history can tell us about the future. *American Journal of Public Health*. American Public Health Association 100(1). 54–63. https://doi.org/10.2105/AJPH.2009.163956.

Flores, Nelson & Jonathan Rosa. 2015. Undoing Appropriateness: Raciolinguistic Ideologies and Language Diversity in Education. *Harvard Educational Review* 85(2). 149–171. https://doi.org/10.17763/0017-8055.85.2.149.

Garfinkel, Harold. 1991. *Studies in ethnomethodology*. Wiley. https://www.wiley.com/en-us/Studies+in+Ethnomethodology-p-9780745600055 (2 November, 2021).

Garfinkel, Harold & Harvey Sacks. 1986. On formal structures of practical actions. In *Ethnomethodological Studies of Work*. Routledge.

Gostin, Lawrence O. 2001. Public health, ethics, and human rights: a tribute to the late Jonathan Mann. *Journal of Law, Medicine & Ethics* 29(2). 121.

Grin, François. 1998. Language policy in multilingual Switzerland: Overview and recent developments. In. Barcelona.

Hanlon, P., S. Carlisle, M. Hannah, D. Reilly & A. Lyon. 2011. Making the case for a 'fifth wave' in public Health. *Public Health* 125(1). 30–36. https://doi.org/10.1016/j.puhe.2010.09.004.

Helmich, Esther, Sanneke Bolhuis, Tim Dornan, Roland Laan & Raymond Koopmans. 2012. Entering medical practice for the very first time: emotional talk, meaning and identity development. *Medical Education* 46(11). 1074–1086. https://doi.org/10.1111/medu.12019.

Jenkins, Jennifer. 2006. Current perspectives on teaching world Englishes and English as a lingua franca. *TESOL Quarterly* 40(1). 157–181. https://doi.org/10.2307/40264515.

Kachru, Braj B. 1991. Liberation linguistics and the Quirk Concern. *English Today*. Cambridge University Press 7(1). 3–13. https://doi.org/10.1017/S026607840000523X.

Lambek, Michael. 2010. *Ordinary Ethics: Anthropology, Language, and Action*. New York: Fordham Univ Press.

Lynch, Michael. 2019. Garfinkel, Sacks and Formal Structures: Collaborative Origins, Divergences and the History of Ethnomethodology and Conversation Analysis. *Human Studies* 42(2). 183–198. https://doi.org/10.1007/s10746-019-09510-w.

McNaughton, Nancy. 2013. Discourse(s) of emotion within medical education: the ever-present absence. *Medical Education* 47(1). 71–79. https://doi.org/10.1111/j.1365-2923.2012.04329.x.

Michigan Civil Rights Commission. (Feb. 17, 2017). The Flint water crisis: Systemic racism through the lens of Flint. Retrieved from https://www.michigan.gov/documents/mdcr/VFlintCrisisRep-F-Edited3-13-17_554317_7.pdf

Norton, Bonnie. 2013. *Identity and Language Learning: Extending the Conversation*. 2nd edn. Bristol: Multilingual Matters.

Pennycook, Alastair. 2021. *Critical Applied Linguistics: A critical re ^introduction*. 2nd edn. New York: Routledge. https://doi.org/10.4324/9781003090571.

Piller, Ingrid. 2012. Multilingualism and social exclusion. In *The Routledge handbook of multilingualism*, 281–296.

Planetree Foundation. 2013. *The Putting Patients First Field Guide: Global Lessons in Designing and Implementing Patient-Centered Care*. John Wiley & Sons.

Prior, Lindsay, David Hughes & Stephen Peckham. 2012. The discursive turn in policy analysis and the validation of policy stories. *Journal of Social Policy*. Cambridge University Press 41(2). 271–289. https://doi.org/10.1017/S0047279411000821.

Ricento, Thomas. 2006. *An introduction to language policy: Theory and method*. Malden, MA: Blackwell.

Rosenberg, Charles E. 2012. Epilogue: Airs, waters, places. A status report. *Bulletin of the History of Medicine*. The Johns Hopkins University Press 86 (4). 661–670.

Seidlhofer, Barbara. 2001. Closing a conceptual gap: The case for a description of English as a lingua franca. *International Journal of Applied Linguistics* 11(2). 133–158. https://doi.org/10.1111/1473-4192.00011.

Seidlhofer, Barbara (ed.). 2003. *Controversies in Applied Linguistics*. OUP Oxford.

Selinker, Larry. 1972. Interlanguage. *IRAL* 10(1–4). 209–232. https://doi.org/10.1515/iral.1972.10.1-4.209.

Shohamy, Elana G. & Bernard Spolsky. 2000. Language practice, language ideology, and language policy. In *Language policy and pedagogy: Essays in honor of A. Ronald Walton*, 1–41.

Smith, Dorothy E. 2005. *Institutional Ethnography: A Sociology for People*. Rowman Altamira.

Spolsky, Bernard. 2004. *Language Policy*. Cambridge University Press.

Subtirelu, Nicholas Close. 2013. "English . . . it's part of our blood": Ideologies of language and nation in United States Congressional discourse. *Journal of Sociolinguistics* 17(1). 37–65. https://doi.org/10.1111/josl.12016.

Webster, Fiona, Kathleen Rice, Katie N. Dainty, Merrick Zwarenstein, Steve Durant & Ayelet Kuper. 2015. Failure to Cope: The Hidden Curriculum of Emergency Department Wait Times and the Implications for Clinical Training. *Academic Medicine* 90(1). 56–62. https://doi.org/10.1097/ACM.0000000000000499.

Contributor information

Preface

Paul McPherron is a Professor of English at Hunter College of the City University of New York (CUNY), where he is also the Co-PI on the Hunter College AANAPISI Project (HCAP). His research has examined questions about English language learning in relation to identity, globalization, neo-nationalism, and teaching policies in China and the United States. In earlier work, he co-edited the book *Language, Body, and Health* that examined biomedical, societal, and poststructuralist discourses of health and bodies.

Chapter 1

Abigail Konopasky, PhD, is an assistant professor in the Center for Health Professions Education at the Uniformed Services University of the Health Sciences. Her research focuses on critical approaches to diversity, equity, and inclusion; linguistic analyses of learner agency; and qualitative research methods. She received her PhD in linguistics from Princeton University and her PhD in educational psychology from George Mason University.

Anthony R. Artino, Jr., PhD, is a tenured professor and the Associate Dean for Evaluation and Educational Research at the George Washington University School of Medicine and Health Sciences. His research focuses on various aspects of human motivation, learning, and assessment in medicine. Dr. Artino is a member of several editorial review boards and has published widely in medical and health professions education. He received his PhD in educational psychology from the University of Connecticut.

Clara Hua, MD, is a General Surgery intern at the Walter Reed National Military Medical Center. Her research interests include health professional education, biotechnology, and regenerative medicine. She received her MD from Uniformed Services University of the Health Sciences.

Alexis Battista, PhD, is an assistant professor in the Center for Health Professions Education at the Uniformed Services University of the Health Sciences. She specializes in researching, designing, and implementing simulation-based learning for diverse healthcare specializations, including physicians, nurses, and allied health professionals, in the undergraduate and postgraduate setting. She received her PhD in educational psychology from George Mason University.

Chapter 2

Dr. Caroline Vickers is Interim Associate Dean of Graduate Studies and Professor of English with a specialization in Applied Linguistics at California State University, San Bernardino. Her main scholarly interests are related to second language socialization; multilingual interaction in the health care setting; and the integration of multilingual people in schools, universities, and society. She has published on these topics in journals such as *Communication & Medicine*, *Critical Inquiry in Language Studies*, *Health Communication*, *Journal of Language, Identity, and Education*, *Journal of Pragmatics*, *Journal of Sociolinguistics*, and *The Modern Language Journal*. Caroline is the co-author of a book, *Introduction to Sociolinguistics: Society and Identity*. She has also been the recipient of two National Institutes of Health grants.

Ryan Goble is a graduate of the Doctoral Program in Second Language Acquisition at the University of Wisconsin – Madison. His research draws on discourse and narrative analytic methods to investigate bi/multilingual and identity development away in relation to professional life. Recent publications have appeared in *Critical Inquiry in Language Studies* and the *International Journal of Bilingual Education and Bilingualism*. His dissertation examined the affordances of career advising for prolonging collegiate language learners' bi/multilingual development beyond higher education.

Chapter 3

Boyd H. Davis is Cone Professor and Graduate Professor Emerita in linguistics from UNC Charlotte, USA, now living in Taiwan. Her research areas include articles and books on socio- and interpersonal pragmatics in dementia discourse, multilingual caregiver education and post-TBI language. Publications in 2022: with Maclagan & Shu-Chiao Tsai, Meeting demographic changes: Expanding and translating caregiver training to incorporate social aspects of care, in Davis, B., Vicentini, V., Grego, K., (eds.) (2022). *Seniors, foreign caregivers, families, institutions: Linguistic and multidisciplinary perspectives*. Milan: Mimesis. With Maclagan and Pope, C., 2022. Digital outreach in online dementia discourse: A preliminary introduction. *Journal of Interactional Research in Communication Disorders*, *12*(2), 185–211.

Ching-Yi Kuo is a Licensed Professional Counseling Intern at the University of North Texas. Her current research involves the use of sand tray therapy with older adults with and without dementia.

Margaret Maclagan, is a retired linguist from the School of Psychology, Speech and Hearing, University of Canterbury, New Zealand. Her research areas include language change over time including in people with Alzheimer's Disease. Recent (2021–2022) publications with Davis include Signposts, guideposts, and stalls: pragmatic and discourse markers in dementia discourse. In Stickle, T., (ed.) *Learning from the talk of persons with dementia: A practical guide to interaction and interactional research* (Palgrave) and co-editorship, *Dementia caregiving east and west: Issues of communication* (Cambridge Scholars Press). She, Davis and Meredith Troutman-Jordan are developing digital dementia caregiver education materials in five languages, using graphic medicine.

Chapter 4

Robert W. Schrauf, PhD is Professor of Applied Linguistics at Pennsylvania State University. He conducts research in mixed methods, language and dementia, and multilingualism and culture. He is author of *Mixed Methods: Interviews, Surveys, and Cross-Cultural Comparisons* (Cambridge, 2016) and co-editor of *Language Development over the Lifespan* (with Kees de Bot; Routledge, 2009), *Dialogue and Dementia: Communicative Strategies of Engagement* (with Nicole Müller; Taylor and Francis, 2014) and *Multilingual Interaction in Dementia* (with Charlotta Plejert and Camilla Lindholm; Multilingual Matters, 2017).

Chapter 5

Peter Joseph Torres, PhD, is a Heanon Wilkins faculty fellow in the Department of English at Miami University, Ohio. His research interests include applied and interactional sociolinguistics with an emphasis on discourse analysis of policy and health issues. His recent publications tackle language issues surrounding the opioid crisis (2020, Discourse Studies; 2021, Applied Corpus Linguistics).

Chapter 6

Brett A. Diaz, PhD, is a research fellow at the Wilson Centre & University of Toronto, and Post-doctoral Fellow in the Centre for Faculty Development at St. Michael's Hospital. His research focuses on the interplay between emotion discourse and health contexts, and on beliefs expressed during the implementation of policy, using Peircean semiotics, corpus-assisted discourse analysis, and mixed methodology. His current projects center on critically reflective practices, and on policy discourse in Health Professions Education. His publications have appeared in *Applied Corpus Linguistics*, *The Journal of Language & Politics*, *Language & Communication*, and *Language in Society*.

Chapter 7

Patria López de Victoria is an assistant professor in the English department at the University of Puerto Rico, Cayey campus. She conducts research in language, health care practices, caregiving, and ageing in rural Puerto Rico. Her current work on negotiating dementia care by informal caregivers, extended family, and friends of elderly persons diagnosed with Alzheimer's Disease (AD) focuses on how helpseeking dynamics and networks play out over the years among families, friends, and health and social services professionals seeking/delivering comprehensive dementia care for elders diagnosed with AD in the interior of the island post-disaster and other cascading crises.

Elba L. González Márquez has a master's degree in Public Health with a specialty in Gerontology from the University of Puerto Rico, Medical Sciences Campus. Her research interests include the heterogeneity of the elderly population, and medical helpseeking by and for older adults and caregivers in times of sustained crisis and challenge.

Krystal Colon Rivera is a doctoral student in the School Psychology Doctoral Program at University of Puerto Rico (UPR) Mayagüez. She completed her bachelor's in Sociology with a double major in Psychology at UPR Cayey. Her research interests include intergenerational support, the role of play in early childhood cognitive development and learning early childhood. She also creates and designs plain language infographics and digital material on topics ranging from disaster preparedness to health practices and tips for caregivers for the research page, *Estrategias y Redes de Aprendizaje en la Salud*.

Chapter 8

Emily M. Feuerherm, PhD, is an Associate Professor of linguistics in the Department of Language and Communication at the University of Michigan-Flint. Her interests include ESL program and curriculum development, community-based research, and the intersection of language, literacy, and health. Recent publications include a multi-authored chapter "Language as a social determinant of health: Partnerships for health equity" in Warriner and Miller's edited volume *Extending Applied Linguistics for Social Impact* and a co-authored article "Conducting a community-based ESOL programme needs analysis" in the *ELT Journal*.

Bonnie McIntosh, MBA, MPH, BA Community Health, CHES, is an Assistant Professor and Program Chair of Health Care Management in the School of Business at Rochester University, and a Principal Consultant at ACE Community Health. Her interests include curricular design, health care, health communication, and community-based participatory research. Recent presentations and a publication include a co-authored presentation "Health and English as a Second Language Literacy Program (HELP): Bridging Health, Culture, and Linguistics Following a Public Health Crisis" at the *National Public Health Information Coalition and the Centers for Disease Control and Prevention, Health Communication Marketing and Media Forum*; a co-authored presentation "English as a Second Language Health Literacy Program: The Process of Engaging Diverse Stakeholders for a Social Practice" at the *Society for Public Health Education Conference*; and a multi-authored publication "British Columbian Healthcare Providers' Perspectives on Facilitators and Barriers to Adhering to Pediatric Diabetes Treatment Guidelines" in the *Canadian Journal of Diabetes*.

Chapter 9

Lisa Mikesell is an Associate Professor of Communication and Associate Faculty at the Institute for Health, Health Care Policy and Aging Research at Rutgers University with a background in mental health services research. Using mixed methods and working across the life course, her research focuses on how to improve patient and stakeholder engagement, patient-provider communication, and practices of patient-centeredness to foster trusting healthcare relationships. She is co-editor of the book series *Language, Discourse and Mental Health* published by University of Exeter Press.

Index

adult basic skills 234
advisory boards 257
Affordable Care Act 230
Agha 119
Applied Linguistics
– definition 2
– research strands 3
austerity measures 193
Austin 4
automated linguistic analysis 22
autonomous organization 212

Baynham and Lee 129
breast cancer 201

Candlin and Sarangi 2
Centers for Disease Control and
    Prevention 148
code-switching 59
collaboration 3
communication design 259
community advisory board 235
Community-Based Participatory Action
    Research 16, 233
community engagement 269
complex interventions 256
construction
– co-construction 46, 57
– discursive 284
– joint 40
context models 146
Conversation Analysis 4, 65, 249
– activity transitions 268
– applied 268
– foundational applied 268
– institutional applied 268
– institutional talk 268
– interventionist applied 269
– unmotivated looking 255
critical 279
cultural competence 60
– culturally competent 61
cultural logics 197
curriculum 238

debrief 25
Demjén 7
depression 201
design 247
diagnostic reasoning 26
disaster recovery 193, 285
disciplines
– interdiscipline 247
– multidiscipline 247, 276
– transdiscipline 247
Discourse 172
Discourse Analysis 4, 195
– accounts 195
– agency 195
– analysts 174
– corpus-assisted discourse analysis 176, 284
– corpus-based 143
– discourse-oriented 194
– narrative 284
– stance 173
disempowerment 204
dominant language 60

Enfield & Sidnell 4
engaged scholarship 248
English as a second language 234
epistemic asymmetries 251
ethnography 194
– linguistic 195
Extended Lexical Unit 173
– collocation 173
– semantic preference 173
– semantic prosody 173

feedback 26
first responders 212
Fostering Literacy for Good Health Today 239
frames 147
functional linguistics 23

Garfinkel and Sacks 124

Hamilton and Chou 6
Hanks 119

Health Applied Linguistics 5
– future of 275
– linguists 276
health equity 226
health history
– interview 57
– narrative 57
health interventions 247
health outcomes 262
Health Policy Implementation 171
Health Professions Education 21
– linguistic research design 47
health services 169
helpseeking 194
Hurricanes 194
– Maria 202

illness narratives 265
indexicality 131, 194
institutional interactions 251

Jakobson 118
Jones 4

language and social interaction 247
language normativity 61
Language Policy and Planning 143
language policy arbiters 242
lead poisoning 231
learning
– self-regulated 25
– simulated 25
Limited English Proficient 61
Linguistic Inquiry and Word Count 22
linguistic resources 195
– diminutives 207
– extreme case formulations 207
– lists 209
linguistics 4
longitudinal study 198

macro-level 60
mastectomy 203
McGill Illness Narrative Interview 200
medical texts 278
medication titration 263

memoed 40
metafunctions 23
mHealth 263
Michigan Civil Rights Commission 226
micro-interaction 60
modality
– scale 155
– verbs 143
Mondada 124
monolingual 279
multilingual 280

narrative 194
National Standards for Culturally and
  Linguistically Appropriate Services 230
needs assessment 255

older adult 169
older adults 193
opioids 169
– California 144
– crisis 170
– epidemic 169
– opioid crisis 148

paradigms 278
participation framework 59
– bureaucratic side talk 74
– non-participant 59
patient-centered outcomes 257
patient-provider relationship 265
performativity 194
pharmacy 209
– community 211
– prescribers 214
– third-party payers 214
plurilingual 279
policy
– action 155
– amendment 156
– antidiscrimination 229
– enactment 144, 171
– interpretation 145
– stakeholders 154
power 279
practitioner training 267

prescription
- chronic pain 148
- controlled substance 148
- narcotic 148
professional vision 117
Publication 131
- data segments 131
- excerpts 131
public debt 193
public health
- crisis 211
- policy 143

redlining 232
reflection 23
reported speech 119

semiotic productions 196
shifters 197
Silverstein 120
situated practice 124
social determinants of health 227
- evaluating health information 241
- language access 281
- language barrier 61
- language concordance 62
social logics 208
solidarity 208
source languages 117
Spanish 228
- Hispanic people 228

stakeholder engagement 257
stocks of professional knowledge 63
supply chain disruption 211

talk and text 4
talk-in-interaction 194
Transcription 124
- conventions 125
- re-transcribing 130
Translanguaging 128
Translation
- grammar and lexicon 121
- indexical 135
- interlingual 119
- intralingual 118
- lexico-grammatic 131
- transduction 122
translation and interpreting services 226
triangulation 26

US census 232
US Civil Rights Act 229
U.S. Environmental Protection Agency 239

Vive Desarollando Amplia Salud 239
vulnerabilities 204

ways of being 277
white flight 232

www.ingramcontent.com/pod-product-compliance
Lightning Source LLC
Chambersburg PA
CBHW050516170426
43201CB00013B/1979